Infant & Toddler Health Sourcebook

Infectious Diseases Sourcebook

Injury & Trauma Sourcebook

Learning Disabilities Sourcebook,
2nd Edition

Leukemia Sourcebook

Liver Disorders Sourcebook

Lung Disorders Sourcebook

Medical Tests Sourcebook, 2nd Edition

Men's Health Concerns Sourcebook,
2nd Edition

Mental Health Disorders Sourcebook,
3rd Edition

Mental Retardation Sourcebook

Movement Disorders Sourcebook

Muscular Dystrophy Sourcebook

Obesity Sourcebook

Osteoporosis Sourcebook

Pain Sourcebook, 2nd Edition

Pediatric Cancer Sourcebook

Physical & Mental Issues in Aging
Sourcebook

Podiatry Sourcebook, 2nd Edition

Pregnancy & Birth Sourcebook,
2nd Edition

Prostate Cancer Sourcebook

Prostate & Urological Disorders
Sourcebook

Public Health Sourcebook

Reconstructive & Cosmetic Surgery
Sourcebook

Rehabilitation Sourcebook

Respiratory Diseases & Disorders
Sourcebook

Sexually Transmitted Diseases
Sourcebook, 3rd Edition

Sleep Disorders Sourcebook,
2nd Edition

Smoking Concerns Sourcebook

Sports Injuries Sourcebook, 2nd Edition

Stress-Related Disorders Sourcebook

Stroke Sourcebook

Substance Abuse Sourcebook

Surgery Sourcebook

Thyroid Disorders Sourcebook

Transplantation

Traveler's Health Sourcebook

Urinary Tract & Kidney Diseases &
Disorders Sourcebook, 2nd Edition

Vegetarian Sourcebook

Women's Health Concerns Sourcebook,
2nd Edition

Workplace Health & Safety Sourcebook

Worldwide Health Sourcebook

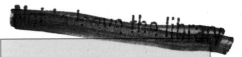

Teen Health Series

Alcohol Information for Teens

Allergy Information for Teens

Asthma Information for Teens

Cancer Information for Teens

Complementary & Alternative
Medicine Information for
Teens

Diabetes Information for Teens

Diet Information for Teens,
2nd Edition

Drug Information for Teens,
2nd Edition

Eating Disorders Information
for Teens

Fitness Information for Teens

Learning Disabilities Information
for Teens

Mental Health Information for
Teens, 2nd Edition

Sexual Health Information for
Teens

Skin Health Information for
Teens

Sports Injuries Information
for Teens

Suicide Information for Teens

Tobacco Information for Teens

Cancer Survivorship SOURCEBOOK

Health Reference Series

First Edition

Cancer Survivorship
SOURCEBOOK

*Basic Consumer Health Information about the Physical,
Educational, Emotional, Social, and Financial Needs of
Cancer Patients from Diagnosis, through Cancer
Treatment, and Beyond, Including Facts about
Researching Specific Types of Cancer and Learning
about Clinical Trials and Treatment Options, and
Featuring Tips for Coping with the Side Effects of Cancer
Treatments and Adjusting to Life after Cancer Treatment
Concludes*

*Along with Suggestions for Caregivers, Friends, and
Family Members of Cancer Patients, a Glossary of
Cancer Care Terms, and Directories of Related Resources*

Edited by
Karen Bellenir

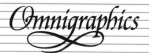

Omnigraphics

615 Griswold Street • Detroit, MI 48226

Bibliographic Note

Because this page cannot legibly accommodate all the copyright notices, the Bibliographic Note portion of the Preface constitutes an extension of the copyright notice.

Edited by Karen Bellenir

Health Reference Series

Karen Bellenir, *Managing Editor*
David A. Cooke, M.D., *Medical Consultant*
Elizabeth Collins, *Research and Permissions Coordinator*
Cherry Stockdale, *Permissions Assistant*
EdIndex, Services for Publishers, *Indexers*

* * *

Omnigraphics, Inc.

Matthew P. Barbour, *Senior Vice President*
Kay Gill, *Vice President—Directories*
Kevin Hayes, *Operations Manager*
David P. Bianco, *Marketing Director*

* * *

Peter E. Ruffner, *Publisher*
Frederick G. Ruffner, Jr., *Chairman*
Copyright © 2007 Omnigraphics, Inc.
ISBN 978-0-7808-0985-7

Library of Congress Cataloging-in-Publication Data

Cancer survivorship sourcebook : basic consumer health information about the physical, educational, emotional, social, and financial needs of cancer patients from diagnosis, through cancer treatment, and beyond, including facts about researching specific types of cancer and learning about clinical trials and treatment options, and featuring tips for coping with the side effects of cancer treatments and adjusting to life after cancer treatment concludes; along with suggestions for caregivers, friends, and family members of cancer patients, a glossary of cancer care terms, and directories of related resources / edited by Karen Bellenir. -- 1st ed.
    p. cm.
  Summary: "Provides basic consumer health information about living with cancer after diagnosis and treatment. Includes index, glossary of related terms, and other resources"--Provided by publisher.
  Includes bibliographical references and index.
  ISBN 978-0-7808-0985-7 (hardcover : alk. paper) 1. Cancer--Popular works. 2. Cancer--Patients--Care. 3. Cancer--Patients--Life skill guides. I. Bellenir, Karen.
  RC263.C296 2007
  616.99'4--dc22
                                                              2007003055

Table of Contents

Visit www.healthreferenceseries.com to view *A Contents Guide to the Health Reference Series*, a listing of more than 13,000 topics and the volumes in which they are covered.

Part III: Clinical Trials and Cancer Research Updates

Part IV: Coping with Side Effects and Complications of Cancer Treatment

Part V: Emotional, Cognitive, and Mental Health Issues in Cancer Care

Part VI: Maintaining Wellness during and after Cancer Treatment

Part VII: Information for Friends, Family Members, and Caregivers

Part VIII: Additional Help and Information

Preface

About This Book

In 1971 there were two million cancer survivors living in the United States. Today, their number has increased to more than 10 million—a number made possible through better and earlier detection of cancer, advances in medical technologies, and improved treatments. The Centers for Disease Control and Prevention estimates that one out of every six people over the age of 65 is a cancer survivor. Statistics also suggest that approximately 65% of people diagnosed with cancer will live at least five years after their diagnosis, and nearly 75% of those with childhood cancer will live at least ten years. Cancer survivorship presents multiple challenges, however. Cancer survivors often lack the information they need to make treatment choices, maintain optimal physical and mental health during and after treatment, prevent disability and late effects associated with cancer, and handle economic issues related to cancer care.

Cancer Survivorship Sourcebook provides information for cancer patients and their family members, friends, and caregivers. It includes tips for researching specific types of cancer, treatment advances, and clinical trials, and it offers suggestions for coping with the side effects and complications of cancer treatments. Facts about emotional, cognitive, and mental health issues in cancer care are included, and a special section focuses on the challenges of maintaining wellness during and after cancer treatment. A glossary of cancer care terms is also provided, along with a directory of resources for cancer patients and information about financial assistance for cancer care.

Readers seeking information about the major forms and stages of cancers affecting specific organs and body systems may wish to consult *Cancer Sourcebook, Fifth Edition* a separate volume within the *Health Reference Series*. In addition, some specific forms of cancer are discussed in a more in-depth manner in other *Health Reference Series* books:

- Breast cancer: *Breast Cancer Sourcebook, Second Edition*
- Childhood cancers: *Pediatric Cancer Sourcebook*
- Gynecological cancers: *Cancer Sourcebook for Women, Third Edition*
- Leukemia: *Leukemia Sourcebook*
- Prostate cancer: *Prostate Cancer Sourcebook* and *Prostate and Urological Disorders Sourcebook*
- Thyroid cancer: *Thyroid Disorders Sourcebook*

How to Use This Book

This book is divided into parts and chapters. Parts focus on broad areas of interest. Chapters are devoted to single topics within a part.

Part I: If Your Doctor Says It's Cancer offers information of immediate concern to the newly diagnosed cancer patient. It describes the process of finding a qualified healthcare provider and getting a second opinion. It also provides facts about the tests that are used to diagnose cancer and to monitor the effectiveness of cancer treatments.

Part II: Making Treatment and Cancer Care Decisions discusses various strategies that can help a cancer patient research and understand issues related to his or her own care. It provides an overview of commonly used cancer treatments, medications, and complementary and alternative medicine (CAM) practices. It also discusses the use of palliative care and describes the transitions that may occur during care if cancer treatments are not effective in halting the advance of the disease.

Part III: Clinical Trials and Cancer Research Updates provides information for cancer patients who are considering participating in cancer-related research studies. It explains the procedures commonly used in clinical trials and explains how to locate one. It also offers updated information about recent research results, new treatments, and current research initiatives that offer hope for the future.

Part IV: Coping with Side Effects and Complications of Cancer Treatment discusses unwanted side effects that often accompany commonly used cancer treatments. It explains why treatments can cause such physical effects as nausea, vomiting, weight loss, hair loss, and fatigue. It also includes practical suggestions for dealing with these types of effects and other medical complications of cancer treatment.

Part V: Emotional, Cognitive, and Mental Health Issues in Cancer Care provides facts about the non-physical effects and complications of cancer and its treatment. These include changes in self-image that result from illness or from body-altering surgical procedures and the ways people adjust to new circumstances. It also describes mental health disorders that may accompany cancer treatment, including depression, anxiety disorders, post-traumatic stress disorder, and substance abuse.

Part VI: Maintaining Wellness during and after Cancer Treatment describes steps cancer survivors can take to achieve optimal health while they are receiving cancer treatments and after their treatments have been completed. These include eating a healthy diet, participating in rehabilitative programs, exercising, and smoking cessation. Additional chapters address concerns related to resuming "normal" life once cancer treatment is over and appropriate follow-up care.

Part VII: Information for Friends, Family Members, and Caregivers offers guidelines for dealing with family matters, life planning, and practical aspects of cancer caregiving. Individual chapters address specific concerns of loved ones, parents, children, and siblings.

Part VIII: Additional Help and Information includes a glossary of cancer care terms and a glossary of terms commonly used by health insurance companies and in medical billing. It also offers directories of resources able to provide services and support to cancer patients and their families.

Bibliographic Note

This volume contains documents and excerpts from publications issued by the following U.S. government agencies: National Cancer Institute; National Library of Medicine; and Surveillance Epidemiology and End Results (SEER).

In addition, this volume contains copyrighted documents from the following organizations: American Institute for Cancer Research; American Society of Clinical Oncology; CancerConsultants.com; Children's Oncology Group; Cleveland Clinic Foundation; Elsevier; eMedicine.com, Inc.; Healthcommunities.com, Inc. (Oncology Channel); Melissa's Living Legacy Foundation; National Academy of Sciences; People Living with Cancer; Teens Living with Cancer; University of Pennsylvania Cancer Center (OncoLink); and Vanderbilt-Ingram Cancer Center.

Full citation information is provided on the first page of each chapter. Every effort has been made to secure all necessary rights to reprint the copyrighted material. If any omissions have been made, please contact Omnigraphics to make corrections for future editions.

Acknowledgements

In addition to the organizations, agencies, and individuals who have contributed to this *Sourcebook*, special thanks go to editorial assistants Nicole Salerno and Elizabeth Bellenir, research and permissions coordinator Liz Collins, and permissions assistant Cherry Stockdale.

About the Health Reference Series

The *Health Reference Series* is designed to provide basic medical information for patients, families, caregivers, and the general public. Each volume takes a particular topic and provides comprehensive coverage. This is especially important for people who may be dealing with a newly diagnosed disease or a chronic disorder in themselves or in a family member. People looking for preventive guidance, information about disease warning signs, medical statistics, and risk factors for health problems will also find answers to their questions in the *Health Reference Series*. The *Series*, however, is not intended to serve as a tool for diagnosing illness, in prescribing treatments, or as a substitute for the physician/patient relationship. All people concerned about medical symptoms or the possibility of disease are encouraged to seek professional care from an appropriate health care provider.

A Note about Spelling and Style

Health Reference Series editors use *Stedman's Medical Dictionary* as an authority for questions related to the spelling of medical terms and the *Chicago Manual of Style* for questions related to grammatical structures, punctuation, and other editorial concerns. Consistent adherence is not always possible, however, because the individual volumes within the *Series* include many documents from a wide variety of different producers and copyright holders, and the editor's primary goal is to present material from each source as accurately as is possible following the terms specified by each document's producer. This sometimes means that information in different chapters or sections may follow other guidelines and alternate spelling authorities. For example, occasionally a copyright holder may require that eponymous terms be shown in possessive forms (Crohn's disease *vs.* Crohn disease) or that British spelling norms be retained (leukaemia *vs.* leukemia).

Locating Information within the Health Reference Series

The *Health Reference Series* contains a wealth of information about a wide variety of medical topics. Ensuring easy access to all the fact sheets, research reports, in-depth discussions, and other material contained within the individual books of the *Series* remains one of our highest priorities. As the *Series* continues to grow in size and scope, however, locating the precise information needed by a reader may become more challenging.

A *Contents Guide to the Health Reference Series* was developed to direct readers to the specific volumes that address their concerns. It presents an extensive list of diseases, treatments, and other topics of general interest compiled from the Tables of Contents and major index headings. To access *A Contents Guide to the Health Reference Series*, visit www.healthreferenceseries.com.

Medical Consultant

Medical consultation services are provided to the *Health Reference Series* editors by David A. Cooke, M.D. Dr. Cooke is a graduate of Brandeis University, and he received his M.D. degree from the University of Michigan. He completed residency training at the University of Wisconsin Hospital and Clinics. He is board-certified in Internal Medicine. Dr. Cooke currently works as part of the University of Michigan Health System and practices in Ann Arbor, MI. In his free time, he enjoys writing, science fiction, and spending time with his family.

Our Advisory Board

We would like to thank the following board members for providing guidance to the development of this *Series*:

- Dr. Lynda Baker,
  Associate Professor of Library and Information Science,
  Wayne State University, Detroit, MI

- Nancy Bulgarelli,
  William Beaumont Hospital Library, Royal Oak, MI

- Karen Imarisio,
  Bloomfield Township Public Library, Bloomfield Township, MI

- Karen Morgan,
  Mardigian Library, University of Michigan-Dearborn,
  Dearborn, MI

- Rosemary Orlando,
  St. Clair Shores Public Library, St. Clair Shores, MI

Health Reference Series *Update Policy*

The inaugural book in the *Health Reference Series* was the first edition of *Cancer Sourcebook* published in 1989. Since then, the *Series* has been enthusiastically received by librarians and in the medical community. In order to maintain the standard of providing high-quality health information for the layperson the editorial staff at Omnigraphics felt it was necessary to implement a policy of updating volumes when warranted.

Medical researchers have been making tremendous strides, and it is the purpose of the *Health Reference Series* to stay current with the most recent advances. Each decision to update a volume is made on an individual basis. Some of the considerations include how much new information is available and the feedback we receive from people who use the books. If there is a topic you would like to see added to the update list, or an area of medical concern you feel has not been adequately addressed, please write to:

Editor
Health Reference Series
Omnigraphics, Inc.
615 Griswold Street
Detroit, MI 48226
E-mail: editorial@omnigraphics.com

Part One

If Your Doctor Says It's Cancer

Chapter 1

Finding a Cancer Doctor

If you have been diagnosed with cancer, finding a doctor and treatment facility for your cancer care is an important step to getting the best treatment possible. Although the health care system is complex, resources are available to guide you in finding a doctor, getting a second opinion, and choosing a treatment facility. Below are suggestions and information resources to help you with these important decisions.

Physician Training and Credentials

When choosing a doctor for your cancer care, you may find it helpful to know some of the terms used to describe a doctor's training and credentials. Most physicians who treat people with cancer are medical doctors (they have an M.D. degree). The basic training for a physician includes four years of premedical education at a college or university, four years of medical school to earn an M.D. degree, and a residency consisting of three to seven years of postgraduate education and training. Physicians must pass an exam to become licensed (legally permitted) to practice medicine in their state. Each state or territory has its own procedures and general standards for licensing physicians.

Specialists are physicians who have completed their residency training in a specific area, such as internal medicine. Independent specialty boards certify physicians after they have fulfilled certain requirements.

"How to Find a Doctor or Treatment Facility If You Have Cancer," a National Cancer Institute (NCI) FactSheet, reviewed October 12, 2006. For additional information, visit the NCI website at http://www.cancer.gov.

These requirements include meeting specific education and training criteria, being licensed to practice medicine, and passing an examination given by the specialty board. Doctors who have met all of the requirements are given the status of "Diplomate" and are board-certified as specialists. Doctors who are board-eligible have obtained the required education and training, but have not completed the specialty board examination.

After being trained and certified as a specialist, a physician may choose to become a subspecialist. A subspecialist has at least one additional year of full-time education in a particular area of a specialty. This training is designed to increase the physician's expertise in a specific field. Specialists can be board-certified in their subspecialty as well.

The following are some specialties and subspecialties that pertain to cancer treatment:

- **Medical oncology** is a subspecialty of internal medicine. Doctors who specialize in internal medicine treat a wide range of medical problems. Medical oncologists treat cancer and manage the patient's course of treatment. A medical oncologist may also consult with other physicians about the patient's care or refer the patient to other specialists.

- **Hematology** is a subspecialty of internal medicine. Hematologists focus on diseases of the blood and related tissues, including the bone marrow, spleen, and lymph nodes.

- **Radiation oncology** is a subspecialty of radiology. Radiology is the use of x-rays and other forms of radiation to diagnose and treat disease. Radiation oncologists specialize in the use of radiation to treat cancer.

- **Surgery** is a specialty that pertains to the treatment of disease by surgical operation. General surgeons perform operations on almost any area of the body. Physicians can also choose to specialize in a certain type of surgery; for example, thoracic surgeons are specialists who perform operations specifically in the chest area, including the lungs and the esophagus.

Information about other specialties that treat cancer is available from the American Board of Medical Specialties® (ABMS) in a booklet called "Which Medical Specialist For You?" This publication is available on the internet at http://www.abms.org/which.asp. It can also be obtained by writing to: American Board of Medical Specialties, Suite 404, 1007 Church Street, Evanston, IL 60201-5913.

Almost all board-certified specialists are members of their medical specialty society. Physicians can attain Fellowship status in a specialty society, such as the American College of Surgeons (ACS), if they demonstrate outstanding achievement in their profession. Criteria for Fellowship status may include the number of years of membership in the specialty society, years practicing in the specialty, and professional recognition by peers.

Finding a Doctor

One way to find a doctor who specializes in cancer care is to ask for a referral from your primary care physician. You may know a specialist yourself, or through the experience of a family member, coworker, or friend.

The following resources may also be able to provide you with names of doctors who specialize in treating specific diseases or conditions. However, these resources may not have information about the quality of care that the doctors provide.

- Your local hospital or its patient referral service may be able to provide you with a list of specialists who practice at that hospital.

- Your nearest National Cancer Institute (NCI)-designated cancer center can provide information about doctors who practice at that center. The NCI is a component of the National Institutes of Health. The NCI fact sheet "The National Cancer Institute Cancer Centers Program" describes and gives contact information, including websites, for NCI-designated cancer centers around the country. Many of the cancer centers' websites have searchable directories of physicians who practice at each facility. The fact sheet is available on the internet at http://www.cancer.gov/cancertopics/factsheet/NCI/cancer-centers.

- The ABMS has a list of doctors who have met certain education and training requirements and have passed specialty examinations. The *Official ABMS Directory of Board Certified Medical Specialists* lists doctors' names along with their specialty and their educational background. The directory is available in most public libraries. Also, ABMS offers this information on the internet at http://www.abms.org (click on "Who's Certified").

- The American Medical Association (AMA) DoctorFinder database on the internet at http://webapps.ama-assn.org/doctorfinder/home.html?aps/amahg.htm provides basic information on licensed physicians in the United States. Users can search for physicians by name or by medical specialty.

- The American Society of Clinical Oncology (ASCO) provides an online list of doctors who are members of ASCO. The member database has the names and affiliations of over 15,000 oncologists worldwide. It can be searched by doctor's name, institution, location, and/or type of board certification. This service is available on the internet at http://www.plwc.org/portal/site/PLWC (click on "Find an Oncologist").

- The American College of Surgeons (ACS) Membership Database is an online list of surgeons who are members of the ACS. The list can be searched by doctor's name, geographic location, or medical specialty. This service is located on the internet at http://web.facs .org/acsdir/default_public.cfm. The ACS can be contacted at 633 North Saint Clair Street, Chicago, IL 60611-3211, or by telephone at 312-202-5000.

- Local medical societies may maintain lists of doctors in each specialty.

- Public and medical libraries may have print directories of doctors' names listed geographically by specialty.

- Your local Yellow Pages or Yellow Book may have doctors listed by specialty under "Physicians."

- The Agency for Healthcare Research and Quality (AHRQ) offers "Your Guide to Choosing Quality Health Care," which has information for consumers on choosing a health plan, a doctor, a hospital, or a long-term care provider. The guide includes suggestions and checklists that you can use to determine which doctor or hospital is best for you. This resource is available on the internet at http:// www.ahrq.gov/consumer/qntool.htm. You can also order the guide by calling the AHRQ Publications Clearinghouse at 800-358-9295.

If you are a member of a health insurance plan, your choice may be limited to doctors who participate in your plan. Your insurance company can provide you with a list of participating primary care doctors and specialists. It is important to ask your insurance company if the doctor you choose is accepting new patients through your health plan. You also have the option of seeing a doctor outside your health plan and paying the costs yourself. If you have a choice of health insurance plans, you may first wish to consider which doctor or doctors you would like to use, then choose a plan that includes your chosen physician(s).

If you are using a federal or state health insurance program such as Medicare or Medicaid, you may want to ask the doctor about accepting patients who use these programs.

Making Your Choice

You will have many factors to consider when choosing a doctor. To make an informed decision, you may wish to speak with several doctors before choosing one. When you meet with each doctor, you might want to consider the following:

- Does the doctor have the education and training to meet my needs?

- Does the doctor use the hospital that I have chosen?

- Does the doctor listen to me and treat me with respect?

- Does the doctor explain things clearly and encourage me to ask questions?

- What are the doctor's office hours?

- Who covers for the doctor when he or she is unavailable? Will that person have access to my medical records?

- How long does it take to get an appointment with the doctor?

If you are choosing a surgeon, you may wish to ask additional questions about the surgeon's background and experience with specific procedures. These questions may include the following:

- Is the surgeon board-certified?

- Has the surgeon been evaluated by a national professional association of surgeons, such as the American College of Surgeons (ACS)?

- At which treatment facility or facilities does the surgeon practice?

- How often does the surgeon perform the type of surgery I need?

- How many of these procedures has the surgeon performed? What was the success rate?

It is important for you to feel comfortable with the specialist that you choose because you will be working closely with that person to make decisions about your cancer treatment. Trust your own observations and feelings when deciding on a doctor for your medical care.

Other health professionals and support services may also be important during cancer treatment. The NCI fact sheet "Your Health Care Team: Your Doctor Is Only the Beginning" has information about these providers and services, and how to locate them. This fact sheet is located at on the internet at http://www.cancer.gov/cancertopics/factsheet/support/healthcare-team.

Getting a Second Opinion

Once you receive your doctor's opinion about the diagnosis and treatment plan, you may want to get another doctor's advice before you begin treatment. This is known as getting a second opinion. You can do this by asking another specialist to review all of the materials related to your case. A second opinion can confirm or suggest modifications to your doctor's proposed treatment plan, provide reassurance that you have explored all of your options, and answer any questions you may have.

Getting a second opinion is done frequently, and most physicians welcome another doctor's views. In fact, your doctor may be able to recommend a specialist for this consultation. However, some people find it uncomfortable to request a second opinion. When discussing this issue with your doctor, it may be helpful to express satisfaction with your doctor's decision and care, and mention that you want your decision about treatment to be as thoroughly informed as possible. You may also wish to bring a family member along for support when asking for a second opinion. It is best to involve your doctor in the process of getting a second opinion, because your doctor will need to make your medical records (such as your test results and x-rays) available to the specialist.

Some health care plans require a second opinion, particularly if a doctor recommends surgery. Other health care plans will pay for a second opinion if the patient requests it. If your plan does not cover a second opinion, you can still obtain one if you are willing to cover the cost.

If your doctor is unable to recommend a specialist for a second opinion, or if you prefer to choose one on your own, the following resources can help:

- Many of the resources listed above for finding a doctor can also help you find a specialist for a consultation.

- The Pediatric Oncology Branch of the NCI's Center for Cancer Research is dedicated to providing the best medical care possible to children, teenagers, and young adults with cancer or HIV disease.

The Pediatric Oncology Branch offers a second opinion service to physicians and to patients and their families. Their website is located on the internet at http://home.ccr.cancer.gov/oncology/pediatric. To request a second opinion from the Pediatric Oncology Branch, you or your physician may call 877-624-4878 or 301-496-4256 Monday to Friday, between 8:30 AM and 5:00 PM, Eastern time.

- The Neuro-Oncology Branch is a joint program of the NCI and the National Institute of Neurological Disorders and Stroke, another component of the National Institutes of Health. This Branch is dedicated to the treatment of adults and children with brain tumors. Staff can provide a second opinion for doctors, patients, and family members who are interested in this service. Specialists can either evaluate the patient in person or review the patient's medical records and scans. To find out more about this service, and what information is needed, contact the Neuro-Oncology Branch at 301-402-6298. The Branch's website can be found on the internet at http://home.ccr.cancer.gov/nob.

- The R. A. Bloch Cancer Foundation, Inc., can refer cancer patients to institutions that are willing to provide multidisciplinary second opinions. A list of these institutions is available on the internet at http://www.blochcancer.org/articles/xtrnew.asp. You can also contact the R. A. Bloch Cancer Foundation, Inc., by telephone at 816-854-5050 (816-WE-BUILD) or 800-433-0464.

Finding a Treatment Facility for Patients Living in the United States

Choosing a treatment facility is another important consideration for getting the best medical care possible. Although you may not be able to choose which hospital treats you in an emergency, you can choose a facility for scheduled and ongoing care. If you have already found a doctor for your cancer treatment, you may need to choose a facility based on where your doctor practices. Your doctor may be able to recommend a facility that provides quality care to meet your needs. You may wish to ask the following questions when considering a treatment facility:

- Has the facility had experience and success in treating my condition?

- Has the facility been rated by state, consumer, or other groups for its quality of care?

- How does the facility check on and work to improve its quality of care?

- Has the facility been approved by a nationally recognized accrediting body, such as the American College of Surgeons (ACS) and/or the Joint Commission on Accreditation of Healthcare Organizations (JCAHO)?

- Does the facility explain patients' rights and responsibilities? Are copies of this information available to patients?

- Does the treatment facility offer support services, such as social workers and resources, to help me find financial assistance if I need it?

- Is the facility conveniently located?

If you are a member of a health insurance plan, your choice of treatment facilities may be limited to those that participate in your plan. Your insurance company can provide you with a list of approved facilities. Although the costs of cancer treatment can be very high, you have the option of paying out-of-pocket if you want to use a treatment facility that is not covered by your insurance plan. If you are considering paying for treatment yourself, you may wish to discuss the possible costs with your doctor beforehand. You may also want to speak with the person who does the billing for the treatment facility. In some instances, nurses and social workers can provide you with more information about coverage, eligibility, and insurance issues.

The following resources may help you find a hospital or treatment facility for your care:

- The NCI fact sheet "The National Cancer Institute Cancer Centers Program" (described above in the section "Finding a Doctor") describes and gives contact information for NCI-designated cancer centers around the country.

- The ACS accredits cancer programs at hospitals and other treatment facilities. More than 1,400 programs in the United States have been designated by the ACS as Approved Cancer Programs. The ACS website offers a searchable database of these programs on the internet at http://web.facs.org/cpm/default.htm. The ACS can be contacted at 633 North Saint Clair Street, Chicago, IL 60611-3211, or by telephone at 312-202-5000.

- The JCAHO is an independent, not-for-profit organization that evaluates and accredits health care organizations and programs in the United States. It also offers information for the general public about choosing a treatment facility. The JCAHO website can be found on the internet at http://www.jointcommission.org. The JCAHO is located at One Renaissance Boulevard, Oakbrook Terrace, IL 60181-4294. The telephone number is 630-792-5000.

- The JCAHO offers an online Quality Check® service that patients can use to determine whether a specific facility has been accredited by the JCAHO and to view the organization's performance reports. This service is located on the internet at http://www.qualitycheck.org.

- The AHRQ publication "Your Guide to Choosing Quality Health Care" (described above in the section "Finding a Doctor") has suggestions and checklists for choosing the treatment facility that is right for you.

Finding a Treatment Facility for Patients Living Outside the United States

If you live outside the United States, facilities that offer cancer treatment may be located in or near your country. Cancer information services are available in many countries to provide information and answer questions about cancer; they may also be able to help you find a cancer treatment facility close to where you live. A list of these cancer information services is available on the International Cancer Information Service Group's (ICISG) website on the internet at http://www.icisg.org/meet_memberslist.htm, or may be requested by writing to the NCI Public Inquiries Office, Cancer Information Service, Room 3036A, 6116 Executive Boulevard, MSC 8322, Bethesda, MD 20892–8322, USA. The ICISG is an independent international organization composed of cancer information services. Their mission is to provide high-quality cancer information services and resources to those concerned about, or affected by, cancer throughout the world.

The International Union Against Cancer (UICC) is another resource for people living outside the United States who want to find a cancer treatment facility. The UICC consists of international cancer-related organizations devoted to the worldwide fight against cancer. UICC membership includes research facilities and treatment centers and, in some countries, ministries of health. Other members include volunteer cancer leagues, associations, and societies. These organizations serve as resources for the public and may have helpful information about cancer and treatment facilities. To find a resource in or near your country, contact the UICC at this address:

International Union Against Cancer (UICC)

62 route de Frontenex
1207 Geneva
Switzerland
Telephone: + 41 22 809 18 11
Web site: http://www.uicc.org

Some people living outside the United States may wish to obtain a second opinion or have their cancer treatment in this country. Many facilities in the United States offer these services to international cancer patients. These facilities may also provide support services, such as language interpretation, assistance with travel, and guidance in finding accommodations near the treatment facility for patients and their families.

If you live outside the United States and would like to obtain cancer treatment in this country, you should contact cancer treatment facilities directly to find out whether they have an international patient office. The NCI fact sheet "The National Cancer Institute Cancer Centers Program" (described above in the section "Finding a Doctor") offers contact information for NCI-designated cancer centers throughout the United States. This fact sheet is located on the internet at http://www.cancer.gov/cancertopics/factsheet/NCI/cancer-centers.

Citizens of other countries who are planning to travel to the United States for cancer treatment generally must first obtain a nonimmigrant visa for medical treatment from the U.S. Embassy or Consulate in their home country. Visa applicants must demonstrate that the purpose of their trip is to enter the United States for medical treatment; that they plan to remain for a specific, limited period; that they have funds to cover expenses in the United States; that they have a residence and social and economic ties outside the United States; and that they intend to return to their home country.

To determine the specific fees and documentation required for the nonimmigrant visa and to learn more about the application process, contact the U.S. Embassy or Consulate in your home country. A list of links to the websites of U.S. Embassies and Consulates worldwide can be found on the internet at http://usembassy.state.gov. More information about nonimmigrant visa services is available on the U.S. Department of State's website on the internet at http://travel.state.gov/visa/temp/temp_1305.html.

Chapter 2

Getting a Second Opinion

Cancer can be a confusing and frightening diagnosis, and it is hard to make decisions about possible treatment. Because cancer today is more often found at an early stage, and because treatments are continually improving, it may be valuable to seek the knowledge and advice of more than one doctor. This is called a second opinion. A second opinion is helpful when a doctor suspects or diagnoses cancer, or recommends a specific treatment plan.

Asking for a second opinion is common practice. Many people request a second opinion and some insurance providers require one in order for services to be covered. In all cases, the more knowledge you have about a particular diagnosis and the treatment options available, the more comfortable you will be regarding the health-care decisions you will be asked to make.

A second opinion after diagnosis: A second opinion after the diagnosis can provide a great deal of information:

- Confirmation that cancer is present and more detail on the type of cancer involved

- An opportunity for earlier treatment, if cancer is found where it was suspected, but not originally diagnosed

- Evidence that a disease other than cancer is present, preventing unnecessary treatment

A second opinion before treatment: Seeking a second opinion before beginning treatment can also provide a great deal of information:

- More information on the type of cancer, especially if the cancer is rare and knowledge is limited about the particular cancer or treatment

- Access to recognized experts and specialists (such as radiologists or surgeons), especially at a major cancer center

- Increased access to potentially promising new treatments not yet available to the public through participation in clinical trials, especially if the doctor providing a second opinion is affiliated with a major cancer center

Paying for a Second Opinion

Most insurance companies and health maintenance organizations (HMOs) pay for a second opinion when cancer is suspected or diagnosed. However, it's recommended that you inquire about payment before seeking a second opinion. Be sure to also ask if patients are required to select from a specific group of doctors when seeking a second opinion. Some insurers even require a second opinion before they will pay for cancer treatment.

Finding a Doctor for a Second Opinion

Patients should let their doctors know they are seeking a second opinion. Most doctors fully understand the value of a second opinion and are not offended when patients seek one. They may even be able to suggest another doctor. If you need an oncologist in your area to consult for a second opinion, you can search the Find an Oncologist database at the People Living with Cancer website, www.plwc.org, which includes American Society of Clinical Oncology members in the United States and abroad who have made their contact information public.

In some cases, seeking a second opinion from a specialist is very helpful, as there are many different types of oncologists. Possible sources for finding a doctor are listed below:

- Local hospitals, medical clinics, or cancer centers
- Medical schools and medical associations

- Friends and family
- Patient information or support organizations

Once a person locates a source for a second opinion, ask about the doctor's area of specialty and credentials, such as board certification, training, and experience, and bring all relevant medical records, including test results, x-rays, and any related materials to the appointment. Often, the doctor providing a second opinion will request the results of any tests or procedures you have already had performed, eliminating much of the need for repeat testing. It may also help to bring a notebook to the appointment to write down the recommendations provided.

Chapter 3

Tests Used to Diagnose and Monitor Cancer

What Is the Purpose of Diagnostic Tests?

Cancer patients undergo many different types of tests in order to accurately diagnose their disease, determine their prognosis, and monitor their cancer for progression or recurrence.

The term "diagnostic test" can be misleading, as these tests are not used only for diagnosing cancer, but also for monitoring cancer progression. There are many reasons for employing diagnostic tests depending on whether the disease is active or progressing, being treated, or in remission. Diagnostic tests may be used for the following purposes:

- **Diagnose primary disease:** Identify the disease the first time it occurs.

- **Identify cancer subtype:** Some cancers are divided into subtypes that are more or less aggressive; identification of a more aggressive subtype may influence the type of treatment proposed.

- **Predict prognosis:** Test results may indicate chance of cure, based on outcomes of other patients with similar results.

- **Direct treatment:** Cancer is many different diseases, all of which respond differently to various treatments. A diagnosis

This chapter includes the following "Diagnostic and Monitoring Tests" documents: "What Is the Purpose of Diagnostic Tests?" "Pathology Tests," "Diagnostic Imaging," "Blood Tests," "Tumor Marker Tests," and "The Emerging Role of Genomics in Diagnosing and Monitoring Cancer," © 2006 CancerConsultants .com. All rights reserved. Reprinted with permission.

that accurately identifies the type of cancer and predicts prognosis will also help to identify the type of treatment that maximizes chance of cure.

- **Evaluate response to treatment:** Some tests show whether the cancer is responding to treatment.

- **Detect minimal residual disease (MRD):** Cancer cells that remain after treatment is completed are called MRD. Detection of MRD may indicate a higher likelihood of recurrence.

- **Monitor remission or progression:** If a cancer is in remission, frequent tests may help detect the cancer if it returns or determine whether it is progressing.

- **Screen at-risk individuals:** Identifying abnormalities in cells or the DNA of cells of asymptomatic (healthy) individuals may indicate an increased risk (although not a certainty) of developing disease.

Pathology tests: Pathology tests involve microscopic evaluation of abnormal cells.

Diagnostic imaging: Diagnostic imaging involves visualization of abnormal masses using high-tech machines that create images. Examples of diagnostic imaging include x-rays, computed tomography (CT) scans, positron emission tomography (PET) scans, magnetic resonance imaging (MRI), and combined PET/CT scans.

Blood tests: Blood tests measure substances in the blood that may indicate how advanced the cancer is or other problems related to the cancer.

Tumor markers: Tumor marker tests detect substances in blood, urine, or other tissues that occur in higher than normal levels with certain cancers.

Genomics: Special laboratory evaluation of DNA involves the identification of the genetic make-up of the DNA of the abnormal cells.

Pathology Tests

Pathology is still the gold standard for the diagnosis of cancer, meaning it has been the most important diagnostic tool to date. A pathologist is a physician specializing in the diagnosis of disease based on examination of tissues and fluids removed from the body. Pathology tests involve evaluation of a small sample of cells under a microscope to determine whether they are cancerous by identifying structural abnormalities.

Tissue Samples

Most cancer patients will undergo a biopsy or other procedure to remove a sample of tissue for examination by a pathologist in order to diagnose their disease. There are a variety of methods used to obtain samples, including a typical biopsy, fine needle aspiration, or a biopsy with the use of an endoscope. The method used to gain a tissue sample depends on the type of mass and location in the body.

A typical biopsy involves the surgical removal of a mass of abnormal cells. Fine needle aspiration involves guiding a thin needle into the cancer and gently sucking out cells for microscopic evaluation. An endoscope is a lighted tube that can be guided into the body through an orifice, such as the mouth or anus, and is used to perform a biopsy. It allows the physician to see the cells in question and then "scrape" the abnormal cells in order to get a sample. For example, throat cells may be sampled in this way.

A physician may also perform a bone marrow biopsy, which uses a large needle to remove a sample of the bone marrow. The purpose of this procedure is to diagnose lymphoma and leukemia or determine whether certain types of cancer, such as breast or prostate, have spread to the bones. Bone marrow biopsies are usually performed in the bones of the rear hip. This procedure may also be called a bone marrow aspiration.

Once a tissue sample is obtained, it is then "fixed", meaning it is treated in a way that stops degradation and prevents the cells in the sample from changing characteristics. Next, the sample is stained so that the pathologist can see the cell structure under a microscope and determine whether the cells are exhibiting cancerous characteristics.

The Pathology Report

Once a tissue sample is obtained, the pathologist will examine the tissue sample under the microscope in order to determine if it contains normal, pre-cancerous or cancerous cells. The pathologist then writes a pathology report summarizing his or her findings.

The pathology report is a critical component of the diagnostic process. The primary doctor will use this report in conjunction with other relevant test results to make a final diagnosis and develop a treatment strategy.

After any biopsy or excision, you should request a copy of the pathology report for your records so that you have documentation of your pathologic diagnosis. In addition, it is helpful to have a copy of the pathology report to refer to when you are researching your disease.

By having a basic understanding of what the pathologist is looking for and the structure of the report, you may better understand your pathology report. Having a copy of your pathology report for your personal records is highly recommended. Your primary doctor should be able to address specific questions you have about your pathology report.

Understanding Your Pathology Report

Although pathology reports are written by physicians for physicians, you may be able to decipher some of the medical jargon provided by the report. Your primary doctor should be able to address specific questions you have about your pathology report; however, it is helpful to have a basic understanding of what the pathologist is looking for. The structure and information provided in your pathology report may vary, but the following sections are usually included.

Demographics: This section includes the patient's name and date of procedure. You should check that this information is correct to ensure that you have the correct pathology report.

Specimen: The specimen section describes the origin of the tissue sample(s).

Clinical history: The clinical history section provides a brief description of the patient's medical history relevant to the tissue sample that the pathologist is examining.

Clinical diagnosis (pre-operative diagnosis): The clinical diagnosis describes what the doctors are expecting before the pathologic diagnosis.

Procedure: The procedure describes how the tissue sample was removed.

Gross description (macroscopic): The gross description refers to the pathologist's observations of the tissue sample using the naked eye.

It may include size, weight, color or other distinguishing features of the tissue sample. If there is more than one sample, this section may designate a letter or number system to distinguish each sample.

Microscopic description: In the microscopic description, the pathologist describes how the cells of the tissue sample appear under a microscope. Specific attributes that the pathologist may look for and describe may include cell structure, tumor margins, vascular invasion, depth of invasion and pathologic stage.

Cell structure: Using a microscope, the pathologist examines the cell structure and microscopic attributes of the tissue sample and assigns a histologic grade to the tumor. The histologic grade helps the pathologist identify the type of tumor. The grade may be described numerically with the Scarff-Bloom-Richardson system (1–3) or as well-differentiated, moderately differentiated or poorly differentiated.

- Grade 1 or well-differentiated: Cells appear normal and are not growing rapidly.
- Grade 2 or moderately differentiated: Cells appear slightly different than normal.
- Grade 3 or poorly differentiated: Cells appear abnormal and tend to grow and spread more aggressively.

Tumor margins: If cancerous cells are present at the edges of the sample tissue, then the margins are described as "positive" or "involved." If cancerous cells are not present at the edges of the tissue, then the margins are described as "clear," "negative" or "not involved."

Vascular invasion: Pathologists will describe whether or not blood vessels are present within the tumor.

Depth of invasion: The depth of invasion may not be applicable to all tumors, but is used to describe invasion of the tumor.

Pathologic stage: The clinical stage is determined from the pathologic stage as well as other diagnostic tests such as x-rays. The pathologic stage, designated with a "p," describes the extent of the tumor as determined from the pathology report only. The staging system most often used by pathologists is based on the American Joint Commission on Cancer's (AJCC) TNM (tumor, node invasion, metastasis) system.

Special tests or markers: Depending on the tissue sample, the pathologist may conduct tests to further determine whether or not specific proteins or genes are present, as well as how fast cells are growing.

Diagnosis (summary): The final diagnosis is the section where the pathologist compiles the information from the entire pathology report into a concise pathologic diagnosis. It includes the tumor type and cell of origin.

Pathologist signature: The report is signed by the pathologist responsible for its contents.

Diagnostic Imaging

Imaging provides a non-invasive and painless way of visualizing tissues and organs in the body so that abnormalities can be identified. There are many different techniques for generating images. Some techniques utilized for detecting or diagnosing cancer include the following:

Radiography (x-ray): Radiography involves the use of radiation (x-rays) to create an image of the body. Radiographs are created by passing small, highly controlled amounts of radiation through the human body, capturing the resulting image on a special type of photographic film. Radiation passes through the various structures of the body differently. For example, very little radiation passes through the bones, leaving white "shadows" on the x-ray film. This is why x-rays are very useful for evaluating bones, as in detecting fractures.

X-rays are useful for determining whether cancer has spread (metastasized) to the bones. Because cancer cells are so dense and metabolically active, tumors, or masses of cancer cells, may also appear white on an x-ray, as is the case with lung cancer.

Bone scan: A type of x-ray called a bone scan may be performed to diagnose cancer in the bones or bone metastases. In this test, low level radioactive particles are injected into a vein. They circulate through the body and are selectively picked up by the bones. A high concentration of these radioactive particles indicates the presence of rapidly growing cancer cells in the bones.

Skeletal survey: A skeletal survey may be performed to diagnose cancer in the bones that causes extra build-up of bone, called blastic lesions. A skeletal survey is a type of x-ray. Conventional x-rays are used to image small sections of the body that may be of concern, such as the spine; whereas skeletal surveys image all areas of the body.

Dual energy x-ray absorptiometry (DEXA) scanning: DEXA scanning is the most widely used method for measuring bone mineral density. Bone density may weaken with bone metastases, cancer that has spread to the bones, or with osteoporosis, a weakening of the bones related to aging. DEXA scanning rapidly directs x-ray energy, alternating from two different sources, through the bone being examined. Once the x-rays have passed through the bone, their strength is recorded. Bone density or bone loss is calculated from the amount of energy that travels through the bone and is picked up by the detector. The minerals in bone, predominantly calcium, weaken the transmission of the x-rays through the bone. The denser the bone is, the less x-rays get through to the detector. The use of two different x-ray energy sources greatly improves the precision and accuracy of the measurement.

Mammography: Mammography uses safe, low doses of x-rays to image the inside of the breast. During a mammogram, the breast tissue will be compressed with a smooth plastic shield in order to help produce a highly detailed image. The x-rays pass through the breast and form an image on the x-ray film. Typically, two or three images are made of each breast.

Ultrasound (sonography): Ultrasound uses high frequency sound waves and their echoes to create an image. The primary advantage of ultrasound is that internal organs and other structures can be observed without using radiation. The ultrasound machine transmits sound pulses into the body using a probe. The sound waves travel through the body until they hit a boundary between tissues (between fluid and soft tissue, soft tissue and bone). At the boundary, some of the sound waves get reflected back to the probe, while some travel on further until they reach another boundary and get reflected. The reflected waves are detected by the probe and relayed to the machine, which calculates the distance from the probe to the tissue or organ. The machine displays the distances and intensities of the echoes on the screen, forming a two-dimensional image.

Newer ultrasound machines are capable of creating three-dimensional images. In these machines, several two-dimensional images are acquired by moving the probes across the body surface or rotating inserted probes. The two-dimensional scans are then combined by specialized computer software to form 3D images. 3D imaging allows the physician to see the organ being examined better, and is often used for early detection of cancer in the prostate, colon, rectum, and breast.

Ultrasound that is enhanced with the use of additional technologies appears to be even more effective for detecting cancer. A new development in ultrasound involves the use of color Doppler imaging. Doppler imaging is a technique that can detect differences in velocity (blood flow versus solid tissue) and transmits these differences in the form of different colors on a screen. This technique allows physicians to better determine the presence and exact location of a mass within the body.

Another type of ultrasound is microbubble-enhanced color Doppler, which has been shown to improve the detection of some cancers and reduce unnecessary biopsies compared to color Doppler that is not enhanced. Microbubbles are tiny bubbles of gas that can permeate through small blood vessels without causing harm. Since blood vessels and blood flow are more prevalent in cancerous tissues than regular tissues, microbubbles tend to concentrate in the cancer, which is revealed on the ultrasound image. This allows physicians to more accurately locate where to do the biopsy.

Positron emission tomography (PET): Unlike techniques that provide anatomical images, such as x-ray, CT and MRI, PET scans show chemical and physiological changes related to metabolism. This is important because these functional changes often occur before structural changes in tissues. PET images may therefore show abnormalities long before they would be revealed by x-ray, CT, or MRI.

Before a PET scan, a patient will receive an injection of a radiopharmaceutical, which is a drug labeled with a basic element of biological substances, called an isotope. These isotopes distribute in the organs and tissues of the body and mimic natural substances such as sugars, water, proteins, and oxygen. This radioactive substance is then taken up by the cancer cells, thereby allowing the radiologist to visualize areas of increased activity.

After the patient has received the injection, a small amount of radiation is passed through the body, which detects the isotopes and reveals details of cellular-level metabolism. Although the radiation is different from that used in radiography, it's roughly equivalent to what is administered in two chest x-rays. After the scan is complete the radiation does not stay in the body for very long.

PET is useful for diagnosing lung and breast cancer, and for monitoring response to therapy. Effective therapy leads to rapid reductions in the amount of glucose that is taken up by tumors. PET imaging can easily reveal this drop in metabolic activity and show—sometimes within minutes or hours—whether a patient is responding positively to a particular course of treatment. PET has been shown effective for predicting outcomes, detecting spread of cancer, and monitoring therapeutic response in a wide range of cancers, including breast, colon, lung, ovarian, head, neck, and thyroid cancers, as well as melanoma and lymphoma.

Magnetic resonance imaging (MRI): MRI uses a strong magnet and radiofrequency waves to produce an image of internal organs and structures. Under the influence of the strong magnet, the hydrogen atoms in the body line up like compass needles. Next, the patient is exposed to radio waves that cause the hydrogen atoms to momentarily change positions. In the process of returning to their orientation under the influence of the magnet, they emit a brief radio signal. The intensity of these radio waves reflects what type of tissue exists in that area of the body. The MRI system goes through the area of the body being imaged, point by point, collecting information from how the radio waves emit. A computer generates an image of organs and structures based on these radio wave recordings.

MRI has proven useful for detecting some types of cancer, and in some cases, may be more effective than biopsy, mammography, or ultrasound.

Computed tomography (CT): A CT scan is a detailed radiograph, or x-ray. The CT imaging system is comprised of a motorized table that moves the patient through a circular opening and an x-ray machine that rotates around the patient as they move through. Detectors on the opposite side of the patient from where the x-ray entered record the radiation exiting that section of the patient's body, creating an x-ray "snapshot" at one position (angle). Many different "snapshots" are collected during one complete rotation of the x-ray machine. A computer then assembles the series of x-ray images into a cross-section, or a picture of one small slice of the body. A CT scan is a series of these cross-sectional images.

PET/CT combination scan: Recent research indicates that a combination PET/CT scan may be more effective than whole body MRI for diagnosing the extent of spread for various cancers. Researchers from Germany conducted both combination PET/CT and MRI on 98 patients with various cancers. Overall, PET/CT scanning was 77% accurate for detecting the original cancer, cancer spread to nearby lymph nodes, and cancer spread to distant sites in the body, compared with only 53% accuracy with MRI.[1]

References

1. Antoch G, Vogt FM, Freudenberg LS et al. Whole-Body Dual-Modality PET/CT and Whole-Body MRI for Tumor Staging in Oncology. *Journal of the American Medical Association* 2003; 290:3199–3206.

Blood Tests

Blood tests are used to measure the number of blood cells in circulation and the levels of chemicals, enzymes, proteins, and organic waste products that are normally found in the blood. The levels of blood cells, such as red blood cells, white blood cells and platelets, may be low in patients receiving treatment for cancer. Also, the levels of some chemicals normally found in the blood may be either too high or too low as a result of the cancer or its treatment. There are two types of blood tests typically performed during cancer treatment: the complete blood count (CBC) and a blood chemistry panel.

Complete Blood Count (CBC)

The CBC measures the levels of the three basic blood cells: red blood cells, white blood cells, and platelets. In the United States, the CBC is typically reported in the format shown in Table 3.1. It is important to understand not only which blood counts are being tested, but also how those results are reported. You will want to pay careful attention to the result column, which shows any results that are normal, and the flag column, which shows any results that are abnormal.

Result column: The result column shows counts that fall within the normal range.

Flag column: The flag column shows counts that are lower ("L") or higher ("H") than the normal range.

Reference interval (or reference range) column: The reference interval shows the normal range for each measurement for the lab performing the test. Different labs may use different reference intervals.

White blood cells: White blood cells help protect individuals from infections. The CBC report in Table 3.1 shows that the patient's total white cell count is 1.5, which is lower than the normal range of 4.0–10.5. The low white cell count increases the risk of infection.

Absolute neutrophil count: Neutrophils are the main white blood cell for fighting or preventing bacterial or fungal infections. In the CBC report, neutrophils may be referred to as polymorphonuclear cells (polys or PMNs) or neutrophils. The absolute neutrophil count (ANC) is a measure of the total number of neutrophils present in the blood. When the ANC is less than 1,000, the risk of infection increases. The ANC can be calculated by multiplying the total WBC by the percent of polymorphonuclear cells. For example, this patient's ANC (Table 3.1) is 0.34, which equals (WBC) 1.5 x 23%.

Red blood cells: Red blood cells carry oxygen from the lungs to the rest of the body. The CBC report in Table 3.1 indicates that the

Table 3.1. CBC with Results and Reference Interval

Test	Result	Flag	Units	Reference Interval
White Blood Count		1.5 L	x 10–3/mL	4.0–10.5
Red Blood Count		3.50 L	x 10–6/mL	4.70–6.10
Hemoglobin		10.8 L	g/dL	14.0–18.0
Hematocrit	31.1 L	%	42.0–52.0	
Platelets	302		x 10–3/mL	140–415
Polys		23 L	%	45–76
Lymphs		68 H	%	17–44
Monocytes	7		%	3–10
Eos	2		%	0–4
Basos	>		%	0.2
Polys (absolute)		.34 L	x 10–3/mL	1.8–7.8
Lymphs (absolute)	1.0		x 10–3/mL	0.7–4.5
Monocytes (absolute)	0.1		x 10-3/mL	0.1–1.0
Eos (absolute)	0.1		x 10–3/mL	0.0–0.4
Basos (absolute)		0.0	x 10–3/mL	0.0–0.2

patient has a red cell count of 3.5, which is lower than the normal range of 4.70–6.10, and therefore, shown in the flag column.

Hemoglobin (Hb or Hgb): Hemoglobin is a protein in the red cell that carries oxygen. The CBC report in Table 3.1 indicates that the patient's Hb count is 10.8, which is below the normal range of 14.0–18.0. The hematocrit (HCT), another way of measuring the amount of Hb, is also low. This means that the patient has mild anemia and may be starting to notice symptoms.

Platelets: Platelets are the cells that form blood clots that stop bleeding. The CBC report in Table 3.1 indicates that the platelet count for this patient is normal.

Blood Chemistry Panel

The blood chemistry panel measures the levels of chemicals, enzymes, and organic waste products that are normally found in the blood. The results of a blood chemistry panel are typically reported with the name of the substance, the result, and the reference interval, as shown in Table 3.2. The reference interval is the normal range for that laboratory. Reference intervals may vary between laboratories. Substances that are typically measured in cancer patients are as follows:

- **Albumin** is the most prevalent protein in the blood. It is synthesized in the liver and removed from circulation by the kidney, which causes it to be excreted in the urine. Albumin is often measured in order to detect liver damage or kidney damage, either of which may be a side effect of cancer or cancer treatment.

- **Alanine aminotransferase (ALT)** is an enzyme in the liver that rearranges the building blocks of proteins. It is released from damaged liver cells. Cancer patients may experience liver damage as a side effect of some cancer treatments or due to spread of cancer to their liver. ALT may also be referred to as SGPT (serum glutamic pyruvic transferase).

- **Aspartate aminotransferase (AST)** is an enzyme in the liver that rearranges the building blocks of proteins. It is released from damaged liver cells. Cancer patients may experience liver damage as a side effect of some cancer treatments or due to spread of cancer to their liver. AST may also be referred to as SGOT (serum glutamic oxaloacetic transaminase).

- **Alkaline phosphatase** is an enzyme is that involved in bone growth. It is processed in the liver and excreted into the digestive tract in the bile. A higher than normal amount of alkaline phosphatase indicates bone or liver problems. In cancer patients, elevated alkaline phosphatase may indicate that cancer has spread to the bones or that liver damage, possibly due to some chemotherapy drugs, has caused problems with bile excretion.

- **Bilirubin** is a substance that is formed from broken down red blood cells. It becomes part of bile, which is produced by the liver. A build-up of bilirubin can cause jaundice and may be measured to test for liver or bile duct function, which may be compromised if there is cancer in the liver or if there is liver damage. Some chemotherapy drugs may cause liver damage.

Table 3.2. Sample Blood Chemistry Panel with Results and Reference Interval

Test	Result	Units	Reference interval
Albumin	3.9	g/dL	3.5–5.0
ALT (SGPT)	19	IU/L	6–31
AST (SGOT)	21	IU/L	11–36
Alkaline phosphatase	57	mg/dL	38–126
Total bilirubin	0.8	mg/dL	0.2–1.3
BUN	11	mg/dL	7–17
Calcium	9.2	mg/dL	8.4–10.2
Chloride	101	mmol/L	98–107
Creatinine	0.8	mg/dL	0.7–1.2
Glucose	98	mg/dL	65–105
Lactate dehydrogenase (LDH)	149	IU/L	100–250
Magnesium	0.89	mmol/L	0.65–1.05
Potassium	4.0	mmol/L	3.6–5.0
Sodium	141	mmol/L	137–145
Total protein	7.0	g/dL	6.3–8.2
Uric Acid	301	mmol/L	227–367/467

- **BUN (blood urea nitrogen)** is a part of urea, the waste product that is left over from the breakdown of protein. Urea circulates in the blood until it is filtered out by the kidneys and excreted in the urine. If the kidneys are not functioning properly, there will be excess urea in the bloodstream, resulting in higher than normal BUN levels. Cancer patients may have elevated BUN if they have been treated with certain chemotherapy drugs that may cause kidney damage.

- **Calcium** is a chemical that is necessary for muscle contraction, nerve function, blood clotting, cell division, healthy bones, and teeth. An increased level of calcium in the bloodstream is a possible complication of cancer and is referred to as hypercalcemia. In its severe form, hypercalcemia may be a life-threatening emergency.

- **Chloride** is a chemical that helps maintain fluid balance in the body. Low chloride levels may be caused by vomiting or diarrhea.

- **Creatinine** is a compound that is produced by the body and excreted in the urine. Compounds that leave the body in the urine are processed by the kidney, therefore creatinine may be used to monitor for kidney function. Some cancer treatments may cause kidney damage.

- **Glucose** is the simplest form of sugar that the body uses for energy. The body requires insulin to move sugar from the bloodstream into the cells for energy production. An abnormal glucose reading may signify a problem with insulin production, which occurs in the pancreas.

- **Lactate dehydrogenase (LDH)** is involved in producing energy and is released from damaged cells in many areas of the body, including the heart and liver. Cancer patients may have an elevated LDH due to spread of cancer to their liver or damage to their liver from certain cancer treatments. LDH is also considered a tumor marker, which is a substance that occurs at higher than normal amounts in the presence of cancer.

- **Magnesium** is a chemical that is necessary for muscle contraction, nerve function, heart rhythm, bone strength, generating energy, and building protein.

- **Potassium** is a chemical that regulates heart contraction and helps maintain fluid balance.

- **Sodium** is a chemical that helps maintain fluid balance and is necessary for muscle contraction and nerve function. Low sodium levels may be caused by vomiting or diarrhea.

- **Uric acid** is the end product of the digestion of certain proteins and is normally eliminated through the urine. Excess uric acid may be a side effect of some cancer treatments, and may lead to a condition called tumor lysis syndrome. When excess uric acid is present, it is converted to crystal. These crystals may be deposited in the tiny tubes that are part of the kidney and cause acute kidney damage, which can ultimately lead to kidney failure.

Additional results that are sometimes included in the blood chemistry panel are measures of the blood's clotting capacity (Table 3.3). Some cancer treatments reduce the number of platelets in circulation, which can cause the blood to clot more slowly so that the patient is more susceptible to excessive bleeding.

Table 3.3. Measures of the Blood's Clotting Capacity

Test	Result	Units	Reference Interval
aPTT	3.9	seconds	24–35
Prothrombin time (PT)/INR	19	seconds	24–35

- **Activated partial thromboplastin time (aPTT)** is a measure of bleeding and clotting and is used to evaluate unexplained bleeding or monitor heparin treatment. Heparin is a drug that is administered to increase the clotting capacity of a patient's blood. Some cancer patients may receive heparin as treatment for a low platelet count, or thrombocytopenia, which is a side effect of some cancer treatments. This condition can lead to more easy bruising and bleeding.

- **Prothrombin time (PT)** is the most common way to express the clotting capacity of blood. PT results are reported as the number of seconds the blood takes to clot when mixed with a thromboplastin reagent. The International Normalized Ratio (INR) was created by the World Health Organization because PT results can vary depending on the thromboplastin reagent used. The INR is a conversion unit that takes into account the different sensitivities

31

of thromboplastins. The INR is widely accepted as the standard unit for reporting PT results. Cancer patients may have an abnormally low PT/INR due to a lower than normal platelet count. Platelets are the components of blood that stop bleeding by clotting the blood. A low platelet count, also called thrombocytopenia, and a low PT may lead to more frequent bruising and bleeding.

Tumor Marker Tests

Tumor markers are substances that can often be detected in higher than normal amounts in the blood, urine, or body tissues of some patients with certain types of cancer. These substances can be proteins, enzymes, biochemicals, or antigens. Tumor markers may either be produced by the cancer itself or by the body in response to the cancer. In general, tumor marker levels are lower in early stage disease (but still higher than normal) and higher with advanced disease. Furthermore, their levels decrease in response to treatment and increase when the cancer progresses.

Tumor markers are often used for these purposes:

- **Monitor response to treatment:** Some tests show whether the cancer is responding to treatment.

- **Monitor for progression:** In general, an increase in some tumor markers indicates disease progression.

- **Detect recurrence:** Regular monitoring of some tumor markers during a remission may help detect recurrence.

- **Detect metastasis:** Metastasis is the spread of cancer from its site of origin to another distant location in the body.

- **Screen at-risk individuals:** Prostate specific antigen is an example of a tumor marker that is specific enough for one condition—prostate cancer—to function as a screening test for asymptomatic, at-risk men, which generally refers to men over 50 years of age with at least a 10-year life expectancy.

- **Identify specific cancer subtype:** Some cancers are divided into subtypes that are more or less aggressive; some tumor marker tests make it possible to distinguish between cancer types.

- **Predict prognosis:** Test results may indicate the chance of a negative or positive outcome, based on outcomes of other patients with similar results.

Tumor markers are not specific enough to be used alone for diagnosing cancer. There are several reasons for this:

- Tumor marker levels can be elevated in people with benign (non-cancerous) disease.

- Tumor markers are not elevated in every person with cancer, particularly those with early stage disease.

- Most tumor markers are not totally specific for a single condition, meaning that many different cancers or diseases can result in a higher than normal level of a particular marker.

For these reasons, tumor markers are not used in isolation; instead, results from tumor marker tests are evaluated in the context of a patient's history, symptoms, and other test results.

Despite these limitations, researchers continue to study the markers listed below, as well as potential new markers to determine whether they may have a role in screening, early detection, and directing treatment.

Tumor Markers by Cancer Type

Bladder Cancer

- *Tumor marker:* Bladder tumor antigen (BTA)
  - *Primary use:* Detect recurrence
  - *Other conditions that cause elevated levels:* recent surgery; genitourinary tract infection; cancer of kidney or ureters
  - *Normal value:* Not detectable
  - *Detected in:* Urine
- *Tumor marker:* Nuclear matrix protein (NMP 22)
  - *Primary use:* Predict prognosis; detect recurrence
  - *Other conditions that cause elevated levels:* Recent surgery; chemotherapy; genitourinary infection or disease; renal or bladder stones; rigorous exercise
  - *Normal value:* <10 U/ml
  - *Detected in:* Urine

Breast Cancer

- *Tumor marker:* CA 15-3

- *Primary use:* Monitor response to treatment; detect metastases
- *Other conditions that cause elevated levels:* Cervical cancer; liver cancer
- *Normal value:* <31 unit/ml
- *Detected in:* Blood

- *Tumor marker:* CA 27.29
  - *Primary use:* Monitor response to treatment; detect metastases
  - *Other conditions that cause elevated levels:* Cervical cancer
  - *Normal value:* <38–40 unit/ml
  - *Detected in:* Blood

- *Tumor marker:* Carcinoembryonic antigen (CEA)
  - *Primary use:* Predict prognosis; monitor response to treatment; detect recurrence; used in combination with CA 15-3
  - *Other conditions that cause elevated levels:* Colorectal cancer; lung cancer; gastric cancer; pancreatitis; hepatitis; COPD; cigarette smoking
  - *Normal value:* <3 ng/ml
  - *Detected in:* Blood

Colorectal Cancer

- *Tumor marker:* Carcinoembryonic antigen (CEA)
  - *Primary use:* Predict prognosis; detect recurrence; monitor response to treatment
  - *Other conditions that cause elevated levels:* Breast cancer; lung cancer; gastric cancer; pancreatitis; hepatitis; COPD; cigarette smoking
  - *Normal value:* <3 ng/ml
  - *Detected in:* Blood

- *Tumor marker:* CA 19-9
  - *Primary use:* Monitor response to treatment; monitor progression
  - *Other conditions that cause elevated levels:* Pancreas cancer; gastric cancer; liver cancer; pancreatitis; ulcerative colitis; inflammatory bowel disease

- *Normal value:* <33 unit/ml
- *Detected in:* Blood

Liver Cancer

- *Tumor marker:* Alpha-fetoprotein (AFP)
  - *Primary use:* Diagnose liver cancer in patients with chronic hepatitis; follow-up after surgery for liver cancer
  - *Other conditions that cause elevated levels:* Germ cell cancer of ovaries/testes; cirrhosis; hepatitis; inflammatory bowel disease; pregnancy
  - *Normal value:* 0–6.4 IU/ml
  - *Detected in:* Blood

Non-Small Cell Lung Cancer (NSCLC)

- *Tumor marker:* Carcinoembryonic antigen (CEA)
  - *Primary use:* Diagnosis, but not very important because lung cancer can be easily seen on an x-ray
  - *Other conditions that cause elevated levels:* Colorectal cancer; breast cancer; gastric cancer; pancreatitis; hepatitis; COPD; cigarette smoking
  - *Normal value:* <3 ng/ml
  - *Detected in:* Blood

Small Cell Lung Cancer (SCLC)

- *Tumor marker:* Neuron-specific enolase (NSE)
  - *Primary use:* Distinguish SCLC from NSCLC; monitor response to treatment; monitor progression
  - *Other conditions that cause elevated levels:* Neuroblastoma; pancreatic cancer; thyroid cancer; chronic bronchitis; COPD
  - *Normal value:* <13 ng/ml
  - *Detected in:* Blood

Lymphoma

- *Tumor marker:* Lactic dehydrogenase (LDH)

- *Other conditions that cause elevated levels:* Hepatitis; myocardial infarction; melanoma metastasis; liver metastases
- *Normal value:* 100–210 unit/l
- *Detected in:* Blood
- *Tumor marker:* Beta-2-microglobulin (B2M)
  - *Primary use:* Predict prognosis; monitor progression
  - *Other conditions that cause elevated levels:* Multiple myeloma
- *Tumor marker:* Gamma globulin
  - *Other conditions that cause elevated levels:* Multiple myeloma
  - *Normal value:* 3.0–13.0 g/L
  - *Detected in:* Blood

Melanoma Skin Cancer

- *Tumor marker:* TA 90
  - *Primary use:* Detect metastasis; predict prognosis
  - *Normal value:* Not detected
  - *Detected in:* Blood

Multiple Myeloma

- *Tumor marker:* Bence Jones protein
  - *Primary use:* Diagnosis; predict prognosis; monitor progression; monitor response to treatment
  - *Other conditions that cause elevated levels:* Non-Hodgkin lymphoma
  - *Normal value:* 0.02–0.5 mg/mL
  - *Detected in:* Urine
- *Tumor marker:* Myeloma protein (M-protein or M-spike)
  - *Primary use:* Diagnosis; predict prognosis
  - *Normal value:* <30 g/L
  - *Detected in:* Blood
- *Tumor marker:* Beta-2-microglobulin (B2M)
  - *Primary use:* Predict prognosis; monitor progression

- *Other conditions that cause elevated levels:* Lymphoma; acute lymphocytic leukemia

- *Tumor marker:* Gamma globulin

  - *Other conditions that cause elevated levels:* Non-Hodgkin lymphoma
  - *Normal value:* 3.0–13.0 g/L
  - *Detected in:* Blood

Ovarian Cancer (epithelial)

- *Tumor marker:* CA 125

  - *Primary use:* Indicates most common form of ovarian cancer, epithelial; monitor response to treatment; detect recurrence
  - *Other conditions that cause elevated levels:* Breast cancer; colorectal cancer; ovarian cysts or fibroids; endometriosis; inflammatory bowel disease; cirrhosis; peritonitis; pancreatitis
  - *Normal value:* 0–35 unit/ml
  - *Detected in:* Blood

Ovarian Cancer (germ cell)

- *Tumor marker:* Alpha-fetoprotein (AFP)

  - *Primary use:* Diagnosis; follow-up after treatment
  - *Other conditions that cause elevated levels:* Germ cell cancer of the testes; cirrhosis; hepatitis; inflammatory bowel disease; pregnancy
  - *Normal value:* 0–6.4 IU/ml
  - *Detected in:* Blood

Pancreatic Cancer

- *Tumor marker:* CA 19-9

  - *Primary use:* Predict prognosis; monitor response to treatment; monitor progression
  - *Other conditions that cause elevated levels:* Colorectal cancer; gastric cancer; liver cancer; pancreatitis; ulcerative colitis; inflammatory bowel disease

- *Normal value:* <37 unit/ml
- *Detected in:* Blood

Prostate Cancer

- *Tumor marker:* Prostate specific antigen (PSA)
  - *Primary use:* Screening; detect early stage disease; monitor progression
  - *Normal value:* <4 ng/ml
  - *Detected in:* Blood
- *Tumor marker:* Prostatic acid phosphatase (PAP)
  - *Primary use:* Rarely used because PSA is more sensitive
  - *Other conditions that cause elevated levels:* Present in many body tissues; enlarged prostate
  - *Normal value:* Varies from lab to lab
  - *Detected in:* Blood
- *Tumor marker:* Prostate-specific membrane antigen (PSMA)
  - *Primary use:* Still under investigation
  - *Other conditions that cause elevated levels:* Age

Testicular Cancer

- *Tumor marker:* Human chorionic gonadotropin (hCG)
  - *Primary use:* Diagnose at-risk individuals; monitor response to treatment; detect metastases
  - *Other conditions that cause elevated levels:* Pregnancy; cirrhosis; duodenal ulcers; benign breast, lung, pancreas, ovary, GI cancers; choriocarcinoma; mediastinal germ cell neoplasms
  - *Normal value:* >31 ng/mL
  - *Detected in:* Blood
- *Tumor marker:* Alpha-fetoprotein (AFP)
  - *Primary use:* Diagnose; follow-up after treatment
  - *Other conditions that cause elevated levels:* Germ cell cancer of the ovaries; cirrhosis; hepatitis; inflammatory bowel disease; pregnancy

- *Normal value:* <40 ng/mL
- *Detected in:* Blood

Thyroid Cancer

- *Tumor marker:* Calcitonin
  - *Primary use:* Diagnose early disease; screening for at-risk individuals
  - *Other conditions that cause elevated levels:* Lung cancer (rarely measured)
  - *Normal value:* <13 pg/ml
  - *Detected in:* Blood
- *Tumor marker:* Thyroglobulin
  - *Primary use:* Monitor response to treatment; monitor progression
  - *Normal value:* >1 mcg/L
  - *Detected in:* Blood

New Advances in Tumor Marker Tests

Most tumor markers are proteins. Since DNA is the code that determines which proteins will be produced by a cell, researchers are developing methods to detect DNA. Even in many early stage diseases, cancer cells may break away from the tissue where they originated and can be detected in the blood or other body substances. For example, researchers have detected abnormal DNA in these conditions:

- Blood of people with breast, liver, lung, ovarian cancer, and melanoma

- Urine of individuals with bladder cancer

- Saliva of individuals with cancers of the oral cavity

This new approach to tumor marker testing can be thought of as measuring the cause (DNA) rather than the effect (protein), and may thus provide even more accurate and useful information for screening, early detection, monitoring, and planning treatment.

Researchers from Italy have found that measuring circulating DNA appears to be an accurate and quick method of detecting lung cancer, even in its earliest stages. This trial involved 100 patients who had been newly diagnosed with lung cancer, with stages I–IV (earliest stage to most advanced stage). Blood was drawn and tested for DNA in 100 patients who had been newly diagnosed with lung cancer (stages I–IV) and compared blood drawn from control groups, which included the following:

- Individuals who were heavy smokers but did not have lung cancer

- Individuals who were not smokers and did not have lung cancer

DNA levels in the blood were eight times higher in patients with lung cancer, compared to the control group. These levels were also detected in individuals with early-stage cancer. Only patients with cancer had high levels of DNA in their blood. Elevated DNA accurately detected lung cancer in 90% of cases.[1]

References

1. Sozzi G, Conte D, Leon M, et al. Quantification of free circulating DNA as a diagnostic marker in lung cancer. *Journal of Clinical Oncology* 2003;21:3902–3908.

The Emerging Role of Genomics in Diagnosing and Monitoring Cancer

Cancer is the result of genetic abnormalities that affect the function of particular genes. Genes determine the form, function, and growth patterns of cells. Those that accelerate or suppress growth are often involved in cancer. For example, many cancers have an abnormality in a gene that is responsible for stimulating cellular growth and the gene that normally prevents cancer is not working properly. Both of these genetic abnormalities can result in uncontrolled and excessive cellular growth, the hallmark trait of cancer. Genomic tests, or assays as they are called by scientists, are a tool for identifying the specific genes in a cancer that are abnormal or are not working properly. In essence, this is like identifying the genetic signature or fingerprint of a particular cancer.

Genomic testing is different from genetic testing. Genetic tests are typically used to determine whether a healthy individual has an inherited trait (gene) that predisposes them to developing cancer. Genomic tests evaluate the genes in a sample of diseased tissue from a patient who has already been diagnosed with cancer. In this way, genes that have mutated, or have developed abnormal functions, are identified in addition to those that may have been inherited.

Genomic testing can help doctors to do the following:

- Determine a patient's prognosis (potential outcome)

- Determine whether a cancer is aggressive/fast growing or slow growing

- Choose the most effective treatment for each individual cancer

- Monitor patients who are undergoing treatment to determine if the treatment is working

- Monitor patients who are in remission to catch a potential disease progression early when it is more treatable

Perhaps the greatest promise of genomic testing is its potential for individualizing treatment. This means that patients with more serious conditions can be identified and offered aggressive and innovative therapies that may prolong their lives, while patients who are diagnosed with a less serious condition may be spared unnecessary treatments. For example, some women with node-negative breast cancer will relapse after being treated with surgery alone. Genomic testing has been shown to differentiate between which node-negative breast cancer patients are more likely to relapse and therefore benefit from additional chemotherapy and which patients may not need chemotherapy.

To appreciate how the science of genetics is applied to the diagnosis and monitoring of cancer, it is helpful to have an understanding of the basic principles of genetics. This includes knowing what DNA, chromosomes, and genes are, how they work, and how the information contained in DNA is transformed, through gene expression, into specific structures that dictate the functions of a cell.

With this background knowledge, it is possible to understand the promise of tests for detecting genetic abnormalities, such as these:

- Fluorescence *in situ* hybridization (FISH)
- Polymerase chain reaction (PCR)
- Reverse transcription PCR
- Microarray technology
- Serum proteomics

Background—Basic Principles of Genetics

The importance of genetics in heredity is well known; however, the role that genetics plays in controlling the structure and function of cells may be even more critical for an individual organism. Heredity assures that humans and all species are able to reproduce and perpetuate their unique traits and directing how cells are built, what work they do, and how they grow is necessary to ensure that an organism will survive to reproduce. An understanding of this critical role that DNA and genes have in determining the minute-by-minute life of a cell is also important for understanding how genetics are involved in cancer.

DNA: The genetic information for an entire organism is contained in the nucleus of every cell in the form of deoxyribonucleic acid, commonly known as DNA. DNA is a double-stranded helical (coiled) molecule. Each strand is composed of a structural backbone plus a sequence of nitrogen-containing compounds called nitrogenous bases, which can be thought of as the alphabet of genetics. There are four bases: adenine, guanine, thymine, and cytosine. The two strands are connected at the bases.

The genetic code, or the genetic information that controls structure and function of the cell, is contained in the sequence of bases. The base sequence eventually controls the sequence of amino acids that are connected together to make a protein molecule. Different sequences make different proteins. The proteins that are synthesized in a cell determine the structure and function of that cell.

Chromosomes: DNA is packaged in a specific number of units called chromosomes. Humans have 46 chromosomes in each cell. Most of the time, the chromosomes are packed tightly around proteins in the nucleus of the cell so that they cannot be seen. However, in the stages of the cell's life just before cell division, the chromosomes become visible with a light microscope. They appear like a capital "H" with four lengths of coiled DNA joined by a protein as the "cross" of the "H".

Genes: DNA is organized into genes, which are long segments of DNA that include regions that contain codes for proteins called exons, as well as non-coding regions called introns. Genes are defined as the basic unit of heredity because they are passed to offspring and then replicated and passed on to individual cells during cell division. Replication involves using both strands of DNA as templates to synthesize complimentary DNA (cDNA), which is a matching strand. The result is two identical copies of DNA for each cell after cell division is complete. Under normal conditions, the structure of DNA, and thus genes, remains relatively constant through replication and cell division.

Gene expression: The genetic information contained in genes is translated into cellular structure and function through a process called gene expression. Genes can be thought of as codes, or recipes, for making proteins. Proteins are the basic component of cell structure and function. When a gene is "expressed," the protein or proteins that it codes for are actively being built in the cell and the function that those proteins serve are being performed. For example, when the HER-2/neu gene is expressed in breast cancer, there are more epidermal growth factor receptors (EGFRs) present, which are proteins on the cell surface that HER-2/neu codes for. Furthermore, the function of EGFR is to stimulate cell growth; so a cell that is expressing HER-2/neu has many EGFRs and is actively growing.

Gene expression occurs through a complex system that involves the following steps:

- Temporary separation of the two strands of the DNA molecule at a particular gene.

- Transcription of the segment of DNA, which is the synthesis of a single-stranded copy of the DNA sequence that is exposed; this copy is called messenger RNA (mRNA).

- Protein synthesis, or building new proteins in the cell, based on the information contained in the mRNA.

Genetic abnormalities: Genetic abnormalities are alterations in the DNA of a cell that may occur by chance or due to an environmental influence. These alterations lend the affected cell some advantage over normal cells that helps them grow. As a result, the cell is able to divide rapidly, becoming a cancer growth. However, this growth advantage only benefits the individual cell, and not necessarily the whole organism (human).

Types of genetic abnormalities include the following:

- **Translocations:** The changing places of a gene from one chromosome with a gene on another chromosome; this type of abnormality defines the many different leukemias

- **Deletions:** A gene or sequence of nucleotides is missing in the DNA

- **Polymorphisms:** Variations in nucleotide sequence

Tests for Detecting Genetic Abnormalities

A variety of new laboratory tests can detect genetic abnormalities. Finding a disease-causing mutation in a gene can confirm a suspected diagnosis of cancer or identify those predisposed to certain cancers. Some of these techniques that are currently used in the clinical setting include these:

- Fluorescence *in situ* hybridization (FISH)

- Polymerase chain reaction (PCR)

- Reverse transcription PCR

Furthermore, the following laboratory technique is being used in cancer research and may be available for clinical use in the future:

- Microarray

Fluorescence In Situ *Hybridization (FISH)*

FISH is a laboratory technique that is used to detect genetic abnormalities at the single-cell and single-gene level, such as numerical abnormalities (gains and losses of nucleotides), and translocations (the changing places of a gene or segment of genes on one chromosome with gene or a segment on another chromosome). These abnormalities play a role in the development and progression of some cancers, such as leukemias and lymphomas.[1]

How does FISH work? FISH is performed on sample cells whose DNA has unraveled so that the individual chromosomes are visible. This happens during cell phases just before cell division, called metaphase or interphase. The sample DNA is first denatured using heat and the chemical formamide so that the individual strands separate, exposing the base sequence. Next, specific DNA sequences, called probes, that are attached to colored fluoros are incubated, or combined, with the sample DNA. The probes hybridize (connect) with the DNA in the chromosomes that is the compliment to the base sequence in the probe. The presence or absence of fluorescence from the hybridized DNA and probe are visible with a specialized microscope and indicate whether the DNA sequence of interest is present in the sample. Furthermore, specialized FISH techniques can be used to detect translocations, inversions, and amplifications that are involved in cancer.[2]

FISH in breast and ovarian cancer: A common use of FISH is to determine whether patients with breast and ovarian cancer overexpress the HER2/neu oncogene, a gene that is commonly involved in cancer. HER2/neu carries the genetic code for the HER2 receptor, a protein on the surface of some cancer cells. HER2 binds with growth factors in the blood, thereby stimulating cancer cells to grow.

HER2/neu is amplified in approximately 20% to 30% of breast and ovarian cancers and this amplification or overexpression indicates a poor prognosis.[3] FISH can be used to observe whether the HER2/neu oncogene is sending multiple signals at the level of the individual cells, which indicates gene amplification.

FISH in hematological (blood) cancers: FISH may also be used to diagnose and manage various hematological malignancies. The genetic abnormality that underlies many hematological malignancies is chromosomal translocation, or the changing places of gene from one chromosome with a gene on another chromosome.

Polymerase Chain Reaction (PCR)

PCR is an in vitro laboratory method that is useful for genetic testing for disease and detecting minimal residual disease, which is a small amount of disease left after treatment that may lead to recurrence and is typically not detectable with other techniques. This procedure amplifies a segment of DNA from a small sample, making it detectable. With PCR, relatively small sequences of known DNA can be replicated into millions of copies over a short period of time.

How does PCR work? This method requires four principle components: the sample DNA, an ample supply of nucleotides, a heat-stable polymerase enzyme which is responsible for copying DNA, and primers, short sequence of nucleotides that lie on either side of the DNA fragment of interest and signal the polymerase to begin replication of the specific DNA segment.

PCR is a three-step process, each occurring at a different temperature. The sample DNA is first heated to approximately 90° C in order to separate the two paired DNA strands. Once separated, it is cooled to a temperature that allows the primers to hybridize to their complementary sequence on the target DNA, approximately 40° C. Lastly,

DNA replication occurs at approximately 70° C, the temperature at which DNA polymerase is most active. This process is repeated 20 to 30 times, resulting in approximately 1 million-fold amplification of the DNA fragment of interest.[4]

Reverse Transcription PCR

Reverse transcription (RT)-PCR is a technique that detects the degree to which genes are expressed. Complicated processes control which segment of DNA separates, gets transcribed (copied) into mRNA, and then expressed as proteins in the cell. Not all genes are transcribed and then expressed equally. Due to many controls in the cell, some genes are over-expressed, which means they are transcribed and expressed at a higher rate than normal, while other genes are now expressed, or "turned off" so that certain functions are not manifested in the cell.

How does RT-PCR work? RT-PCR uses the same steps as PCR to amplify a segment of DNA, but the sample is a complimentary copy of mRNA. By starting with mRNA, this test measures only the DNA that is expressed, making it possible to determine the degree to which certain genes are expressed. Recent uses of RT-PCR in clinical oncology include detection of lymph node micrometastases in prostate cancer and bone metastases in breast cancer.[5]

RT-PCR in breast cancer: The breast cancer test Oncotype DX™ utilizes RT-PCR to determine the individual risk of recurrence in women with node-negative estrogen receptor (ER)-positive breast cancer. This test evaluates expression of 21 genes in breast cancer. Overexpression of some of these genes indicates a worse prognosis, while expression of others may indicate a better prognosis. The expression of all 21 genes is used to calculate a "Recurrence Score™", or the likelihood that that cancer will recur. A large clinical trial showed that Recurrence Score™ was more effective for predicting prognosis of women with node-negative, ER-positive breast cancer than standard measures such as patient age, cancer size, and cancer stage.[6]

Strategies to Improve Detection of Genetic Abnormalities

Several methods for detecting genetic abnormalities are being utilized for cancer research. While they are not yet routinely used in the clinical setting, the following appears to be promising and may be used in the future for diagnosing, testing, and monitoring cancer.

Microarrays: Microarray analysis is a technique that combines biology with computer science to generate a genetic profile for a given tissue sample that reflects the activity of thousands of genes. This technology has advantages over FISH or PCR because, in a single analysis, it can evaluate the expression of all of the genes that may be involved in a cancer, rather than just a few. By graphically showing how all of the genes are involved in a cancer, microarrays can generate a "genetic signature" for a particular cancer. This makes the identification of cancer subtype more precise. The ability to take a snapshot of a cancer's genetic signature may lead to a better understanding of how that cancer develops and how to design individualized treatment.

How do microarrays work? While different microarray methods are utilized, each consists of five basic steps:

- **Preparation of the sample:** In the initial step, cDNA is synthesized from RNA by reverse transcription (remember transcription involves copying DNA to make RNA, so reverse transcription is generating DNA from RNA) from RNA that has been extracted from both a test and a reference sample. The sample DNA segments are labeled with fluorochromes, or radioactive chemicals, so that they can be detected after they combine with the computer chip.

- **Combining the sample with the computer chip:** Next, the sample is combined with the computer chip, which is a rectangular grid of spots. Each spot has many copies of a particular DNA sequence. These sequences are derived from public databases of DNA sequences that were generated through the Human Genome Project, the scientific endeavor that identified virtually all of the DNA sequences in the human species. When the sample is added to the computer chip, a process called hybridization occurs. This means that the sample DNA segment binds (hybridizes) to the segment on the computer chip that has the exact complimentary sequence of nucleotides (the four compounds that are the alphabet of genetics).

- **Scanning the computer chip:** Once hybridization is complete, scanners are used to detect the fluorescence and create a digital image that reflects where the sample DNA combined with spots on the microarray chip.

- **Normalization:** Because raw signal intensities may vary between individual chips from many patients or experiments, individual chip intensity must be adjusted to a common standard, or normalized. For example, subtraction of background noise is a common normalization method that is applied to all samples. Normalization makes it possible to compare gene expression profiles from many patients or experiments.

- **Computer analysis:** The final step in a microarray experiment is computer analysis. The thousands of raw data points that result from microarray analyses are essentially unintelligible unless they are evaluated in the context of other results. For example, the gene expression profile (microarray results) of normal and diseased tissue can be compared to identify genes that vary in their expression and also identify a pattern (profile) that may indicate a distinct class or stage of disease.[7]

Microarrays in oncology: Microarray analysis has contributed to oncology by increasing an understanding of the genetic basis of several types of cancer, including B-cell non-Hodgkin lymphoma (BCNHL), acute leukemia, and breast cancer.

- Considerable knowledge regarding the pathology of BCNHL has been gained by comparing gene expression patterns of diseased and normal tissue. Two different disease categories display distinct gene expression profiles. Microarrays have helped establish these expression profiles and, in the future, they may help accurately classify new cases of BCNHL.

- In the case of acute leukemia, microarrays have helped establish distinct gene expression patterns that have helped differentiate acute lymphocytic leukemia (ALL) and acute myeloid leukemia (AML). Using these profiles, 29 of 34 new cases of leukemia were correctly predicted.

- Furthermore, microarrays have helped identify two distinct gene expression profiles in breast cancer, BCRA1 and BCRA2. This finding suggests different ways that breast cancer develops and provides clues that promote further understanding of the cause of breast cancer.[7]

References

1. Spagnolo SD, Ellis DW, Juneja S, Leong AS, et al. The role of molecular studies in lymphoma diagnosis: a review. *Pathology* 2004; 36 (1)19–44.

2. Spurbeck JL, Adams SA, Stupca PJ, Dewald GW. Primer on Medical Genomics Part XI: Visualizing Human Chromosomes. *Mayo Clinic Proceedings* 2004:79:58–75.

3. Paik S, Hazan R, Fisher ER, et al. Pathological findings from the national surgical adjuvant breast and bowel project: prognostic significance of erb B-2 protein overexpression in primary breast cancer. *J Clin Oncol* 1990;8:103–112.

4. Tefferi A, Wieben ED, Dewald GW, et al. Primer on Medical Genomics Part II: Background Principles and Methods in Molecular Genetics. *Mayo Clinic Proceedings* 2002;77:785–808.

5. Tefferi A, Wieben ED, Dewald GW, et al. Primer on Medical Genomics Part II: Background Principles and Methods in Molecular Genetics. *Mayo Clinic Proceedings* 2002;77:785–808.

6. Paik S, Shak S, Tang G, et al. Multi-gene PT-PCR assay for predicting recurrence in node negative breast cancer patients— NSABP studies B-20 and B-14. *Proc of the 26th Annual San Antonio Breast Cancer Symposium.* December 3-8k, 2003; San Antonio, TX, Abstract #16.

7. Tefferi A, Bolander ME, Ansell SM, et al. Primer on Medical Genomics Part III: Microarray Experiments and Data Analysis. *Mayo Clinic Proceedings* 2002;77:927–940.

Chapter 4

Understanding
Your Cancer Diagnosis

Cancer Diagnosis

The diagnosis of cancer entails an attempt to accurately identify the anatomical site of origin of the malignancy and the type of cells involved. Cancer can arise in any organ or tissue in the body except fingernails, hair, and teeth.

The site refers to the location of the cancer within the body. The body part in which cancer first develops is known as the primary site. A cancer's primary site may determine how the tumor will behave; whether and where it may spread (metastasize) and what symptoms it is most likely to cause. The most common sites in which cancer develops include the skin, lungs, female breasts, prostate, colon and rectum, and corpus uteri.

Secondary site refers to the body part where metastasized cancer cells grow and form secondary tumors. A cancer is always described in terms of the primary site, even if it has spread to another part of the body. For instance, advanced breast cancer that has spread to the lymph

This chapter includes text from "Cancer Diagnosis," "Derivation of Cells and Tissues," "Cancer Classification," educational units produced by the Surveillance, Epidemiology, and End Results Program (SEER), National Cancer Institute (NCI) in 2000. Two additional NCI FactSheets are also included: "Tumor Grade: Questions and Answers," reviewed May 19, 2004; and "Staging: Questions and Answers," reviewed January 6, 2004. For additional information, visit the NCI website at http://www.cancer.gov.

51

nodes under the arm and to the bone and lungs is always considered breast cancer (and the spread to the lymph nodes, bones, and lungs describe the stage of the cancer).

As is the case with other medical conditions, there are many signs and symptoms that may indicate the presence of cancer. These may be observed directly, through imaging technologies, or confirmed by lab tests. However, these signs and symptoms of cancer may resemble those of other conditions. For example, weight loss and abdominal pain can be caused by stomach cancer or an ulcer. Pink or reddish urine can be caused by kidney cancer or a kidney infection. A positive fecal occult blood test can indicate a variety of intestinal problems. A biopsy (removal of tissue for microscopic evaluation) is preferred to establish, or rule out, a diagnosis of cancer.

Tissue samples can be easily retrieved from a tumor near the body's surface. If the mass is inaccessible, an imaging exam that enables a tumor to be located precisely and visualized may be ordered before the biopsy is performed.

The histological type is determined by microscopic examination of suspected tissue that has been excised by biopsy or surgical resection. If the histological type is different from what is usually found in the tissue being examined, it can mean the cancer has spread to that area from some primary site. Metastasis can occur by direct extension, through the blood stream or the lymphatic system, or by seeding or implantation of cancer cells.

A biopsy, together with advanced imaging technologies, may not only confirm the presence of cancer, but may also pinpoint the primary site and secondary site(s).

It is also important to identify the cell types. Various histological types have different growth rates and dissimilar prognoses. More than one histological type of cell may be found in the same site. For example, a tumor whose primary site is skin can be a basal cell carcinoma, a squamous cell carcinoma, or a melanoma.

Once cancer has been confirmed, the pathologist tries to determine how closely the cancer cells resemble healthy, mature cells. Such cells are said to be differentiated. Cancer cells that do not look like their healthy counterparts are called undifferentiated, or, because they often look like very immature cells, primitive. The pathologist assigns a pathological grade to a tumor according to how aggressive the tissue looks under the microscope. Tumor grades can be expressed in words or by a number. One set of terms consists of well differentiated (grade 1), moderately differentiated (grade 2), poorly differentiated (grade 3), or undifferentiated (grade 4). When tumors are graded by number (1 through 4), a grade 1 tumor has a better natural history than a grade 4 tumor does.

Cancers are further classified according to stage. Staging describes how far a cancer has progressed based on the size of the primary tumor and whether it has spread.

In summary, a biopsy is the preferred method to confirm the diagnosis of cancer. Biopsies can provide information about histological type, classification, grade, potential aggressiveness and other information that may help determine the best treatment.

Derivation of Cells and Tissues

Cancers are named according to the organ in which they originate. Even if a cancer metastasizes to another part of the body, it keeps its original name. Cancer names such as breast cancer, brain cancer, lung cancer, and skin cancer are examples. However, cancer names may also be based on the type of tissue affected. This section will introduce you to some basics regarding the derivation of tissues in the context of embryology, which is the study of the development of an organism.

Derivation of Cells

Human beings begin life as a single, newly fertilized cell. Like every cell that contains a nucleus, the fertilized cell holds all the instructions for its growth and development. The characteristics common to all living cells include the ability to reproduce, exchange gases, move, react to external stimuli, and create or utilize energy to perform their tasks.

Shortly after the ovum or egg is fertilized, it divides to form two cells. These two cells then divide to form a total of four; these again divide to form eight, and so on. This group of cells continues dividing; after nine days it attaches to the wall of the uterus and becomes an embryo.

About two weeks after conception, the cells of the embryo continue to divide, changing their shape and structure. This process is known as differentiation. The cells arrange into distinct layers called germ layers: an outer ectoderm and inner endoderm (entoderm). A third embryonic layer, the mesoderm, develops between the ectoderm and the endoderm. All the organs of the body develop or differentiate in an orderly fashion from these three primary germ layers.

Derivation of Tissue

Cells that are similar in structure tend to group themselves together and form tissues. A tissue, then, is composed of a group of cells that are similar in structure and perform one or more common functions. Some tissues contain intercellular material which is very important in the performance of a particular function belonging to that tissue.

The body tissues and organs develop from the three primary germ layers that form during the growth process of the human embryo.

The tissues derived from the ectoderm are: some epithelial tissue (epidermis or outer layer of the skin, the lining for all hollow organs which have cavities open to a surface covered by epidermis), modified epidermal tissue (fingernails and toenails, hair, glands of the skin), all nerve tissue, salivary glands, and mucous glands of the nose and mouth.

In fact, epithelial tissue can be derived from either the ectoderm or endoderm. The epithelial tissue derived from the endoderm includes the epithelial lining of the digestive tract, except at the open ends, and the epithelial lining of all hollow structures formed as outpockets in the digestive tract. This includes the following:

- The parenchyma of the liver including communicating or connecting ducts

- The lining of the pharynx and respiratory tract (except the nose). This includes the lungs and the passageways leading from the pharynx to the lungs.

- The epithelium of the bladder and urethra

- Glands that form secretions in the digestive tract

Epithelial tissue derived from ectoderm is generally squamous epithelium; epithelial tissue derived from endoderm is essentially glandular epithelium.

There are a variety of body tissues derived from the third or middle primary germ layer known as the mesoderm. These body tissues include the following:

- Muscles
- Fibrous tissue
- Bone and cartilage
- Fat or adipose tissue
- Blood and lymph vessels
- Blood cells

In the early embryo the first cavity that develops is the coelomic cavity; this is derived from mesoderm. Parts of the urinary and genital systems are derived as outpouchings of the coelomic cavity. Later this coelomic cavity divides into the pleural cavity and the pericardial cavity. The linings of these cavities are composed of a single layer of cells called mesothelium. A few epithelial cells are of mesodermal origin, for example endometrium of the uterus, vaginal epithelium, and mucosa of the bladder.

Endothelium derived from mesoderm lines the blood and lymphatic vessels and the walls of the heart. In the capillaries where the endothelium is covered only by a basement membrane, diffusion takes place. It is surrounded elsewhere by supportive layers of connective tissue and smooth muscle. This is necessary because the endothelium is so thin that diffusion would occur otherwise. Many authorities classify this endothelium as connective tissue.

Cancer Classification

Cancers are classified in two ways: by the type of tissue in which the cancer originates (histological type) and by primary site, or the location in the body where the cancer first developed. This section introduces you to the first method: cancer classification based on histological type. The international standard for the classification and nomenclature of histologies is the *International Classification of Diseases for Oncology, Third Edition (ICD-O-3)*.

From a histological standpoint there are hundreds of different cancers, which are grouped into five major categories: carcinoma, sarcoma, myeloma, leukemia, and lymphoma. In addition, there are also some cancers of mixed types.

Carcinoma

Carcinoma refers to a malignant neoplasm of epithelial origin or cancer of the internal or external lining of the body. Carcinomas, malignancies of epithelial tissue, account for 80 to 90 percent of all cancer cases.

Epithelial tissue is found throughout the body. It is present in the skin, as well as the covering and lining of organs and internal passageways, such as the gastrointestinal tract.

Carcinomas are divided into two major subtypes: adenocarcinoma, which develops in an organ or gland, and squamous cell carcinoma, which originates in the squamous epithelium.

Adenocarcinomas generally occur in mucus membranes and are first seen as a thickened plaque-like white mucosa. They often spread easily through the soft tissue where they occur. Squamous cell carcinomas occur in many areas of the body.

Most carcinomas affect organs or glands capable of secretion, such as the breasts, which produce milk, or the lungs, which secrete mucus, or colon or prostate or bladder.

Sarcoma

Sarcoma refers to cancer that originates in supportive and connective tissues such as bones, tendons, cartilage, muscle, and fat. Generally occurring in young adults, the most common sarcoma often develops as a painful mass on the bone. Sarcoma tumors usually resemble the tissue in which they grow.

Examples of sarcomas include the following:

- Osteosarcoma or osteogenic sarcoma (bone)
- Chondrosarcoma (cartilage)
- Leiomyosarcoma (smooth muscle)
- Rhabdomyosarcoma (skeletal muscle)
- Mesothelial sarcoma or mesothelioma (membranous lining of body cavities)
- Fibrosarcoma (fibrous tissue)
- Angiosarcoma or hemangioendothelioma (blood vessels)
- Liposarcoma (adipose tissue)
- Glioma or astrocytoma (neurogenic connective tissue found in the brain)
- Myxosarcoma (primitive embryonic connective tissue)
- Mesenchymous or mixed mesodermal tumor (mixed connective tissue types)

Myeloma

Myeloma is cancer that originates in the plasma cells of bone marrow. The plasma cells produce some of the proteins found in blood.

Leukemia

Leukemias ("liquid cancers" or "blood cancers") are cancers of the bone marrow (the site of blood cell production). The word leukemia means "white blood" in Greek. The disease is often associated with the overproduction of immature white blood cells. These immature white blood cells do not perform as well as they should, therefore the patient is often prone to infection. Leukemia also affects red blood cells and can cause poor blood clotting and fatigue due to anemia. The following are examples of leukemia:

- Myelogenous or granulocytic leukemia (malignancy of the myeloid and granulocytic white blood cell series)

- Lymphatic, lymphocytic, or lymphoblastic leukemia (malignancy of the lymphoid and lymphocytic blood cell series)

- Polycythemia vera or erythremia (malignancy of various blood cell products, but with red cells predominating)

Lymphoma

Lymphomas develop in the glands or nodes of the lymphatic system, a network of vessels, nodes, and organs (specifically the spleen, tonsils, and thymus) that purify bodily fluids and produce infection-fighting white blood cells, or lymphocytes. Unlike the leukemias which are sometimes called "liquid cancers," lymphomas are "solid cancers." Lymphomas may also occur in specific organs such as the stomach, breast, or brain. These lymphomas are referred to as extranodal lymphomas. The lymphomas are subclassified into two categories: Hodgkin lymphoma and non-Hodgkin lymphoma. The presence of Reed-Sternberg cells in Hodgkin lymphoma diagnostically distinguishes Hodgkin lymphoma from non-Hodgkin lymphoma.

Mixed Types

The type components may be within one category or from different categories. Here are some examples:

- Adenosquamous carcinoma
- Mixed mesodermal tumor
- Carcinosarcoma
- Teratocarcinoma

Tumor Grade: Questions and Answers

What is a tumor?

In order to understand tumor grade, it is helpful to know how tumors form. The body is made up of many types of cells. Normally, cells grow and divide to produce new cells in a controlled and orderly manner.

Sometimes, however, new cells continue to be produced when they are not needed. As a result, a mass of extra tissue called a tumor may develop. A tumor can be benign (not cancerous) or malignant (cancerous). Cells in malignant tumors are abnormal and divide without control or order. These cancerous cells can invade and damage nearby tissue, and spread to other parts of the body (metastasize).

What is tumor grade?

Tumor grade is a system used to classify cancer cells in terms of how abnormal they look under a microscope and how quickly the tumor is likely to grow and spread. Many factors are considered when determining tumor grade, including the structure and growth pattern of the cells. The specific factors used to determine tumor grade vary with each type of cancer.

Histologic grade, also called differentiation, refers to how much the tumor cells resemble normal cells of the same tissue type. Nuclear grade refers to the size and shape of the nucleus in tumor cells and the percentage of tumor cells that are dividing.

Tumor grade should not be confused with the stage of a cancer. Cancer stage refers to the extent or severity of the cancer, based on factors such as the location of the primary tumor, tumor size, number of tumors, and lymph node involvement (spread of cancer into lymph nodes).

How is tumor grade determined?

If a tumor is suspected to be malignant, a doctor removes a sample of tissue or the entire tumor in a procedure called a biopsy. A pathologist (a doctor who identifies diseases by studying cells under a microscope) examines the tissue to determine whether the tumor is benign or malignant. The pathologist can also determine the tumor grade and identify other characteristics of the tumor cells.

What do the different tumor grades signify?

Based on the microscopic appearance of cancer cells, pathologists commonly describe tumor grade by four degrees of severity: Grades 1, 2, 3, and 4. The cells of Grade 1 tumors resemble normal cells, and tend to grow and multiply slowly. Grade 1 tumors are generally considered the least aggressive in behavior.

Conversely, the cells of Grade 3 or Grade 4 tumors do not look like normal cells of the same type. Grade 3 and 4 tumors tend to grow rapidly and spread faster than tumors with a lower grade.

The American Joint Commission on Cancer recommends the following guidelines for grading tumors:[1]

Table 4.1. Grading Tumors

Grade

GX	Grade cannot be assessed (Undetermined grade)
G1	Well-differentiated (Low grade)
G2	Moderately differentiated (Intermediate grade)
G3	Poorly differentiated (High grade)
G4	Undifferentiated (High grade)

Does the same grading scale apply to all tumors?

Grading systems are different for each type of cancer. For example, pathologists use the Gleason system to describe the degree of differentiation of prostate cancer cells. The Gleason system uses scores ranging from Grade 2 to Grade 10. Lower Gleason scores describe well-differentiated, less aggressive tumors. Higher scores describe poorly differentiated, more aggressive tumors. Other grading systems include the Bloom-Richardson system for breast cancer and the Fuhrman system for kidney cancer.

Does tumor grade affect a patient's treatment options?

Doctors use tumor grade and many other factors, such as cancer stage, to develop an individual treatment plan for the patient and to predict the patient's prognosis. Generally, a lower grade indicates a better prognosis (the likely outcome or course of a disease; the chance of recovery or recurrence). However, the importance of tumor grade in planning treatment and estimating a patient's prognosis is greater for certain types of cancers, such as soft tissue sarcoma, primary brain tumors, lymphomas, and breast and prostate cancer. Patients should speak with their doctor about tumor grade and how it relates to their diagnosis and treatment.

References

1. American Joint Committee on Cancer. *AJCC Cancer Staging Manual.* 6th ed. New York, NY: Springer, 2002.

Staging: Questions and Answers

What is staging?

Staging describes the extent or severity of an individual's cancer based on the extent of the original (primary) tumor and the extent of spread in the body. Staging is important for these reasons:

- Staging helps the doctor plan a person's treatment.

- The stage can be used to estimate the person's prognosis (likely outcome or course of the disease).

- Knowing the stage is important in identifying clinical trials (research studies) that may be suitable for a particular patient.

Staging helps researchers and health care providers exchange information about patients. It also gives them a common language for evaluating the results of clinical trials and comparing the results of different trials.

What is the basis for staging?

Staging is based on knowledge of the way cancer develops. Cancer cells divide and grow without control or order to form a mass of tissue, called a growth or tumor. As the tumor grows, it can invade nearby organs and tissues. Cancer cells can also break away from the tumor and enter the bloodstream or lymphatic system. By moving through the bloodstream or lymphatic system, cancer can spread from the primary site to form new tumors in other organs. The spread of cancer is called metastasis.

What are the common elements of staging systems?

Staging systems for cancer have evolved over time. They continue to change as scientists learn more about cancer. Some staging systems cover many types of cancer; others focus on a particular type. These are the common elements considered in most staging systems:

- Location of the primary tumor

- Tumor size and number of tumors

- Lymph node involvement (spread of cancer into lymph nodes)

- Cell type and tumor grade (how closely the cancer cells resemble normal tissue)

- Presence or absence of metastasis

What is the TNM system?

The TNM system is one of the most commonly used staging systems. This system has been accepted by the International Union Against Cancer (UICC) and the American Joint Committee on Cancer (AJCC). Most medical facilities use the TNM system as their main method for cancer reporting. PDQ®, the National Cancer Institute's (NCI) comprehensive cancer database, also uses the TNM system.

The TNM system is based on the extent of the tumor (T), the extent of spread to the lymph nodes (N), and the presence of metastasis (M). A number is added to each letter to indicate the size or extent of the tumor and the extent of spread.

For example, breast cancer T3 N2 M0 refers to a large tumor that has spread outside the breast to nearby lymph nodes, but not to other

Table 4.2. Primary Tumor (T)

TX	Primary tumor cannot be evaluated
T0	No evidence of primary tumor
Tis	Carcinoma in situ (early cancer that has not spread to neighboring tissue)
T1, T2, T3, T4	Size and/or extent of the primary tumor

Table 4.3. Regional Lymph Nodes (N)

NX	Regional lymph nodes cannot be evaluated
N0	No regional lymph node involvement (no cancer found in the lymph nodes)
N1, N2, N3	Involvement of regional lymph nodes (number and/or extent of spread)

Table 4.4. Distant Metastasis (M)

MX	Distant metastasis cannot be evaluated
M0	No distant metastasis (cancer has not spread to other parts of the body)
M1	Distant metastasis (cancer has spread to distant parts of the body)

parts of the body. Prostate cancer T2 N0 M0 means that the tumor is located only in the prostate and has not spread to the lymph nodes or any other part of the body.

For many cancers, TNM combinations correspond to one of five stages. Criteria for stages differ for different types of cancer. For example, bladder cancer T3 N0 M0 is stage III; however, colon cancer T3 N0 M0 is stage II.

Table 4.5. Definitions of Stages

Stage	Definition
Stage 0	Carcinoma in situ (early cancer that is present only in the layer of cells in which it began).
Stage I, Stage II, and Stage III	Higher numbers indicate more extensive disease: greater tumor size, spread of the cancer to nearby lymph nodes, or organs adjacent to the primary tumor.
Stage IV	The cancer has spread to another organ.

Are all cancers staged with TNM classifications?

Most types of cancer have TNM designations, but some do not. For example, cancers of the brain and spinal cord are classified according to their cell type and grade. Different staging systems are also used for many cancers of the blood or bone marrow, such as lymphoma. The Ann Arbor staging classification is commonly used to stage lymphomas and has been adopted by both the AJCC and the UICC. However, other cancers of the blood or bone marrow, including most types of leukemia, do not have a clear-cut staging system. Another staging system, developed by the International Federation of Gynecology and Obstetrics, is used to stage cancers of the cervix, uterus, ovary, vagina, and vulva. This system uses the TNM format. Additionally, childhood cancers are staged using either the TNM system or the staging criteria of the Children's Oncology Group, a group that conducts pediatric clinical trials.

Many cancer registries, such as the NCI's Surveillance, Epidemiology, and End Results Program (SEER), use summary staging. This system is used for all types of cancer. It groups cancer cases into five main categories:

- In situ is early cancer that is present only in the layer of cells in which it began.

- Localized is cancer that is limited to the organ in which it began, without evidence of spread.

- Regional is cancer that has spread beyond the original (primary) site to nearby lymph nodes or organs and tissues.

- Distant is cancer that has spread from the primary site to distant organs or distant lymph nodes.

- Unknown is used to describe cases for which there is not enough information to indicate a stage.

What types of tests are used to determine stage?

The types of tests used for staging depend on the type of cancer. Tests include the following:

- Physical exams are used to gather information about the cancer. The doctor examines the body by looking, feeling, and listening for anything unusual. The physical exam may show the location and size of the tumor and the spread of the cancer to the lymph nodes or to other organs.

- Imaging studies produce pictures of areas inside the body. These studies are important tools in determining stage. Procedures such as x-rays, computed tomography (CT) scans, magnetic resonance imaging (MRI) scans, and positron emission tomography (PET) scans can show the location of the cancer, the size of the tumor, and whether the cancer has spread.

- Laboratory tests are studies of blood, urine, other fluids, and tissues taken from the body. For example, tests for liver function and tumor markers (substances sometimes found in increased amounts if cancer is present) can provide information about the cancer.

- Pathology reports may include information about the size of the tumor, the growth of the tumor into other tissues and organs, the type of cancer cells, and the grade of the tumor (how closely the cancer cells resemble normal tissue). A biopsy (the removal of cells or tissues for examination under a microscope) may be performed to provide information for the pathology report. Cytology reports also describe findings from the examination of cells in body fluids.

- Surgical reports tell what is found during surgery. These reports describe the size and appearance of the tumor and often include observations about lymph nodes and nearby organs.

How can a patient find more information about staging?

The doctor most familiar with a patient's situation is in the best position to provide staging information for that individual. For background information, PDQ, the NCI's cancer information database, contains cancer treatment summaries that describe the staging of each type of cancer. PDQ treatment summaries are available at http://www.cancer.gov/cancerinfo/pdq on the NCI's website.

Staging information can also be obtained by calling the NCI's Cancer Information Service (CIS) toll-free at 800-4-CANCER (800-422-6237). For deaf and hard of hearing callers with TTY equipment, the toll-free number is 800-332-8615. CIS information specialists also offer immediate online assistance through the Help link on the internet at http://www.cancer.gov.

Part Two

Making Treatment and Cancer Care Decisions

Chapter 5

Learning about Your Cancer and Treatment Choices

Making Decisions about Cancer Treatment

After a diagnosis of cancer, patients and their families must make a number of decisions about cancer treatment, some of which are more difficult than others. These decisions are complicated by unfamiliar words, various statistics, and a sense of urgency. However, it is important to allow time to research your options and ask questions. Decisions about cancer treatment are personal, and it is important that you feel comfortable about your decisions.

Learn about your cancer. Try to understand as much as you can about your cancer, such as where it is located and how advanced it is (called cancer stage). If you are unfamiliar with certain words, ask your doctor or nurse or use a medical dictionary. Some people find it helpful to take notes during a doctor's visit or bring a friend along to help keep track of all the information.

Know your options. Talk to your doctor about treatment options for your type and stage of cancer. Some of these options may include surgery, radiation treatment, chemotherapy, hormone therapy, delaying treatment, enrolling in a clinical trial, and not receiving treatment. People are often surprised to learn that they may have different treatment options.

This chapter includes "PLWC Feature: Making Decisions about Cancer Treatment," reprinted with permission from the American Society of Clinical Oncology. © 2005. All rights reserved. And, "Questions to Ask the Doctor," reprinted with permission from the American Society of Clinical Oncology. © 2004. All rights reserved.

Understand the goals of treatment. Often, cancer can be cured with treatment, called curative treatment. However, there are times when treatment is only used to relieve side effects, such as pain, called palliative treatment. Knowing the goals of treatment helps people evaluate which risks are acceptable. For example, people who know their treatment is curative may be more willing to face potentially unpleasant side effects.

Learn about the risks and benefits of each treatment option. Different treatments have different risks, as well as potential side effects. An important part of making a decision is weighing the positives and negatives of each treatment option, including your ability to manage the side effects that are more common for the specific type of treatment. Factors to consider include the likelihood that the cancer will recur (come back) after treatment, the chances of living longer with or without treatment, the possibility of side effects, and your personal and family preferences.

Obtain a second opinion. Many people find that it helps to get a second or even third opinion from another doctor, particularly an oncologist, and many doctors encourage it. Different oncologists may have different experiences with various treatments, and seeking multiple opinions may help you make a decision. Read more about types of oncologists. Also, learn more about seeking a second opinion.

Consult guidelines or other decision-making tools. Many cancer organizations such as the American Society of Clinical Oncology (ASCO) and the National Comprehensive Cancer Network (NCCN) publish guidelines and treatment decision-making tools to help doctors and people with cancer understand various treatment options. Some cancer centers offer sophisticated statistical tools you can use with your doctor to help determine the best treatment option based on your personal medical information. Always use treatment guidelines and other programs with the help and interpretation of your doctor.

Talk about your decision with people you trust. Talk to your family, friends, a member of the clergy or spiritual advisor, and other people with cancer who have been through the treatment. What you decide is ultimately up to you, but some people find it helpful to talk through their concerns with other people. Many patient support organizations can help locate other people who have coped with similar experiences.

The role of statistics: Your doctor will probably mention many statistics when describing treatment options, including relative survival rates, disease-free survival rates, and progression-free survival rates. This may be a good way to learn about how the treatment options differ, but it is also important to remember that cancer statistics are generated with large populations of people with cancer, and should only be used as one part of a comprehensive treatment plan designed by a doctor who is familiar with a person's situation.

Questions to Ask the Doctor

Studies show that people with cancer who are fully informed about their disease and treatment options usually tend to fare better and experience fewer side effects than those who simply follow doctors' orders. Being informed gives you some control over your disease and encourages a positive outlook. Some people, however, tend to be overwhelmed by too much information or do not want to know as many details about their condition. It is important for you to identify how much information is right for you.

Getting answers to your questions: Your doctor should make time to answer your questions and explain various treatment options. Because you may feel overwhelmed by your cancer diagnosis, here are some tips to help you communicate with your doctor.

• Tell your doctor if you are having trouble understanding an explanation, description, or unfamiliar medical words. Sometimes, the doctor may be able to draw a picture or give an example.

• Consider writing your questions down in advance of a visit to reduce your level of stress and pressure for time.

• Bring a notebook or a tape recorder to the appointment. During the appointment, write down your doctor's answers, or ask a family member to write them down for you. This way, you can read or listen to the information later.

• Be patient. It may take a few meetings with the doctor before you begin to understand each other.

• Ask your doctor where you can find printed material about your condition. Many doctors have this information readily available.

The internet can be very helpful to people who are seeking information about their type of cancer, or those who are making decisions about their treatment. However, it is important to consider the reputation of the organization posting information, as not all information on the internet is accurate. Like cancer information found in books, magazines, or newspaper articles, information on the internet should be used for informational purposes only. If you have questions about the information you find, please talk with your doctor.

- If you are interested in seeking a second opinion, let your doctor know. Most doctors fully understand the value of a second opinion and are not offended when patients seek one. They may even be able to suggest another doctor.

Suggested questions to ask the doctor: An important part of managing your care is knowing what questions to ask of your doctor. Every person's needs are unique, and your questions will change during the different phases of your disease.

Below are some examples of the types of questions you may want to ask your doctor.

General Information

- What causes this type of cancer?
- What are the risk factors for this disease?
- Is this type of cancer caused by genetic factors? Are other members of my family at risk?
- How many people are diagnosed with this type of cancer each year?
- What lifestyle changes (diet, exercise, rest) do you recommend I make to best manage my disease?

Symptoms

- What are some common symptoms of this type of cancer?
- How can I avoid symptoms and/or reduce their impact on my daily activities?
- Is there anything I can do to make my symptoms better?
- Are there activities I should avoid that may make the symptoms worse?
- If new symptoms arise or existing symptoms worsen, what do you recommend I do?

Diagnosis

- What diagnostic tests or procedures are necessary? How often?
- What will these tests tell me about my cancer?
- How can I prepare myself for any tests or procedures?
- Is this test done in a doctor's office, or do I need to go to the hospital?
- How much information concerning my diagnosis should I share, and at what time, with my friends and loved ones?
- If I seek a second opinion, will I have to repeat any tests or procedures?

Staging

- How is staging used to determine cancer treatment?
- What is the stage of my cancer? What does this mean?
- Is my disease expected to progress?
- What is my prognosis (chance of recovery)?
- What are the cure rates for my disease?
- What are the survival rates for my disease?
- Could my disease go into remission?

Treatment

Keep in mind that all treatments offer risks and benefits. Discuss these with your doctor and consider your medical history and current condition in deciding whether the treatment approach is appropriate for you.

- What is the recommended treatment for my disease?
- Is this a standard treatment?
- Are there treatment options beyond the standard treatment for this disease?
- How often and how long will I have to undergo treatment?
- Are there any side effects of treatment?
- What are the benefits versus the risks of treatment?
- Has my cancer spread? If so, how does this affect treatment decisions?

- What are the expected results of treatment?
- How long does each treatment take?
- Is the treatment painful? What can you do to make it less painful?
- What will be involved in recovery? How long will I have to stay in the hospital?
- When can I resume my normal activities?

Clinical Trials

- What are clinical trials?
- How do clinical trials help people with cancer?
- Am I eligible for any clinical trials for this type of cancer?
- How will my progress be tracked while participating in a clinical trial?
- What happens if my disease progresses or is not treated effectively while participating in a clinical trial?
- How is treatment paid for if I participate in a clinical trial?
- Where can I get more information on clinical trials?

Support

- Is there a social worker that I can talk to?
- Where can I find information on coping with my diagnosis?
- Where can I find emotional, psychological, and spiritual support?
- Where can I find financial support?
- How can I best minimize the psychological impact of this disease on my family and myself?
- Where can I find resources for children? For teenagers?

Follow-up Care

- Who should I call with questions or concerns during non-business hours?
- Where can I find more information about my cancer?
- May I contact you or the nurse to talk about additional information I find?
- Is there anything else I should be asking?

Chapter 6

Understanding Prognosis and Cancer Statistics

People facing cancer are naturally concerned about what the future holds. Understanding cancer and what to expect can help patients and their loved ones plan treatment, think about lifestyle changes, and make decisions about their quality of life and finances. Many people with cancer want to know their prognosis. They may ask their doctor or search for statistics on their own.

A prognosis gives an idea of the likely course and outcome of a disease—that is, the chance that a patient will recover or have a recurrence (return of the cancer). Many factors affect a person's prognosis. Some of the most important are the type and location of the cancer, the stage of the disease (the extent to which the cancer has metastasized, or spread), or its grade (how abnormal the cancer cells look and how quickly the cancer is likely to grow and spread). Other factors that may also affect the prognosis include the person's age, general health, and response to treatment. When doctors discuss a person's prognosis, they carefully consider all factors that could affect that person's disease and treatment, and then try to predict what might happen. The doctor bases the prognosis on information researchers have collected over many years about hundreds or even thousands of people with cancer. When possible, the doctor uses statistics based on groups of people whose situations are most similar to that of an individual patient.

"Understanding Prognosis and Cancer Statistics," a National Cancer Institute (NCI) FactSheet, reviewed December 4, 2003. For more information, visit the NCI website at http://www.cancer.gov.

The doctor may speak of a favorable prognosis if the cancer is likely to respond well to treatment. The prognosis may be unfavorable if the cancer is likely to be difficult to control. It is important to keep in mind, however, that a prognosis is only a prediction. The doctor cannot be absolutely certain about the outcome for a particular patient.

Survival rates indicate the percentage of people with a certain type and stage of cancer who survive the disease for a specific period of time after their diagnosis. Often, statistics refer to the 5-year survival rate, which means the percentage of people who are alive five years after diagnosis, whether they have few or no signs or symptoms of cancer, are free of disease, or are having treatment. Survival rates are based on large groups of people. They cannot be used to predict what will happen to a particular patient. No two patients are exactly alike, and treatment and responses to treatment vary greatly.

Cancer patients and their loved ones face many unknowns. Some people find it easier to cope when they know the statistics. Other people find statistical information confusing and frightening, and they think it is too impersonal to be of use to them. The doctor who is most familiar with a patient's situation is in the best position to discuss the prognosis and to explain what the statistics may mean for that person. At the same time, it is important to understand that even the doctor cannot tell exactly what to expect. In fact, a person's prognosis may change if the cancer progresses, or if treatment is successful.

Seeking information about the prognosis is a personal decision. It is up to each patient to decide how much information he or she wants and how to deal with it.

Chapter 7

Researching Medical Literature about Your Cancer

Information about cancer is available in libraries, on the internet, and from many government and private sector organizations. Most libraries have resources to help people locate cancer-related articles in the medical and scientific literature, as well as cancer information written specifically for patients and the public. Information may also be accessed through the internet using a computer, and many libraries offer public access to computers.

National Cancer Institute

The National Cancer Institute's (NCI) website, http://www.cancer.gov, is a one-stop resource for cancer information. This website provides immediate access to critical information and resources about cancer, helping people with cancer become better informed about their disease and play a more active role in their treatment and care. The site's information is arranged by topic, and a search function allows convenient text-word searching across all NCI web pages. Search results often include "Best Bets" at the top of the search results pages. Best Bets are editorially selected web pages that are judged to be most pertinent to the search term(s) used. NCI's website is a comprehensive

Text in this chapter includes text excerpted from "Cancer Information Sources," National Cancer Institute, May 2005; "Questions about Using Libraries" is excerpted from "National Library of Medicine Guide to Finding Health Information," National Library of Medicine (NLM), April 2006; "PubMed Quick Start" and "How to Get the Journal Article" are NLM fact sheets dated August 2006.

resource that enables users to quickly find accurate and up-to-date information about all types of cancer, clinical trials (research studies with people), research programs, funding opportunities, cancer statistics, and the Institute itself.

Many of the NCI's cancer information resources are accessible through the cancer topics section of the Institute's website at http://www.cancer.gov/cancertopics. This section contains information from PDQ®, NCI's cancer information database, including information about ongoing clinical trials. Over 160 PDQ information summaries about cancer treatment, supportive care, screening, prevention, genetics, and complementary and alternative medicine are available. Written by experts and updated regularly, these summaries are based on current standards of care and the latest research. Most of the cancer information summaries are available in both a technical version for health professionals and a nontechnical version for patients, their families, and the general public. Many are also available in Spanish. In addition, the cancer topics section offers fact sheets and patient-oriented publications on a range of topics. A dictionary of cancer terms, prepared literature searches on specific cancer topics, and slide show tutorials about cancer-related science concepts are also available.

NCI's website provides comprehensive information about clinical trials at http://www.cancer.gov/clinicaltrials. Information is available about recent advances in cancer research, what clinical trials are and how they work, and points to consider when deciding whether to participate in a clinical trial. A simple-to-use search tool is available for those interested in finding trials for a specific type of cancer, in a certain geographic region, or for a particular type of treatment.

The NCI NewsCenter web page at http://www.cancer.gov/newscenter/ provides background information about many of the Institute's programs and resources, as well as an NCI News distribution list that allows individuals to receive NCI news updates as soon as they are posted to the Cancer.gov website. The Institute also offers the NCI Cancer Bulletin at http://www.cancer.gov/ncicancerbulletin. The Bulletin provides useful and authoritative news about cancer research, including important NCI programs and initiatives.

Up-to-date, accurate cancer information is available to patients and their families, the public, and health professionals through the NCI's Cancer Information Service (CIS). The CIS, a national information and education network, also serves as a resource for education and outreach to minority audiences and people with limited access to health care information or services. The CIS responds to calls in English and Spanish. The toll-free telephone number for the CIS is 800-4-CANCER

(800-422-6237). Deaf and hard of hearing callers with TTY equipment may call 800-332-8615. Hours of operation are Monday through Friday, 9:00 AM to 4:30 PM local time. The CIS website provides background information on the CIS and links to NCI resources and other cancer-related government websites. The CIS website is located at http://www.cancer.gov/cis.

The NCI also offers additional websites and services, described below, that are accessible directly or through NCI's main website (http://www.cancer.gov).

- The NCI's Publications Locator website can be used to order or view publications online at http://www.cancer.gov/publications. NCI materials may be identified by topic or searched by keyword, type of cancer, subject, audience, and/or language. The site includes instructions and Frequently Asked Questions. Currently, only internet users within the United States can use the Publications Locator to order NCI publications.

- The NCI's LiveHelp service, which is available through the Help link on the NCI's website, provides internet users with the ability to chat online with an information specialist in English. The service is available Monday through Friday, 9:00 AM to 11:00 PM Eastern time. Information specialists can help internet users navigate NCI websites, search for clinical trials, and find answers to questions about cancer.

Healthfinder

Healthfinder® is a website created by the U.S. Department of Health and Human Services to provide a free gateway to reliable online consumer health information. It offers information from selected online publications, clearinghouses, databases, and websites, as well as support and self-help groups. Healthfinder also provides links to the websites of government agencies and nonprofit organizations that provide health information for the public. Healthfinder is located at http://www.healthfinder.gov.

Public, University, and Medical Libraries

Books and articles about cancer are available in public, university, hospital, and medical school libraries. However, not all hospital and medical school libraries are open to the public, so it is advisable to ask about their policies and to find out whether particular journals or books are available. If materials cannot be borrowed, most libraries have photocopying facilities; they usually charge a fee for this service. Librarians can provide help with locating and using resources. If journals are not available at a particular library, the staff can usually arrange an interlibrary loan.

The *Reader's Guide to Periodical Literature* is an index of articles in over 225 popular, nontechnical magazines. This publication is available in most public libraries in print or electronically.

Questions about Using Libraries

Why should I go to a public library, and what can I find there?

A local public library is a good place to start your research. A public library can provide services such as these:

- provide individualized reference help
- tell you about other local or regional resources
- help you get materials
- provide internet access to health resources

Library resources may include the following:

- Basic medical reference sources: These may include medical or nursing textbooks, dictionaries or encyclopedias, drug information handbooks, and current therapy books.

- Medical and health directories: Directories of doctors and medical specialists in your area; and health information directories to find consumer health resources, support groups, and organizations.

- Other library resources: Many libraries have databases that index magazines and newspapers, as well as some medical journals. These special resources identify journal articles written for health professionals. They are often the most current source of information on medical topics.

If your library does not own the magazines or journals with the articles you want, ask about getting copies of articles through interlibrary loan. Some libraries may charge a fee for this service.

If you want to get articles cited in PubMed, a search tool for locating medical information, ask a local library about a Loansome Doc®

account. [Additional information about PubMed and how to use it is included below under the headings "National Library of Medicine," and "PubMed Quick Start."] Loansome Doc allows you to order articles directly from PubMed. The articles are sent to you (for a fee set by the library you use). To find a local library that is a Loansome Doc supplier, call your Regional Medical Library at 800-338-7657.

What other resources might I find at a medical library, and how do I find one that is open to me?

Medical libraries are usually found at medical, nursing, and dental schools; large medical centers; and community hospitals. They have textbooks (medical, dental, nursing, and other specialties), health-related journals, and other material used by health care professionals.

- Call your Regional Medical Library at 800-338-7657 to find the closest medical library open to the public.

- Find a library you can use in the list of Medical Research Libraries by State online at http://nnlm.gov/members.

- Ask what services are available to you: interlibrary loan, answering reference questions, and performing bibliographic searches.

- Ask if there is a fee for photocopies or services.

National Network of Libraries of Medicine

The National Network of Libraries of Medicine (NN/LM) directs health professionals, educators, and the general public to health care information resources. Inquirers are directed to medical libraries in their region, which can provide assistance with research. Further information about the Network is available by calling 800-338-7657, or by visiting the NN/LM website at http://nnlm.gov.

Federal Depository Library Program

The Federal Depository Library Program (FDLP) was established by the U.S. Congress to ensure that the American public has permanent access to government publications and information free of charge. The program disseminates information products to federal depository libraries in the 50 states, the District of Columbia, and the U.S. territories. Inquirers can search for federal publications and federal depository libraries in their state or region on the program's website at http://www.gpoaccess.gov/libraries.html.

The National Library of Medicine

The National Library of Medicine (NLM) is the world's largest medical library. The NLM is open to the public, and its databases can be used to search for journal article references and abstracts (summaries of articles) without charge or registration. The NLM's databases can be accessed on the internet and may also be available through some local university, public, and medical libraries.

MEDLINE®, the NLM's premier bibliographic database, contains over 12 million references to articles published since 1966. It is the computerized version of Index Medicus, with entries and references from more than 4,000 medical journals published worldwide. MEDLINE covers all aspects of the life sciences and medicine, including complementary and alternative medicine and toxicology (the biological effects of drugs and other chemicals). By searching MEDLINE, readers can find journal articles about specific topics (such as cancer) and, in many cases, can retrieve abstracts of the articles included in the databases.

The NLM allows free access to MEDLINE through PubMed®. PubMed is an easy-to-use search tool for finding journal articles of interest in the health and medical sciences. It was developed by the National Center for Biotechnology Information (NCBI) at the NLM. PubMed provides links to the full text of articles and other resources at the websites of participating publishers. User registration, a subscription fee, or other fees may be required to access the full text of articles in some journals. PubMed is also linked to molecular biology databases and to PubMed Central, an electronic archive of life sciences journal literature. PubMed can be found at http://pubmed.gov. Guidance on how to use this service is given below under the heading "PubMed Quick Start."

The NLM Gateway is another way to access information from the NLM. The NLM Gateway is designed to provide an overview of the NLM's resources, including journal articles, books, serials, audiovisuals, meeting abstracts, databases, and consumer health information. This resource allows users to search several of the NLM's databases at once. However, users may find that one resource, such as PubMed or MedlinePlus® (see below), has the information they need. They may then choose to go to that resource for a more focused search. The NLM Gateway is available at http://gateway.nlm.nih.gov.

MedlinePlus is the NLM's website for consumer health information. This site includes links to information on more than 650 health topics, the latest health news, a medical encyclopedia, medical dictionaries, databases (including MEDLINE), interactive health tutorials, drug information, directories, organizations, publications, and consumer health libraries. People can access MedlinePlus at http://medlineplus .gov.

Loansome Doc® is an NLM service that allows users to order full-text copies of articles found in MEDLINE. Users must establish an agreement with a library that uses DOCLINE®, the NLM's automated interlibrary loan request and referral system, and register to use Loansome Doc. A fee is usually charged by the ordering library. Charges for copies of articles and other services may vary from library to library. Access to Loansome Doc is available through the PubMed and NLM Gateway websites.

For more information on NLM programs, services, and hours of operation, individuals may contact the Office of Communications and Public Liaison at 888-FIND-NLM (888-346-3656) or 301-594-5983. The address is 8600 Rockville Pike, Bethesda, MD 20894. Online assistance is available on the NLM's website at http://www.nlm.nih.gov through the Contact NLM link on each page, and by e-mail from custserv@nlm.nih.gov.

PubMed Quick Start

How do I search PubMed?

First, identify the key concepts for your search. For example: In the question, "What role does pain have in sleep disorders?" the key concepts are: pain and sleep disorders.

Enter the terms (or key concepts) in the search box. Click Go.

How do I search by author?

Enter the author's last name plus initials without punctuation in the search box and click Go. (Examples: Watson JD; Lederberg J)

If you only know the author's last name, use the author search field tag [au]; for example, brody[au].

Click the Limits tab to use the author search builder that includes an autocomplete feature. For example, to search for citations to articles written by Bonnie Ramsey about gene therapy for cystic fibrosis patients enter the following search terms into the search box: cystic fibrosis gene therapy ramsey bw.

Full author names may be searched for citations published from 2002 forward if the full author name is available in the article (for example: Joshua Lederberg or Garcia Algar, Oscar).

How do I search by journal name?

Enter the journal name or title abbreviation in the search box. Add any additional search terms. Click Go. Click the Limits tab to use the journal search builder that includes an autocomplete feature. Here's an example: To search for citations to articles about Drosophila in the journal *Molecular Biology of the Cell* enter the following in the search box: molecular biology of the cell drosophila.

How do I find a specific citation? I have some information such as the author, journal name, and the year the article was published.

Use the Single Citation Matcher to find citations with a fill-in-the-blank format: Click Single Citation Matcher from the PubMed sidebar. Enter the information you have in the fill-in-the-blank boxes. Click Go.

Is there anything special for clinical searches?

From the Clinical Queries page you can search by a clinical study category, find systematic reviews, and run medical genetics searches.

The Clinical Study Categories use built-in search filters that will limit retrieval to citations to articles reporting research conducted with specific methodologies, including those that report applied clinical research. To find citations for a specific clinical study category:

- Click Clinical Queries from the PubMed sidebar.
- Click Search by Clinical Study Category.
- Enter your search terms in the search box.
- Select a category: therapy, diagnosis, etiology, or prognosis.
- Select a scope: narrow, specific search or broad, sensitive search.
- Click Go.

Here's an example: If you are researching the clinical aspect of gene therapy for cystic fibrosis, from the Clinical Queries page, select the category "therapy" and the Scope "narrow, specific search" and enter the following search terms in the search box: cystic fibrosis gene therapy.

How do I find systematic reviews or medical genetic searches?

In PubMed, Systematic Reviews cover a broad set of articles that build consensus on biomedical topics and Medical Genetics Searches find citations related to topics in medical genetics.

- Click Clinical Queries from the PubMed sidebar.
- Select either Find Systematic Reviews or Medical Genetics Searches.
- Enter search terms in the search box.
- For Medical Genetics Searches, change the search categories, if applicable.
- Click Go.

Here's an example: If you are researching systematic reviews on inhalation therapy for pneumonia from the Clinical Queries page click Systematic Reviews and enter the following search terms in the search box: inhalation therapy pneumonia.

Here's another example: To find information on sickle cell anemia and genetic counseling from the Clinical Queries page click Medical Genetic Search, click the All checkbox to deselect all the categories and click the Genetic Counseling checkbox. Enter the following search terms in the search box: sickle cell anemia.

Can you explain the search results?

PubMed search results are displayed in a summary format. Citations are initially displayed 20 per page with the most recently entered citations displayed first. You can mouse over a journal's title abbreviation to display the full journal name.

How do I display an abstract?

Click on the authors' names in a citation to see the abstract if it is available.

How can I get a copy of the article?

PubMed search results do not include an electronic copy of the journal article. However, the abstract display of PubMed citations may provide links to electronic copies from non-PubMed sources, such as directly from the publisher's website. These electronic journals may require a subscription (which you may access through your local medical library). Sometimes electronic journals have free access. Visit your local medical library if there is not an electronic copy available. For more information on obtaining the article, see "How to Get the Journal Article" below.

How can I save my results?

There are several ways to save PubMed search results including using the Clipboard to save citations temporarily.

- Click the check box on the left of the citations you want to save.
- From the Send to pull-down menu, select Clipboard.
- To view your selections, click Clipboard from the Feature tabs.

Additional information about other options for saving results, including using My NCBI Collections to save indefinitely, is available online.

I retrieved too many citations. How can I focus my search?

Try these suggestions to limit the number of search results:

- Replace general search terms with more specific ones (for example, use low back pain instead of back pain).
- Add more search terms.
- Use PubMed's Limits feature to restrict citations by age group, language, publication type, date, human studies, etc.
- The tool symbol to the right of the filter tabs links you to My NCBI where you can change your filter selections.

I retrieved too few citations. How can I expand my search?

- Click the Related Articles link next to a relevant citation. The link displays a pre-calculated set of PubMed citations closely related to the selected article.
- Remove extraneous or specific terms from the search box.
- Try using alternative terms to describe the concepts you are searching.

I'm not finding what I need. How does a PubMed search work?

PubMed may modify your search terms to enhance your retrieval. Sometimes these changes may not match what you have in mind. To see how PubMed modified your search, click Details from the Feature Tabs. You can edit your search in Details.

Here's an example: If you search for cystic fibrosis by its abbreviation cf, the cf search retrieves some citations that do not discuss cystic fibrosis. To see why PubMed retrieved these citations, click Details. This will tell you that PubMed translated cf to search for citations about cerebrospinal fluid or cf.

How can I get further assistance and training?

Contact customer support:

- E-mail the PubMed pubmednew@ncbi.nlm.nih.gov
- Call the NLM Customer service desk: 888-FIND-NLM (888-346-3656) Monday through Friday 8:30 AM – 8:45 PM EST and Saturday 9:00 AM – 5:00 PM EST.

How to Get the Journal Article

PubMed does not include copies of journal articles. Here are some tips for obtaining articles.

PubMed Central: PubMed Central is a free digital archive of full-text journal articles maintained by the U.S. National Institutes of Health. To access the article, click the icon to go to the abstract display and then click the "Free full text article in PubMed Central" icon.

Free from the publisher: On the summary results, look for a special icon that indicates the full-text article is available from the publisher's website free-of-charge. To access the article, click the icon to go to the abstract display and then click the free full text article icon. In other situations, some publishers will provide free access to articles after you register as a guest. Please note, however when you click a full text link in PubMed, you leave PubMed and are directed to the full text at an external provider's site. NLM/NCBI does not hold the copyright to this material, and cannot give permission for its use. (Users should review all copyright restrictions set forth by the full text provider before reproducing, redistributing, or making commercial use of material accessed through LinkOut.)

Local library: Some local libraries have copies of medical journals or can get a copy of an article for you. Ask your local librarian about interlibrary loan options and if there will be a charge.

You can also ask your local library about a Loansome Doc® account which will allow you to order articles directly from PubMed (for a fee set by the library you use). Call your Regional Medical Library at 800-338-7657 to find a local library that is a Loansome Doc supplier.

Direct from publisher: Journal publishers or related organizations may provide access to articles for a fee or sometimes free following your registration as an individual or guest. When available, icons to these sources can be found on the Abstract and Citation displays in your. Additional links to articles may be available on the LinkOut display.

Chapter 8

Which Study Results Are the Most Helpful in Making Cancer Care Decisions?

Clinical trials are research studies in which people help doctors find ways to improve health and cancer care. Each study tries to answer scientific questions and to find better ways to prevent, diagnose, or treat cancer.

If you or someone you know has cancer, you might want to learn what the best research has to say about its prevention, diagnosis, or treatment. But what constitutes the "best" research? If it's well designed, any clinical trial can produce reliable findings. But reliable findings aren't always definitive.

Research findings that are most likely to set the standard of cancer care usually come from phase III clinical trials that have been randomized and controlled, and that have enrolled enough participants to yield statistically significant results.

This chapter explains what these terms mean, and why a phase III randomized, controlled clinical trial with a specific number of participants is considered the gold standard in cancer research. With this knowledge, you'll be better able to tell which cancer studies are the most definitive, and therefore the most helpful, in guiding your medical decisions.

"Which Study Results Are the Most Helpful in Making Cancer Care Decisions," a National Cancer Institute (NCI) FactSheet, June 12, 2003. For more information, visit the NCI website at http://www.cancer.gov.

Clinical Trials Are Experimental and Prospective

The first thing to realize is that there are different kinds of cancer studies. A clinical trial is a particular kind of cancer study, one that is both experimental and prospective.

What's an experimental study?

Experimental studies can be understood in contrast to observational studies.

In an experimental study, investigators ask participants to take something (such as a drug) or do something (such as attend a support group). Investigators then record what happens to the participants as a result. The "something" that participants take or do is called an intervention.

In an observational study, by contrast, there is no intervention. Investigators simply observe and record naturally occurring events: for example, the number of lung cancer cases that occur within a group of people who live or work in cities along the East Coast.

Observational studies are important and can provide useful information about many issues such as risk factors for cancer. For example, the link between smoking and lung cancer was established through observational studies.

Observational studies, however, cannot be used to draw conclusions about how best to prevent or treat cancer. Prevention and treatment strategies need to be tested in experimental studies.

What's a prospective study?

Prospective studies can be understood in contrast to retrospective studies. In a prospective study, investigators follow participants forward in time for weeks, months, or years and record what happens to them.

In a retrospective study, by contrast, investigators look back at what happened to a group of people in the past. For example, they may take information from participants' medical records or ask participants to recall what they ate or did during a defined period of time.

Retrospective studies, while helpful in cancer research, are of limited use in determining new medical care because information about what happened to participants in the past is often incomplete.

Prospective studies don't rely on the reconstruction of past events, so they are generally considered to produce more reliable results than retrospective studies.

Phase III Clinical Trials

Most clinical research that involves the testing of a new intervention progresses in an orderly series of steps, called phases. Clinical trials are usually classified into one of three phases:

- **Phase I trials:** These are the first studies to look at how a new intervention works in people—the manner and frequency of its application and, if it's a drug, what dose is safe. A phase I trial usually enrolls only a small number of participants, sometimes as few as a dozen.

- **Phase II trials:** A phase II trial continues to test the safety of the intervention, and begins to evaluate how well it works. Phase II studies usually focus on a particular type of cancer.

- **Phase III trials:** These studies test a new intervention in comparison to the current standard of care. Phase III trials often enroll large numbers of people and may be conducted at many doctors' offices, clinics, and cancer centers nationwide.

Because they build on reliable findings from earlier clinical trials, phase III trials are usually considered to be the ultimate test of a new intervention.

Controlled Studies Allow Comparisons

In trying to judge how definitive a clinical trial's results are, note whether it was a controlled or uncontrolled trial. In a controlled clinical trial, one group of participants serves as a control group. These participants do not receive the intervention being studied.

Having a control group in a clinical trial enables investigators to answer the question "Compared to what?" Do participants receiving the intervention (the investigational group) fare better, worse, or the same as those who get standard therapy or a placebo?

In an uncontrolled study, which has no comparison group, investigators cannot be sure whether the outcomes they observe are caused by the intervention, by chance, or by unknown factors.

In a cancer treatment trial, participants in the control group usually receive the current standard treatment for their disease. Only when no standard treatment exists for that particular kind of cancer would participants in the control group receive a placebo, or dummy treatment.

In a cancer prevention trial, participants in the control group may receive an intervention known to help in the prevention of cancer.

Those in the experimental group receive the new intervention. In those cases where no proven intervention exists, participants in the control group would receive a placebo.

Randomization: Chance, Not Choice

Randomization is an important way of minimizing bias in a clinical trial. In a randomized trial, participants are assigned by chance, rather than choice, to either the investigational group or the control group. Random assignment is the most reliable way of ensuring that participants in the two groups are similar and therefore comparable.

If a trial is not randomized, investigators might unconsciously assign participants with a better prognosis to the investigational group, making the intervention seem more effective than it really is. Conversely, participants with a poorer prognosis might be more likely to choose the investigational group, making the intervention look less effective than it really is.

To Blind or Not to Blind

When possible, medical researchers like to blind, or mask, their clinical trials. In a single-blinded trial, participants do not know whether they are in the intervention group or the control group until the trial ends. In a double-blinded trial, neither investigators nor participants know which group a participant is assigned to until the trial's conclusion.

Blinding is another way of reducing bias that may distort a study's results. For example, investigators may behave differently toward participants whom they know are receiving the experimental intervention.

However, blinding is not always feasible. In a trial comparing surgery with chemotherapy, for example, blinding would be impossible—both doctors and participants would know which intervention was being applied.

Cancer prevention clinical trials are sometimes blinded, but cancer treatment trials rarely are.

Study Size Matters

Finally, the size of a clinical study is important when weighing how definitive the study's results are likely to be. Investigators try to enroll as many participants as they need to get a statistically significant result—that is, a result that is not due to chance. The total number of participants needed to get such a result varies depending on what questions the trial's researchers are hoping to answer.

In a very small study, the participants may not be representative of all people with the disease being studied. When a study involves a larger number of participants, there's a better chance those participants are a representative subset of the population with the disease. So in a broad sense, the most definitive studies tend to have a larger number of participants.

But again, what matters is not whether the number of participants is small or large, but whether they are the right number to get a statistically significant result.

Cancer prevention trials are usually much larger than treatment trials. Participants in prevention trials are healthy, although they may be at higher risk for a particular type of cancer than the general population. To be able to detect a significant difference between an intervention group and a control group in the number of cancer cases or cancer deaths, investigators need to enroll thousands of people and, usually, follow them for many years.

Example 1: A Cancer Treatment Trial

Cancer researchers theorized in the 1980s that "dose-dense" chemotherapy—given at two-week instead of conventional three-week intervals—would be a more effective way of killing cancer cells and extending patients' lives. But there was a problem: chemotherapy, which suppresses the immune system, usually made patients too prone to infections to tolerate treatment every two weeks.

In the 1990s, however, a drug called filgrastim became available. Filgrastim promotes the growth of white blood cells and helps patients receiving chemotherapy to withstand infections. With support from filgrastim, researchers thought patients might better tolerate dose-dense chemotherapy.

Researchers also wanted to know whether concurrent chemotherapy—giving more than one drug at a time—resulted in better outcomes than sequential chemotherapy—giving one drug after another. They designed a large phase III, controlled and randomized clinical trial for women with breast cancer to try to answer two questions: Is dose-dense chemotherapy superior to conventional chemotherapy? And is concurrent therapy superior to sequential therapy?

Like all clinical trials, this one was both prospective—it followed patients forward in time—and experimental—it tested an intervention:

schedules of chemotherapy that were more intense than the standard of care.

Between 1997 and 1999, the trial enrolled 2,005 women whose breast cancer had spread to their lymph nodes. After surgery to remove the tumor either by mastectomy (removal of the entire breast) or lumpectomy (removal of the tumor and some nearby breast tissue), participants were assigned at random to one of four treatment groups.

- Group I received the conventional sequential therapy: the drug doxorubicin every three weeks for four cycles, followed by paclitaxel (also called Taxol) every three weeks for four cycles, followed by cyclophosphamide every three weeks for four cycles. All together, this treatment lasted 36 weeks.

- Group II received the same regimen as Group I, but at two-week intervals, along with filgrastim to reduce infection risk. This dose-dense sequential therapy lasted 24 weeks.

- Group III, the control group, received the conventional concurrent therapy every three weeks for four cycles, followed by paclitaxel every three weeks for four cycles. This treatment lasted 24 weeks.

- Group IV received the same regimen as Group III, but at two-week intervals with the support of filgrastim. This dose-dense, concurrent therapy lasted 16 weeks.

In June 2002, after three years of following how patients fared post-treatment, the researchers were able to report statistically significant findings: Patients in the two dose-dense chemotherapy groups lived longer, and experienced fewer recurrences of their cancer, than women in the conventional dose groups. This was true regardless of whether the dose-dense therapy was given sequentially or concurrently.

Specifically, 85 percent of the women who received dose-dense chemotherapy were alive and disease-free after three years, compared with 81 percent of those treated at the conventional three-week intervals. At three years, overall survival (that is whether disease-free or not) was 92 percent in patients who received the dose-dense regimen, compared with 90 percent in conventionally treated patients.

Concurrent therapy produced no better results than sequential therapy, but women receiving sequential therapy suffered slightly fewer side effects. These findings were eventually published in the April 15, 2003, issue of the *Journal of Clinical Oncology*.

Cancer researchers generally prefer to have five-year follow-up data before they consider a study's results to be definitive enough to change the standard of care. If this study's findings are confirmed after two more years of follow-up, sequential dose-dense chemotherapy is likely to become the new standard of care for breast cancer patients whose disease has spread to the lymph nodes.

Example 2: A Cancer Prevention Trial

Findings from observational studies in the 1980s led researchers to wonder whether supplements of beta carotene and vitamin A (also called retinol) might reduce the incidence of cancer, particularly lung cancer. The body converts beta carotene, which is found in plants, to vitamin A, and vitamin A is known to play a part in preventing the uncontrolled growth of cells. The phase III Beta Carotene and Retinol Efficacy Trial (CARET) was designed to test whether supplements of these nutrients could prevent lung cancer in people at high risk for the disease.

CARET was a clinical trial because it was both experimental and prospective. It was experimental in that it was studying the effects of an intervention—in this case, vitamin supplements. And it was prospective in that researchers tracked the health of participants forward in time, after they enrolled in the trial.

The multicenter trial was both controlled and randomized. Between 1983 and 1994, 18,314 men and women who were smokers, former smokers, or workers exposed to asbestos were randomly assigned to one of two groups: the control group received dummy pills (placebos) each day; the intervention group received daily supplements of beta carotene and vitamin A.

The trial was also double-blinded, meaning neither participants nor their doctors knew who was taking the supplements and who was taking the dummy pills.

In January 1996, researchers reported that a preliminary analysis found 28 percent more lung cancer cases and 17 percent more lung cancer deaths in the intervention group than in the placebo group. In other words, there was "clear evidence of no benefit and substantial evidence of possible harm" with regard to the supplements.

Though researchers had planned to continue the experiment for another two years, the trial had progressed far enough and had enrolled enough participants for these early findings to be statistically significant. Researchers immediately told participants to stop taking both the supplements and the placebos, but kept following the participants' health for the next several years. The initial findings were subsequently published in the November 6, 1996, issue of the *Journal of the National Cancer Institute*.

The CARET results confirmed the findings of an earlier phase III, randomized, controlled clinical trial, the Alpha-Tocopherol and Beta Carotene (ATBC) trial, published in 1994 (follow-up data were published in 2003). The ATBC trial, conducted in Finland, involved more than 29,000 male smokers. Participants taking beta carotene supplements experienced 16 percent more cases of lung cancer than those taking either a vitamin A supplement or a placebo.

On the strength of the ATBC and CARET findings, current medical consensus is that taking beta carotene supplements does not help to prevent lung cancer, and may in fact be harmful.

Questions to Ask about a Cancer Study

The questions described in Table 8.1 may help as you look through various cancer studies, looking for the most medically definitive findings.

Table 8.1. Questions About Cancer Studies

Question	Look For
Was the study a clinical trial? In other words, was the study experimental (there was an intervention that people were asked to take or do) and prospective (investigators followed study participants forward in time)?	A study that is both experimental and prospective
What phase was the trial—phase I, phase II or phase III?	A phase III study
Did the clinical trial have a control group? That is, did one group of participants receive the experimental intervention while another did not?	A controlled study
Were participants randomly assigned to either the investigational group or the control group?	A randomized study
How many participants were enrolled in the study?	A study that is large enough for the results to be statistically significant; not due to chance

Chapter 9

Types of Cancer Treatment

The most common types of cancer treatment include surgery, radiation therapy, and chemotherapy. These therapies may be used either alone or in combination with other therapies. More recent treatment options include targeted therapies and biologic treatments. The first treatment that a person is given is called first-line therapy. Adjuvant therapy is treatment that is given after the first treatment (such as chemotherapy after surgery). Neoadjuvant therapy is treatment that is given before the primary treatment (such as hormone therapy before surgery). Most experimental therapies are tested in clinical trials.

As cancer care becomes more specialized, many people are now treated by a team of doctors, nurses, and other health-care specialists. Usually one doctor, often the medical oncologist, will help coordinate the person's care.

Before beginning treatment, people should consider asking the doctor about the goals of treatment, how long the treatment will take, and the potential side effects.

It is also important that people with cancer and their families feel comfortable about their doctor and his or her recommended therapy. It is always appropriate to ask for a second opinion.

Surgery

Surgery involves the removal of cancerous tissue from the body. It is the primary treatment for many types of cancer, and some cancers can be cured with surgery. Surgery can also confirm a diagnosis (biopsy), determine how far a person's cancer has advanced (staging), relieve side effects (such as an obstruction), or ease pain (palliative surgery).

Some types of surgery can be performed in a clinic or doctor's office instead of the hospital. This is called outpatient surgery. Most cancer surgeries, though, will be performed in a hospital. Before surgery, consider preparing a list of questions for the surgeon. Carefully review with your doctor any preparation you may need before surgery.

The side effects of surgery depend on the type of surgery and the health of the person before surgery. One of the more common side effects is pain, which can be successfully treated in most people.

Chemotherapy

Chemotherapy is the use of drugs to destroy cancer cells. Chemotherapy drugs fight cancer by interfering with the growth process of cancer cells, eventually causing the cells to die. Chemotherapy is used to shrink or eliminate the tumor, keep the tumor from spreading, destroy any cancer cells that have spread to other areas in the body, or relieve symptoms. Chemotherapy is called a systemic treatment, because it affects the entire body.

Chemotherapy is given by a medical oncologist, which is a doctor who specializes in treating cancer with medication. Some people may receive chemotherapy in their doctor's office; others may go to the hospital. A chemotherapy regimen usually consists of a specific number of cycles given over a period of time. Some drugs are given continuously over several days; some are given several times a week.

Side Effects of Chemotherapy

Chemotherapy can damage healthy cells along with cancer cells, which may cause side effects, including nausea, vomiting, and fatigue. Depending on the drug, some people may also experience tingling or numbness in the arms and legs, hair loss, and mouth sores. Because some drugs can damage blood cells, a person may experience anemia (low red blood cell counts) or an increased risk of infection (low white blood cell counts). Side effects can usually be treated and go away once treatment is finished. The occurrence of side effects is not related to whether the cancer drug is working or not.

During chemotherapy, a person may lose his or her appetite or develop an aversion to the taste or smell of food. Consider talking to a registered dietitian who can give suggestions about meal planning and managing side effects through simple diet changes.

Many people are concerned about the side effects of chemotherapy, and children and young adults should ask about long-term side effects of chemotherapy. Fortunately, many new drugs do not cause the same, severe side effects as some older chemotherapy drugs. And, there are many effective medications that help reduce side effects, caused by chemotherapy.

Radiation Treatment

Radiation therapy uses high-energy x-rays to destroy cancer cells. Radiation therapy is considered a local treatment, as it only affects one part of the body. The goals of radiation therapy include shrinking the tumor before surgery, keeping the tumor from returning after surgery, eliminating cancer cells in other parts of the body, and relieving pain (palliation).

Radiation therapy can be given two ways: externally and internally. With external-beam radiation therapy, a machine directs the radiation at the tumor from outside the body. With internal radiation therapy, also called brachytherapy, small tubes or implants (also called seeds) containing radioactive materials are placed in the body near the tumor. With internal radiation therapy, the person does not need to come to the hospital every day to be treated, and the doctor can use a higher dose of radiation. However, internal radiation therapy can only be used if the tumor is in a location where the doctor can place the implant.

Before beginning external-beam radiation therapy, the doctor will plan where to aim the radiation. The goal is to hit as much of the tumor as possible, while minimizing the exposure of healthy tissue. A person's skin may be marked to show where the radiation will be directed. New computerized techniques help pinpoint the best place to give the radiation.

Side Effects of Radiation Treatment

Like chemotherapy, radiation therapy can also damage normal cells, causing side effects. These include tiredness (fatigue), swelling, redness or irritation of the skin, hair loss, cough or shortness of breath (if the radiation is given to the neck or chest area), mouth sores (if the radiation is given to the head), and digestive problems (if the radiation is given to the abdominal area). These side effects go away once treatment is finished. Internal radiation therapy may cause bleeding, infection, or irritation after the implant is removed. Radiation treatment does not make a person radioactive.

External-beam radiation therapy may have long-term side effects that can affect a person for many years. For this reason, children and young adults who receive radiation therapy should keep a record of their radiation treatment schedule (including the dose and location of the radiation) and report it as part of their medical history. Long-term side effects can include the risk of a second cancer, the inability to have children (infertility), heart problems (from radiation to the chest), gastrointestinal problems (from radiation to the abdominal area), lung fibrosis (scarring or thickening of the lung tissue), neurologic problems, thyroid problems, or osteoporosis. Also, people who have had previous radiation to the chest should be aware that they are at higher risk of developing breast and lung cancers. Today, most people who receive radiation therapy now receive smaller doses than what was given in years past. Each individual considering radiation therapy should discuss the risks versus benefits of the treatment with his or her doctor.

Hormone Therapy

Several types of cancer, including some breast and prostate cancers, can only grow and spread in the presence of natural chemicals in the body called hormones. Hormone therapy fights cancer by changing the amounts of hormones in the body, and is used to treat cancers of the prostate, breast, and reproductive system. For example, tamoxifen (Nolvadex) is an anti-estrogen drug used to treat some hormone-responsive breast cancers.

Hormone therapy does have potential side effects, but most side effects go away once treatment is finished. The side effects depend on the drug and affect men and women differently.

Biologic Therapy

Biologic therapy, also called immunotherapy, stimulates the disease-fighting mechanisms within the body to fight the cancer. Interferon and colony-stimulating factor are two examples of biologic therapy. These substances help restore functioning of the immune system. Researchers are developing specific types of biologic therapy, such as monoclonal antibodies and vaccines. The side effects of biologic therapy generally include flu-like symptoms, such as chills, nausea, and fever.

Monoclonal antibodies. Monoclonal antibodies are laboratory-produced substances that find and attach themselves to specific places on the surface of cancer cells. When they attach to a protein, they effectively stop the protein from doing its job (such as making cancer cells grow). For example, trastuzumab (Herceptin) is a monoclonal antibody therapy for breast cancers that have too much of a protein called HER2/neu. The antibody binds, or attaches to, the HER2/neu protein on the outer surface of tumor cells, preventing the growth and division of cancer cells. Other examples of monoclonal antibody therapies include cetuximab (Erbitux), rituximab (Rituxan), and bevacizumab (Avastin). Monoclonal antibodies can be used alone, in combination with other therapies, or to deliver drugs, toxins, or radioactive material.

Cancer vaccines. Cancer vaccines are another specific type of biologic therapy. Unlike vaccines that can prevent diseases such as chicken pox, cancer vaccines attempt to treat the cancer by training the immune system to recognize cancer cells and attack them. In some cases, doctors take tumor cells from the patient to make a vaccine. Cancer vaccines are being tested for many types of cancer, but are still highly experimental.

Targeted Treatments

This general term describes drugs that "target" various proteins that can contribute to cancer. Unlike chemotherapy drugs that kill both healthy and cancerous cells, these drugs selectively kill cancer cells, which helps to reduce side effects. For example, imatinib mesylate (Gleevec) selectively blocks a protein that helps cancer cells grow. Other targeted treatments include gefitinib (Iressa) and erlotinib (Tarceva). Most targeted treatments are still experimental and are used along with other types of therapy. The benefits of these drugs can vary depending on a person's response to previous treatment and overall health. Generally, targeted treatments do not have the same side effects as traditional chemotherapy. Depending on the drug and the dosage, a person may experience nausea, vomiting, muscle cramps, rash, or diarrhea.

Anti-angiogenesis drugs: The formation of new blood vessels that feed tumors is known as angiogenesis. Some scientists think that by cutting off a tumor's blood supply, it may be possible to starve the tumor, and prevent it from growing and spreading. Anti-angiogenesis drugs are considered experimental at this time.

Antisense therapy: This therapy utilizes small, chemically modified strands of DNA that block gene expression by binding to messenger RNA before it can produce a protein. Essentially, the technology acts to selectively "knock out" the production of a single protein.

Gene therapy: This therapy is used to repair or replace damaged genetic material or add new genetic material.

Chapter 10

Understanding Cancer Medications

Your Medications

Drugs, drugs, and more drugs! Your head will spin trying to remember all the drugs you will be taking. This chapter will list the most common, how they are given, and the most common side effects.

Chemotherapy Drugs

If your treatment plan includes chemotherapy, you'll get to know some of these drugs, often given in various combinations.

Adriamycin (Doxorubicin): Given through IV. This kind of chemo (anthracycline) may affect your heart muscle. Check with your doctor before exercising and weightlifting. Most common side effects:

- Hair loss
- Nausea, vomiting, and diarrhea
- Bone marrow depression (lowering counts)
- Mouth sores
- Discolored urine
- Skin and nail changes
- Sensitivity to the sun

Asparaginase: Given by injection. Most common side effects:

- Changes in blood clotting
- Fever and chills
- Allergic reaction
- Lethargy, sleepiness and confusion

Bleomycin (Blenoxane): Given through IV or injection. Most common side effects:

- Fever and chills
- Skin and nail changes
- Loss of appetite
- Nausea and vomiting
- Changes to the lungs

Busulfan (Myleran): Given through IV or taken by mouth. Most common side effects:

- Bone marrow depression (lowering counts)
- Nausea, vomiting, and diarrhea
- Hair loss
- Mouth sores
- Seizures
- Skin changes

Carboplatin (Paraplatin): Given through IV. Most common side effects:

- Bone marrow depression (lowering counts)
- Nausea and vomiting

- Poor appetite
- May affect your kidneys
- Will lower your pH
- Hearing loss

Carmustine (BCNU): Given through IV. Most common side effects:

- Nausea and vomiting
- Bone marrow depression (lowering counts)
- Changes to the skin

Cis-Platinum (Cisplatin): Given through IV. Drink lots of fluid while on this drug. Keep anti-nausea medication nearby. Most common side effects:

- Nausea and vomiting (may get worse after a few days)
- Your kidneys may be affected
- Changes to your skin
- Hearing loss
- May cause numbness or tingling in hands or feet

Cyclophosphamide (Cytoxan): Given through IV or taken by mouth. Most common side effects:

- Bone marrow depression (lowering counts)
- Hair loss
- Bladder irritation
- Nausea and vomiting
- Poor of appetite

Cytarabine (ARA-C; Cytosar): Given by injection, IV or intrathecal (injected into fluid around spinal cord). Most common side effects:

- Bone marrow depression (lowering counts)
- Nausea/vomiting/diarrhea
- Eye irritation
- Mouth sores
- Rash
- A flu-like effect

Dacarbazine (DTIC-Dome): Given through IV. Most common side effects:

- Nausea and vomiting, poor appetite
- Bone marrow depression (lowering counts)
- Flu-like effect
- Hair loss

Daunorubicin (Daunomycin): Given through IV. This kind of chemo (anthracycline) may affect your heart muscle. Check with your doctor before exercising or weightlifting. Most common side effects:

- Nausea and vomiting
- Hair loss
- Bone marrow depression (lowering counts)
- Mouth sores
- Discolored urine

Etoposide (VP-16): Given through IV or taken by mouth. Most common side effects:

- Bone marrow depression (lowering counts)
- Hair loss
- Nausea and vomiting, and diarrhea
- Temporary taste alterations
- Mouth sores
- Skin changes

5-Fluorouracil (5-FU): Given through IV or taken by mouth. Most common side effects:

- Mouth sores
- Diarrhea
- Eye sensitivity
- Skin changes
- Bone marrow depression (lowering counts)
- Nausea and vomiting
- Hair loss
- Sensitivity of the skin to sunlight
- Rashes

Fludarabine (Fludara): Given through IV or taken by mouth. Most common side effects:

- Bone marrow depression

Hydroxyurea (Hydrea): Taken by mouth. Most common side effects:

- Bone marrow depression (lowering counts)
- Skin changes

Idarubicin (Idamycin): Given through IV or taken by mouth. This kind of chemo (anthracycline) may affect your heart muscle. Check with your doctor before exercising or weightlifting. Most common side effects:

- Bone marrow depression (lowering counts)
- Nausea and vomiting
- Mouth sores and ulcers
- Hair loss

Ifosfamide (Ifex): Given through IV. Most common side effects:

- Bone marrow depression (lowering counts)
- Nausea and vomiting
- Hair loss
- Irritation of the bladder
- Changes to nails

Lomustine (CCNU; CeeNU): Taken by mouth. Most common side effects:

- Nausea and vomiting
- Bone marrow depression (lowering counts)
- Mouth sores

Mechlorethamine (Nitrogen Mustard): Given through IV. Most common side effects:

- Nausea and vomiting
- Hair loss
- Rash

Melphalan (Alkeran): Given through IV or taken by mouth. Most common side effects:

- Bone marrow depression (lowering counts)
- Nausea and vomiting
- Mouth sores
- Diarrhea
- Hair loss
- Skin changes

Mercaptopurine (Purinethol): Taken by mouth. Most common side effects:

- Bone marrow depression (lowering counts)
- Mouth sores
- Skin changes

Methotrexate (Mexate): Given by mouth, injection, IV or intrathecal (injected into fluid around spinal cord). Most common side effects:

- Bone marrow depression (lowering counts)
- Mouth sores
- Diarrhea, nausea, vomiting
- Skin changes, rash, hair loss

Mitoxantrone (Novantrone®): Given through IV. This is a blue colored medicine. This kind of chemo (anthracycline) may affect your heart muscle. Check with your doctor before exercising or weightlifting. Most common side effects:

- Bone marrow depression (lowering counts)
- Discolored urine
- Nausea and vomiting
- Mouth sores
- Hair loss
- Whites of eyes may have a slight blue tint

Paclitaxel (Taxol®): Given through IV. Most common side effects:

- Bone marrow depression (lowering counts)

- Mouth sores
- Diarrhea, nausea, vomiting
- Hair loss
- Aching or pain in joints and muscles (usually after 2–3 days. Gets better within 5–7 days)
- Skin changes
- Numbness or tingling in hands or feet
- Allergic reaction

Procarbazine (Matulane): Given through IV or taken by mouth. Most common side effects:

- Bone marrow depression (lowering counts)
- Nausea and vomiting
- Alcohol should be avoided while taking this drug
- Delayed low pH

Teniposide (Vumon): Given through IV. Most common side effects:

- Nausea, vomiting, or diarrhea
- Fever, chills
- Allergic reaction

6-Thioguanine (6-TG): Taken by mouth. Most common side effects:

- Bone marrow depression (lowering counts)
- Raised levels of uric acid in the blood
- Skin changes
- Mouth sores

Vinblastine (Velban): Given through IV. Most common side effects:

- Bone marrow depression (lowering counts)
- Nausea, vomiting, and diarrhea
- Hair loss
- Mouth sores
- Constipation
- Numbness or tingling in hands or feet

Vincristine (Oncovin; VCR): Given through IV. Most common side effects:

- Abdominal cramps and constipation
- Numbness or tingling in hands or feet
- Jaw pain

Anthracyclines

Anthracyclines are a group of chemotherapy drugs used to treat a variety of childhood cancers. There is both good and bad news associated with anthracyclines. The good news: significantly increased survival rates. The bad news: possible heart problems that may not show up for 10–15 years.

Anthracyclines include the following:

- Adriamycin
- Daunomycin
- Idarubicin
- Mitoxantrone

If anthracyclines are part of your treatment plan, it is important that you know it so you can take the necessary precautions.

The problem with anthracyclines: We know that these drugs can effect the functioning of your heart's left ventricle. This is a problem when your heart needs to work harder, like during exercise or strenuous activity. The weakened left ventricle—responsible for pumping oxygen-rich blood back into your body—may not be capable of this heavy duty pumping action.

If you are going to be taking anthracyclines, you will probably have some baseline tests (EKG and ECHO cardiogram) done before you start taking the drug. These tests will be repeated throughout your treatment and then annually or as often as your doctor suggests.

You also have to restrict activities that put a heavy strain on your heart. Two sports in particular should be avoided: football and weight lifting.

You can still participate in many other sports and are encouraged to do so. You can still dance, swim, and play tennis, basketball, soccer, and baseball.

Just remember that the effects of anthracyclines are long lasting and need life-long attention. As you get older, you should always take these precautions to stay on the safe side.

Anti-Nausea Drugs

Anti-nausea (or anti-emetic) drugs will become your best friends during your chemotherapy treatment. Your medical team is the best source of information about which drugs will work best for you.

Most people going through chemotherapy will take one or the other of the following two drugs for nausea: Ondansetron (Zofran) or Granisetron (Kytril). These are both given through IV or by mouth.

Depending on your response to the chemo, you may also take some of the following drugs to prevent or treat nausea. You will come to learn which ones work best for you:

- Diphenhydramine (Benadryl)
- Promethazine (Phenergan)
- Metoclopramide (Reglan)
- Prochlorperazine (Compazine)
- Dexamethasone (Decadron)
- Dronabinol (Marinol)
- Lorazepam (Ativan)
- Droperidol (Inapsine)

Most common side effects are dry mouth and drowsiness and light-headedness.

Pain Medications

Your medical team is the best source of information about which pain medications will best control your pain, if you have any.

One goal is to be as pain free as possible when you are in treatment. You have enough other things to worry about without trying to deal with unnecessary pain. You may feel that you have to be totally brave and completely stoic. You don't.

You might be hesitant to take pain medication because you—or your parents—are afraid you will become addicted to them. When given in a controlled manner for short periods of time, addiction to these drugs is not a worry. If you are on a certain drug for a longer period of time, your body may become tolerant to it and you may need to gradually taper off.

Don't be afraid to ask for pain medication if you need them.

Commonly used pain medications include these:

- Morphine (Morphine)

- Hydromorphone (Dilaudid)
- Oxycodone (Percocet)
- Codeine (Codeine)
- Methadone (Dolophine)
- Meperidine (Demerol)
- Fentanyl (Fentanyl)

These are usually given by injection, liquid, pill or IV. Sometimes they are given as a rectal suppository. Common side effects include sedation, light-headedness, dizziness, constipation, and sometimes nausea or vomiting.

Local anesthetic EMLA: EMLA is an anesthetic cream that numbs your skin. It's great if you need to have a needle stick for an IV, access your medi-port, or have an injection. It can also be used for procedures like spinal taps and bone marrow aspirations.

All you have to do is apply it to your skin about 1–2 hours before the procedure, cover it with an airtight dressing, and it will numb the area. You don't feel a thing (if you wait long enough). EMLA is only sold with a prescription.

Anti-Depressants

The use of anti-depressants by patients with cancer is not uncommon. Depression or feelings of sadness, disruption in your eating or sleeping patterns, or having trouble coping with all that is going on can occur anytime during or after your treatment.

Depression is caused by a lack of a chemical in your brain called serotonin. Anti-depressant medication helps increase your serotonin levels. You need to take these drugs for a few weeks before you feel any change. Commonly used anti-depressants include the following:

- Sertraline (Zoloft)
- Paroxetine (Paxil)
- Fluoxetine (Prozac)
- Citalopram (Celexa)

Most common side effects are drowsiness or agitation, dry mouth, nausea, constipation, and headache.

Steroids

This type of medication is often used in the treatment of several different kinds of cancers and other diseases. Don't confuse this kind of steroid with the illegal, anabolic type that have been used to bulk muscles.

Your body normally produces a natural form of steroid called cortisol. You will make less cortisol while you're taking steroid medication. This is why you always taper off this medication—so you own body starts making the normal amounts of cortisol again. Commonly used steroids include the following:

- Prednisone: Taken by mouth.
- Methylprednisolone (Solu-Medrol): Taken through IV.
- Hydrocortisone: Taken through IV, by mouth, or in a cream for the skin.
- Cortisone: Taken by injection into the muscle.

Here is a list of common side effects:

- Increased appetite
- Weight gain
- Mood swings
- Fullness in cheeks
- High blood pressure
- Stomach upset or ulcers
- Osteoporosis (weakens bones)

All Hooked Up: Central Lines

As your treatment continues, you will often need medications, blood products, and possibly nutrients given intravenously. You will also have endless blood tests. Having a central line eliminates the need for repeated needle sticks to start an IV line or draw blood. Even though surgery is required, it will be worth it.

All central lines work on the same general principle. A small tube or catheter is surgically implanted and then fed into the superior vena cava—a major vein in the right ventricle of your heart. Your medications and other supplements can be infused directly into your system. A central line not only avoids needle sticks, it also prevents possible tissue damage caused by leakage of corrosive chemotherapy drugs (it's rare, but it can happen).

Your central line can also be used to draw blood for testing, again eliminating the need for painful needle pokes.

There are two main types of central lines: external and subcutaneous (under the skin). You may have a PICC (peripherally inserted central catheter) line inserted temporarily. You and your medical team will discuss which type is best for you.

External Lines

The two most common types of external central lines are the Broviac and Hickman (refers to the company that makes them). Central lines are almost always surgically implanted while you are under general anesthesia. First, a small incision is made in the area under your collarbone. One end of the catheter is fed into a large vein (the superior vena cava) leading directly into your heart.

The other end of the catheter is "tunneled" under your skin for a short distance, where it exits through another small incision at a spot near your breastbone. The catheter branches out into one or more smaller tubes called lumens that hang on the outside of your body. A sterile dressing covers the exit site at all times.

All chemotherapy drugs, transfusions, and fluids are infused through these lumens or "ports". Depending on your treatment plan, you may have several different types of fluids or medication being infused at the same time through different ports. Sometimes, if the drugs are compatible, you might have two different drugs going through the same lumen at the same time.

Subcutaneous (under the skin) or implantable lines: This type of central line is usually referred to as a medi-port or Port-A-Cath. Unlike a Broviac or Hickman, an implantable port is completely under the skin.

This type of catheter is surgically implanted, usually in your chest but some teens have them in their arms. Most teens have general anesthesia for this procedure. One end of the catheter is fed into a large vein leading directly into your heart. The other end is attached to a small chamber called a portal. The portal is made of either metal or plastic with a rubber top that seals it and is placed under your skin.

You will feel a small bump under your skin where the portal has been placed. When you need to use your port, it is accessed with a special needle (a Huber needle) that has a tube attached to it, much like the lumen on a Broviac. Your medication or whatever will flow through the needle, into the catheter and then into your bloodstream.

After a while, the skin over your port becomes very tough and insensitive. You can also use EMLA cream to numb the area.

Caring for external and subcutaneous lines: External lines are more difficult to take care of than under-the-skin ports. Special care must be taken while bathing to avoid getting the exit site wet and it may be recommended that you don't go swimming.

A Broviac or Hickman must always have a sterile dressing covering it. Check with your medical team to learn their requirements about changing the dressing. Most hospitals will have a special teaching sheet to show you how to change your dressing. You can always have a nurse or your parent do it for you, but many teens prefer to do it themselves. It's usually more convenient and much more private.

Your lines need be flushed daily to prevent clotting and the caps on the ends of the line need to be changed regularly. Your individual situation will determine how often. Check with your medical team about how to specifically care for your central line.

Subcutaneous catheters (or medi-ports, Port-A-Caths) are easier to maintain than external lines. They too need to be flushed with a heparin solution to prevent clotting but usually only once a month or after each use. There is no worry about swimming, bathing or showering with this system. Normal activities can be continued.

You will more fully discuss how to care for your line with your medical team.

PICC line: You may have a PICC line—peripherally inserted central catheter—inserted for some of your treatment. Often a PICC line is used when treatment is short term or until a more durable central line can be surgically implanted. These are simpler and less invasive than other central catheters and can be inserted by a nurse.

The PICC is a thin flexible catheter, about 60 cm long, which is inserted in your upper arm. It then feeds into the superior vena cava—the big vein just above the heart.

PICC lines are easier to maintain than some others. You medical team will give you specific instructions how to care for your PICC line.

All Hooked Up: IV's (Intravenous)

IV, or intravenous, simply means in a vein. Many medications and fluids need to go directly into your vein in order to be most effective.

If you are going through chemotherapy, you will probably have a central line (either external or under the skin) to more easily get IV medications and blood transfusions, as well as have blood drawn. Everything you need is connected to your central line.

Most of your drugs and fluids go in (are infused) over a period of time through an IV line (tubing) that connects to an infusion pump. The pump keeps things flowing at a specific rate to ensure effective dosing. Your medication, fluids, and blood for transfusions are usually hung on an IV pole to which the pump or pumps are connected.

Depending on what you need, several different things may hang on an IV pole at the same time—chemo drugs, antibiotics, fluids, blood products, nutritional supplements, etc. The tricky part is maneuvering around with all this stuff attached to your body. You will soon get the hang of it—knowing just how to move so all your lines don't get tangled up.

One more thing about the pumps: Get used to the beeping and learn how to use the silence button. The pumps 'beep' when the infusion is completed. They also beep if there is air in the line (potentially serious) or if the battery is low. But beware—they often beep for no reason—very annoying especially when you're trying to sleep. You can hit the silence button while you're waiting for your nurse to adjust the pump. In the meantime—just grin and bear it.

Venipuncture

If you don't have a central line yet (and some kids, depending on their treatment plan, never have one), you may need to have some IV procedures done with a venipuncture. This means a needle is inserted into a vein usually in your arm or your hand. If you are having blood drawn, a tube is attached to the needle to collect your blood sample. If you are having drugs or fluids infused, IV tubing is attached through which the substance flows. The same is true for a blood transfusion.

Getting stuck with needles for an IV is not usually real painful, but it's not exactly comfortable either. Some technicians and nurses are really good at it—others are not quite so adept. Whenever possible, use a good dose of EMLA cream before the poke (it takes at least an hour to work). Also, if you are having routine IV's without a central line, try to keep switching veins (if you can remember). It will give them a little time to recover.

Chapter 11

Complementary and Alternative Medicine in Cancer Care

You have many choices to make before, during, and after your cancer treatment. One choice you may be thinking about is complementary and alternative medicine. We call this CAM, for short.

People with cancer may use CAM for the following purposes:

- Help cope with the side effects of cancer treatments, such as nausea, pain, and fatigue
- Comfort themselves and ease the worries of cancer treatment and related stress
- Feel that they are doing something more to help with their own care
- Try to treat or cure their cancer

It's natural to want to fight your cancer in any way you can. There is a lot of information available, and new methods for treating cancer are always being tested, so it may be hard to know where to start.

This chapter may help you understand what you find and make it easier to decide whether CAM is right for you. Many people try CAM therapies during cancer care. CAM does not work for everyone, but some methods may help you manage stress, nausea, pain, or other symptoms or side effects.

"Thinking about Complementary and Alternative Medicine," a National Cancer Institute (NCI) FactSheet, June 8, 2005. For additional information, visit the NCI website at http://www.cancer.gov.

The most important message of this chapter is to talk to your doctor before you try anything new. This will help ensure that nothing gets in the way of your cancer treatment.

What Complementary and Alternative Medicine (CAM) Is

CAM is any medical system, practice, or product that is not thought of as standard care. Standard medical care is care that is based on scientific evidence. For cancer, it includes chemotherapy, radiation, biological therapy, and surgery.

Complementary Medicine

- Complementary medicine is used along with standard medical treatments.

- One example is using acupuncture to help with side effects of cancer treatment.

Alternative Medicine

- Alternative medicine is used in place of standard medical treatments.

- One example is using a special diet to treat cancer instead of a method that a cancer specialist (an oncologist) suggests.

Integrative Medicine

- Integrative medicine is a total approach to care that involves the patient's mind, body, and spirit. It combines standard medicine with the CAM practices that have shown the most promise.

- For example, some people learn to use relaxation as a way to reduce stress during chemotherapy.

Types of Complementary and Alternative Medicine (CAM)

We are learning about CAM therapies every day, but there is still more to learn. Consumers may use the terms "natural," "holistic," "home remedy," or "Eastern medicine" to refer to CAM. However, experts use five categories to describe it. These are listed below with a few examples for each.

Mind-Body Medicines

These are based on the belief that your mind is able to affect your body. Here is a list of some examples:

- **Meditation:** Focused breathing or repetition of words or phrases to quiet the mind

- **Biofeedback:** Using simple machines, the patient learns how to affect certain body functions that are normally out of one's awareness (such as heart rate)

- **Hypnosis:** A state of relaxed and focused attention in which the patient concentrates on a certain feeling, idea, or suggestion to aid in healing

- **Yoga:** Systems of stretches and poses, with special attention given to breathing

- **Imagery:** Imagining scenes, pictures, or experiences to help the body heal

- **Creative outlets:** Such as art, music, or dance

Biologically Based Practices

This type of CAM uses things found in nature. This includes dietary supplements and herbal products, such as the following examples:

- Vitamins
- Herbs
- Foods
- Special diets

A note about nutrition: It's common for people with cancer to have questions about different foods to eat during treatment. Yet it's important to know that there is no one food or special diet that has been proven to control cancer. Too much of any one food is not helpful, and may even be harmful. Because of nutrition needs you may have, it's best to talk with the doctor in charge of your treatment about the foods you should be eating.

Manipulative and Body-Based Practices

These are based on working with one or more parts of the body. Here are some examples:

- **Massage:** Manipulation of tissues with hands or special tools
- **Chiropractic care:** A type of manipulation of the joints and skeletal system
- **Reflexology:** Using pressure points in the hands or feet to affect other parts of the body

Energy Medicine

Energy medicine involves the belief that the body has energy fields that can be used for healing and wellness. Therapists use pressure or move the body by placing their hands in or through these fields. Examples include the following:

- **Tai chi:** Involves slow, gentle movements with a focus on the breath and concentration
- **Reiki:** Balancing energy either from a distance or by placing hands on or near the patient
- **Therapeutic touch:** Moving hands over energy fields of the body

Whole Medical Systems

These are healing systems and beliefs that have evolved over time in different cultures and parts of the world:

- **Ayurvedic medicine:** A system from India emphasizing balance among body, mind, and spirit
- **Chinese medicine:** Based on the view that health is a balance in the body of two forces called yin and yang. Acupuncture is a common practice in Chinese medicine that involves stimulating specific points on the body to promote health, or to lessen disease symptoms and treatment side effects.
- **Homeopathy:** Uses very small doses of substances to trigger the body to heal itself
- **Naturopathic medicine:** Uses different methods that help the body naturally heal itself

Talk with Your Doctor before You Use CAM

Some people with cancer are afraid that their doctor won't understand or approve of the use of CAM. But doctors know that people with

118

cancer want to take an active part in their care. They want the best for their patients and often are willing to work with them.

Talk to your doctor to make sure that all aspects of your cancer care work together. This is important because things that seem safe, such as certain foods or pills, may interfere with your cancer treatment.

The following is a list of question that you should ask your doctor about CAM:

- What types of CAM might...
  - help me cope, reduce my stress, and feel better?
  - help me feel less tired?
  - help me deal with cancer symptoms, such as pain, or side effects of treatment, such as nausea?
- If I decide to try a CAM therapy...
  - will it interfere with my treatment or medicines?
  - can you help me understand these articles I found about CAM?
  - can you suggest a CAM practitioner for me to talk to?
  - will you work with my CAM practitioner?

A Natural Product Does Not Mean a Safe Product

Here are some important facts about dietary supplements such as herbs and vitamins:

They may affect how well other medicines work in your body: Herbs and some plant-based products may keep medicines from doing what they are supposed to do. These medicines can be ones your doctor prescribes for you, or even ones you buy off the shelf at the store. For example, the herb St. John's wort, which some people with cancer use for depression, may cause certain anticancer drugs not to work as well as they should.

Herbal supplements can act like drugs in your body: They may be harmful when taken by themselves, with other substances, or in large doses. For example, some studies have shown that kava, an herb that has been used to help with stress and anxiety, may cause liver damage.

Vitamins can also take strong action in your body: For example, high doses of vitamins, even vitamin C, may affect how chemotherapy and radiation work. Too much of any vitamin is not safe—even in a healthy person.

Tell your doctor if you are taking any dietary supplements, no matter how safe you think they are. This is very important. Even though there are ads or claims that something has been used for years, they do not prove that it is safe or effective. It is still important to be careful.

Supplements do not have to be approved by the federal government before being sold to the public. Also, a prescription is not needed to buy them. Therefore, it's up to consumers to decide what is best for them.

Choose Practitioners with Care

CAM practitioners are people who have training in the therapies previously listed. Choosing one should be done with the same care as choosing a doctor. Here are some things to remember when choosing a practitioner:

- Ask your doctor or nurse to suggest someone or speak with someone who knows about CAM.

- Ask whether someone at your cancer center or doctor's office can help you find a CAM practitioner. There may be a social worker or physical therapist who can help you.

- Ask whether your hospital keeps lists of centers or has staff who can suggest people.

- Contact CAM professional organizations to get names of practitioners who are certified. This means that they have proper training in their field.

- Contact local health and wellness organizations.

- Ask about each practitioner's training and experience.

- Ask whether the practitioner has a license to practice in your state. If you want to confirm the answer, ask what organization gives out the licenses. Then, you may choose to follow up with a phone call.

- Call your health care plan to see if it covers this therapy.

General Questions to Ask the CAM Practitioner

- What types of CAM do you practice?
- What are your training and qualifications?

- Do you see other patients with my type of cancer?
- Will you work with my doctor?

Questions about the Therapy

- How can this help me?
- Do you know of studies that prove it helps?
- What are the risks and side effects?
- Will this interfere with my cancer treatment?
- How long will I be on the therapy?
- What will it cost?
- Do you have information that I can read about it?
- Are there any reasons why I should not use it?

Other Questions to Ask Yourself

- Do I feel comfortable with this person?
- Do I like how the office looks and feels?
- Do I like the staff?
- Does this person support standard cancer treatments?
- How far am I willing to travel for treatment?
- Is it easy to get an appointment?
- Are the hours good for me?
- Will insurance cover the cost of CAM?

Call your health plan or insurer to see whether they cover CAM therapies. Many are not covered.

Getting Information from Trusted Sources

Government Agencies

There is a lot of information on CAM, so it's important to go to sources you can trust. Good places to start are the government agencies. They offer lots of information about CAM that might be helpful to you. They may also know of universities or hospitals that have CAM resources.

Be careful of products advertised by people or companies that raise warning flags such as the following:

- Make claims that they have a "cure"

- Do not give specific information about how well their product works

- Make claims only about positive results that have few side effects

- Say they have clinical studies, but provide no proof or copies of the studies

Just remember, if it sounds too good to be true, it probably is. For ways to find out more about CAM, see the resources section.

Websites

Patients and families have been able to find answers to many of their questions about CAM on the internet. Many websites are good resources for CAM information. However, some may be unreliable or misleading. Questions to ask about a website:

- Who runs and pays for the site?

- Does it list any credentials?

- Does it represent an organization that is well-known and respected?

- What is the purpose of the site, and who is it for?

- Is the site selling or promoting something?

- Where does the information come from?

- Is the information based on facts or only on someone's feelings or opinions?

- How is the information chosen? Is there a review board or is the content reviewed by experts?

- How current is the information?

- Does the site tell when it was last updated?

- How does the site choose which other sites to link you to?

Books

A number of books have been written about different CAM therapies. Some books are better than others and contain trustworthy content, while others do not.

If you go to the library, ask the staff for suggestions. Or if you live near a college or university, there may be a medical library available. Local bookstores may also have people on staff who can help you.

It's important to know that information is always changing and that new research results are reported every day. Be aware that if a book is written by only one person, you may only be getting that one person's view.

Questions to ask include the following:

- Is the author an expert on this subject?
- Do you know anyone else who has read the book?
- Has the book been reviewed by other experts?
- Was it published in the past five years?
- Does the book offer different points of view, or does it seem to hold one opinion?
- Has the author researched the topic in full?
- Are the references listed in the back?

Magazine Articles

If you want to look for articles you can trust, ask your librarian to help you look for medical journals, books, and other research that has been done by experts.

Articles in popular magazines are usually not written by experts. Rather, the authors speak with experts, gather information, and then write the article. If claims about CAM are made in magazine articles, remember these points:

- The authors may not have expert knowledge in this area
- They may not say where they found their information
- The articles have not been reviewed by experts
- The publisher may have ties to advertisers or other organizations; therefore, the article may be one-sided

When you read these articles, you can use the same process that the magazine writer uses:

- Speak with experts
- Ask lots of questions
- Then decide if the therapy is right for you

Resources

National Cancer Institute (NCI)
Office of Cancer Complementary and Alternative Medicine (OCCAM)

- Oversees NCI's projects in CAM
- Funds cancer CAM research
- Provides information about CAM to health providers and the public.

  Visit: http://cancer.gov/cam

Cancer Information Service (CIS)

- Provides help finding NCI information on the internet
- Answers questions about cancer
- Provides printed materials from NCI
- Gives referrals to clinical trials and other cancer-related services

  Visit: http://cis.nci.nih.gov

  Chat online: http://www.cancer.gov Click on "Need Help?" then click on "LiveHelp."

  Toll-free: 800-4-CANCER (800-422-6237)

  TTY: 800-332-8615

PDQ®

- Provides regularly updated information on most types of cancer and many related topics

  Visit: http://www.cancer.gov/cancertopics/pdq

National Center for Complementary and Alternative Medicine (NCCAM)

- Funds CAM research
- Evaluates and provides information about CAM to health providers and the public

  Visit: http://nccam.nih.gov

  Toll-free: 888-644-6226

  TTY: 866-464-3615

National Library of Medicine

- The Directory of Information Resources Online (DIRLINE) contains locations of and information about a number of health organizations, including those that focus on CAM

    Visit: http://dirline.nlm.nih.gov

- Medline Plus provides access to reliable health information, including articles, organizations, directories, and answers to health questions

    Visit: http://medlineplus.gov

- PubMed has a free and easy-to-use search tool for finding scientific articles on CAM

    Visit: http://www.ncbi.nlm.nih.gov/PubMed

Food and Drug Administration (FDA)

- Oversees safety of drugs and medical devices
- Provides information on many issues, including vitamins and pills
- Informs people about how to look for health fraud

    Visit: http://www.fda.gov

    Toll-free: 888-463-6332

Federal Trade Commission (FTC)

- Provides information about consumer protection laws
- Provides information about false advertising for foods and drugs

    Visit: http://www.ftc.gov

    Toll-free: 877-FTC-HELP (877-382-4357)

    TTY: 866-653-4261

National Cancer Institute-Sponsored Cancer Centers

- Many National Cancer Institute-sponsored cancer centers have CAM information available to you

    Visit: http://www3.cancer.gov/cancercenters/centerslist.html

    Toll-free: 800-4-CANCER (800-422-6237) Ask for the cancer center list fact sheet

Chapter 12

Palliative Care

Today, doctors are able to cure many people diagnosed with cancer. Others are treated for several years with successive therapies, although they are not cured. Some experience unwanted side effects from treatment or discomfort due to either the cancer or the treatment. Helping people with cancer live well at every stage of their illness is the overall goal of palliative care. In fact, it is one of the most important goals of cancer treatment throughout the course of the disease (called the disease trajectory).

Defining Palliative Care

Palliative care includes treating the physical, spiritual, psychological, and social needs of a person with cancer. It starts at the beginning of the cancer process and may change over time to reflect each person's priorities and needs. Palliative care is not giving up on treatment. In fact, people with cancer may receive anticancer (curative) therapy and palliative care at the same time. In some settings, people switch and experience a transition from cure-oriented care to palliative, or symptom-oriented, care. In others, both forms of treatment are delivered simultaneously (at the same time), although the emphasis may shift toward comfort measures as the disease progresses.

Palliative care and hospice care: Although the terms palliative care and hospice care are sometimes used interchangeably, they have different meanings. Palliative care applies to every step of the cancer process, whereas hospice care in the United States is used when the life expectancy is six months or less.

Purpose of Palliative Care

Five goals of palliative care include the following:

- To treat pain and all other physical symptoms caused by cancer or its treatment

- To address a person's spiritual needs or concerns

- To address a person's social needs, including financial concerns, and practical needs, such as transportation

- To treat a person's psychosocial needs, such as mood changes and depression

- To provide support for the patient's family, friends, and caregivers, which continues beyond the patient's death

Children can also receive palliative care. The World Health Organization (WHO) defines palliative care for children as the "total care of the child's mind, body, and spirit." Parents usually work with the health-care team to help their children feel as comfortable as possible. Care is also provided to other children in the family and counseling remains available for the entire family for many months afterwards.

The Palliative Care Team

A variety of health professionals may participate as part of a team to give palliative care.

- **Doctor:** Usually acts as the care team leader; makes treatment plans and decides on medication and dosing; may consult with other doctors such as pain specialists or radiation oncologists. The doctor may be available to make home visits or may supervise the care plan without actually seeing the patient.

- **Nurse:** Gives direct care to the patient; can also assist with managing pain and other side effects of cancer or its treatment; may act as a liaison with the rest of the team. When people are enrolled in home hospice programs, nurses visit them at home several times a week and sometimes more than once a day.

- **Social worker:** Helps with financial issues; arranges family meetings; assists with the discharge from the hospital to home or hospice care.

- **Hospital chaplain or other spiritual advisor:** Counsels the patient and family members on religious and spiritual matters.

- **Dietitian:** Helps with nutritional concerns.

- **Physical therapist:** Helps maintain movement and assists when mobility is impaired or there are concerns regarding safety in the home.

- **Grief and bereavement coordinator:** Helps with planning memorial services and counseling for the patient as well as family members.

The Role of Communication

Communication is a central element of palliative care as it helps to clarify needs and expectations. The following are some practical tips to help promote good communication with the health-care team:

- Find doctors who are willing to answer questions and listen to your symptoms and your concerns.

- Ask questions about the diagnosis and treatment. Listen to the answers and ask the doctor to explain things that are not clear.

- Tell the doctor and nurse about pain, discomfort, or other side effects, such as mouth sores, nausea, vomiting, and constipation.

It is important for patients and caregivers to understand the diagnosis and prognosis (chance of recovery) and to participate in the medical decision-making process.

End-of-Life Considerations

Often, people with cancer or their families find it too painful to think about the possibility that the treatment won't cure the person's cancer. Sometimes, though, curative treatment will no longer slow or halt the growth of cancer or may be too toxic. The doctor and his or her patient may then decide to focus only on treatment aimed at maximizing comfort.

Talking about how to comfort a dying person is not easy for most people, and sometimes friends and relatives are afraid that if they mention death, they are giving up. In fact, most people, especially those with an incurable illness, have probably already thought about death. Discussing advance directives (instructions for medical care in the event that the person cannot communicate his or her wishes), hospice care, or memorial services can give the dying person some control over the situation and may help the grieving process for friends and family. It may also afford the family the opportunity to reaffirm love and promote a special closeness, which may help to ease the pain of separation. A social worker or chaplain may be able to help facilitate discussion of these issues. In addition, some palliative care services offer bereavement counseling to help friends and family members cope with loss.

Chapter 13

Transitional Care Planning

Planning for the Care Continuum

Transitional care planning helps the patient's cancer care continue without interruption through different phases of the cancer experience.

Transition means passage from one phase to another. Transitional care planning is the bridge between two phases of care. As the cancer patient's treatment goals change or the place of care changes, the patient may encounter problems during the transition. Patients will need to make decisions that balance disease status and treatment options with family needs, finances, employment, spiritual or religious beliefs, and quality of life. There may be practical problems such as finding an appropriate rehabilitation center, obtaining special equipment, or paying for needed care. There may be mental health problems such as depression or anxiety. Transitional care planning helps identify and manage these problems so the transition can go smoothly, without interruption of care. This can reduce stress on the patient and family and improve the patient's health outcome.

Transitional care planning may include support and education for the patient and family and referral to resources. Ideally, it involves a team approach by the patient's health care providers. It is important that there be close communication between members of the team and that this communication include the patient and family.

PDQ® Cancer Information Summary. National Cancer Institute; Bethesda, MD. Transitional Care Planning (PDQ®): Supportive Care - Patient. Updated 06/2006. Available at http://cancer.gov. Accessed November 10, 2006.

Changing Goals

Each type of cancer requires different care and the goals of a patient's treatment may change as his or her disease gets better or worse. Cancer care may include any of the following:

- **Active treatment:** Treatment given to cure the cancer

- **Supportive care:** Care given to prevent or treat as early as possible the symptoms of the disease; side effects caused by treatment of the disease; and psychological, social, and spiritual problems related to the disease or its treatment

- **Palliative therapy:** Treatment given to relieve symptoms and improve the patient's quality of life. Palliative care may be given along with other cancer treatments or when treatment is no longer curative, to make the patient comfortable at the end of life.

Transitional care planning can help the patient and family with medical, practical, and emotional issues that arise as they adjust to these different levels and goals of care.

Changing Settings

Most of the care received by people with cancer is provided in places other than a hospital. The place where the patient receives treatment may change several times during the course of the illness. Patients may go from receiving care in a hospital or as an outpatient to receiving care at home, in a nursing home, at a rehabilitation center (a place for special training, such as help in regaining strength or movement), or from a hospice team for end-of-life care. When a patient moves from one place of care to another, the process of planning for the move is often called discharge planning. This may involve a case manager who acts on the patient's behalf when dealing with the hospital, visiting nurses, health care companies, rehabilitation facilities, nursing homes, and other groups that provide the care needed. The case manager is a link to resources and services in the community and can arrange for the provision of services, including patient and family education and referrals.

Transitional Care Planning Assessments

An assessment collects information that helps the health care team identify and manage problems a patient may have in adjusting to a change in care.

Having cancer affects more than the patient's physical condition. It also affects mental health, family life, ability to work, financial planning, social relationships, and faith. Many patients will encounter problems in one or more of these areas as they transfer from one level of care to another. For example, a patient's family may have problems obtaining special home equipment or learning to use special equipment. Another patient may have a difficult time accepting the change from anticancer care to symptom relief alone, such as that provided with some types of palliative or hospice care. Transitional care planning is unique to each patient and family. Assessments help identify patients who may have problems during the transition and help determine the kind of support they will need to make the change go smoothly. The assessments may include a complete medical history; a physical exam; a test of learning skills; tests to determine ability to perform activities of daily living; a mental health evaluation; a review of social support available to the patient; and referral to community resources as needed to assist with issues such as transportation, home care, healthy eating, and medication management.

Assessments Are a Routine Part of Care

Assessments are done when the patient moves from one facility to another, such as from hospital to home. They are also done at regular times during the course of the disease, usually at the time of diagnosis, after completing a course of treatment, when there is a relapse, when curative treatment stops, and when treatment is discontinued (end-of-life care begins). The patient may feel added emotional stress at these times. Regular assessments can identify these and other causes of distress in the patient, such as job loss or the death or illness of a patient's loved one or caretaker.

Because no one knows what the patient's needs will be in the future, assessments are done many times during the cancer experience as a routine part of care. This is helps ensure the patient receives the right services at the right times.

The Assessment Process

In planning for a change in cancer care, doctors, nurses, and other members of the patient's health care team will consider all the areas of a patient's life that may be affected. The following professionals may each conduct different parts of the transitional care planning assessment:

- Doctor

133

- Nurse
- Dietitian
- Social worker
- Psychologist
- Chaplain
- Physical therapist
- Occupational therapist

The following types of assessments will be done for transitional care planning:

Physical assessment: Physical assessment will look at the patient's general health, treatment plan, and changes in disease status, including the following factors:

- Type and stage of the cancer
- Symptoms of the cancer
- Side effects of treatment
- Whether the patient smokes
- Nutrition-related side effects and complications
- Ability to perform activities of daily living

Family and home assessment: Factors such as the patient's age and living arrangements may affect how easily a change in level of care can be accomplished. The assessment will look at the following:

- Age of the patient and family members
- Living arrangements
- Whether the patient has a spouse or children
- Level of education of the patient and family
- Language spoken in the home
- Cultural beliefs and practices
- Whether family and friends are able to help during treatment
- The age and floor plan of the home. Will medical equipment (such as a hospital bed, oxygen tank, or portable monitor) fit in the bedroom, if needed, and is wiring adequate? Can a person in a wheelchair move through the house easily?

Mental health assessment: Change can be a stressful time for both the patient and family. The nature of the relationship between the patient and his or her family and others helps determine the kinds of services the family may need to cope with the transition. The following questions may be asked:

- How do the patient and family feel about the cancer, the treatment, and the treatment goals? Sometimes patients develop serious problems such as depression or anxiety. Family members also may need help dealing with their feelings. These problems are often treatable. The doctor or health care professional can make referrals to a support group, counselor, or mental health care worker.

- What beliefs and values are important to the patient and do they affect the patient's treatment decisions?

- How has the family coped with stress and crisis in the past? This may be helpful in predicting how they will react to the stress caused by the changes in the patient's treatment.

- Are there problems in the home that are unrelated to the cancer but may affect how well the patient and family can handle the change?

- Are there current or past mental health problems in the family?

- Has there been physical or sexual abuse in the patient's past?

- In the case of a patient considering home care, does the patient or any family member smoke or use drugs or alcohol? Smoking is not safe around oxygen equipment. Family members responsible for giving the patient medicines or other care must be clear-headed and not under the influence of any substance that could affect their ability to provide care in the prescribed way.

Social assessment: Doctors and other health care professionals can provide referrals to supportive services available to the patient. A review of the kinds of social services already available to the patient will be done:

- What kind of support is available in the home and community? How will the patient travel to medical appointments or other places? Who can the patient call on for help if necessary? Where the patient lives may affect what services are available and how the patient can get to appointments. Referrals can be made to

135

local providers of services such as home nursing, food and medication delivery, and transportation to and from treatment centers.

- Does the patient understand hospice care and palliative care and know about available programs in the community?

- Before home care is considered, the availability of in-home help must be determined. Is there someone at home who can help the patient or will outside help be needed?

- Will the primary caregiver have anyone to help with the caregiving duties and make it possible to take time off?

- How will the change affect the patient's ability to work?

- Does the patient have insurance coverage (group coverage from a job, Medicare, Medicaid, veteran's benefits, or other)?

- What are the patient's financial resources? How will the cost of care be paid?

Spiritual assessment: Knowing the role that religion and spirituality play in the patient's life help the health care team understand how these beliefs may affect the patient's transition to a new level of care. A spiritual assessment may include the following questions:

- Does the patient consider himself or herself to be a spiritual person?

- What is the importance of religion to the patient?

- Is the cancer or its treatment causing spiritual distress?

- Is support available from the patient's religious group? Many patients find visits from members of their religious group valuable. A patient may want to talk to a spiritual advisor (for example, a priest, rabbi, or minister) during treatment.

Most hospitals, especially larger ones, employ hospital chaplains who are trained to work with medical patients and their families. Hospital chaplains are trained to be sensitive to a range of religious and spiritual beliefs and concerns.

Legal assessment: Advance directives and other legal documents can help doctors and family members make decisions about treatment should the patient become unable to communicate his or her wishes.

The patient may be asked if he or she has prepared any of the following documents:

- **Advance directive:** A general term for different types of documents that state what an individual's wishes are concerning certain medical treatments when the patient can no longer communicate those wishes. The patient may declare the wish to be given all possible treatments that are medically appropriate, only some treatments, or no treatment at all.

- **Health care proxy (HCP):** A document in which the patient identifies a person (called a proxy) to make medical decisions if the patient becomes unable to do so. The form may not need to be notarized, but it must be witnessed by two other people. The patient does not have to state specific decisions about individual treatments, only that the proxy may make medical decisions for him or her. HCP is also known as durable power of attorney for health care (DPOAHC) or medical power of attorney (MPOA).

- **Living will:** A living will is a legal document in which a person states that they want certain life-saving medical treatments to be either withheld or withdrawn under certain circumstances. A living will is a type of advance directive. Living wills are not legal in all states.

- **Durable power of attorney:** A document in which the patient names another person to make legal decisions for him or her.

- **Do not resuscitate (DNR) order:** A document in which the patient instructs doctors not to perform cardiopulmonary resuscitation (restart the heart) at the moment of death, so that the natural process of dying occurs. A DNR order may be medically appropriate when cardiopulmonary resuscitation is not likely to save the patient's life.

Transitional Care Options

Different types of care are available for different types of needs. Transitional care may include management of the patient's medical condition and rehabilitation, plus supportive services to ensure basic needs such as comfort, hygiene, safety, and nutrition. It may also include supportive services for educational, social, spiritual, and financial needs. The following is a list of some of the care options that meet the assessed needs of patients during transition:

Place of Care

- Hospital
- Nursing home
- Rehabilitation unit or facility
- Patient's home
- Home of family caregiver
- Hospice (may be in an inpatient setting specified by the hospice or in the patient's home)

Caregivers

Health care specialists and other caregivers work as a team, providing services to patients in their homes, clinics, and other settings. These may include the following:

- Doctor
- Nurse
- Dietitian
- Physical therapist
- Occupational therapist
- Social worker
- Mental health professional
- Clergy or other religious leader
- Companions
- Home care aides

Programs

Programs that provide care may include the following:

- Bereavement programs
- Community support groups
- Employment counseling agencies
- Home health agencies
- Home infusion agencies
- Hospice programs

- Legal aid organizations
- Palliative care programs

Medication Support

- Pain and symptom management
- Chemotherapy
- Blood transfusions
- Medications that cause blood cells to grow and mature
- Antibiotics (drugs used to treat infections)
- Treatments that help improve or restore lung function
- Wound and skin care

Nutrition Support

The patient may be able to eat normally or may need supplemental nutrition by mouth, by tube-feeding, or by delivery into a vein.

Special Equipment

The type of equipment needed, if any, will depend on the patient's condition. Some commonly needed devices include the following:

- Medical appliances (such as catheters, tubes for drainage, and bags for colostomies)
- Assistive devices (wheelchairs, walkers, special beds and mattresses)
- Pumps to deliver medication into the body
- Respirators (machines that help the patient breathe)

Special Considerations

Caring for a patient at home can increase the physical and emotional burdens on the patient's caregivers. The stress and responsibility of in-home care can be hard on family relationships and should be carefully considered. Day-to-day routines may change for everyone. Many families have trouble getting used to the role changes that result. Patients and families may be referred to counseling to help them with these issues.

Pain control is a key factor in successful home care. Pain medications are given to help patients feel better and are often a part of cancer care. Controlling the patient's symptoms, especially pain, can make things easier on both the patient and the caregivers. It is important that the family and caregivers understand the use of pain control medications and other treatments that keep the patient comfortable.

If home care is to be considered, the following factors and others will be assessed:

- The kind of care to be given

- The decision-making skills required by the patient and caregiver

- Whether equipment needed will fit in the home

- The family's ability and desire to provide the care, alone or with the aid of home care workers

This assessment will help determine if care at home is a workable option for the patient.

Paying for Services and Care Needed

Medical insurance, Medicare, veteran's benefits, and/or Medicaid may pay some of a patient's medical expenses. These have limits to their coverage, however, and patients may need to find other ways to pay for costs not covered. The costs of home care, for example, are usually covered only under certain conditions and for a limited time.

Transitional care planning will include referrals to community resources that can help the patient plan for treatment costs not met by insurance. Social service agencies may be available to help with certain care needs. Some organizations lend medical equipment (such as wheelchairs and hospital beds), provide short-term assistance with a nursing aid or housekeeper, or provide transportation to and from the doctor's office or clinic.

For more information about financial resources, contact the National Cancer Information Service (CIS) at 800-4-CANCER. The CIS offices have information about cancer-related services and resources that are available in different parts of the country.

Counseling for the Patient

People with cancer often want to get back to work. Their jobs give them not only an income but also a sense of routine. Some people feel well enough to work while they are having treatment. Others need to wait until their treatments are over. Patients who have disabilities or other special needs after treatment may not be able to return to their old jobs at all.

Referrals can be made to services that help the patient with job-related issues. These services may include employment counseling, education and skills training, and help in obtaining and using assistive technology and tools.

If a patient does return to work, co-workers may not know what to say or may not know if the patient wants to talk about the cancer. Education of the patient's co-workers about the cancer can help ease this transition.

Advance Directives

During transitions in care, the patient's advance directives, health care proxy form, and durable power of attorney document need to be given to the appropriate caregivers. This step will ensure that the patient's wishes are known through all disease stages and places of care.

End-of-Life Decisions

Caring for a person with cancer starts after symptoms begin and the diagnosis is made and continues until the patient is in remission, is cured, or has died. End-of-life decisions should be made soon after the diagnosis, before there is a need for them. These issues are not pleasant or easy to think about, but planning for them can help relieve the burden on family members to make major decisions for the patient at a time when they are likely to be emotionally upset.

A patient's views may reflect his or her philosophical, moral, religious, or spiritual background. If a person has certain feelings about end-of-life issues, these feelings should be made known so that they can be carried out. Since these are sensitive issues, they are often not discussed by patients, families, or doctors. People often feel that there will be plenty of time to talk later about the issues. Many times, though, when the end-of-life decisions are necessary, they must be made by people who do not know the patient's wishes. A patient should talk with the doctor and other caregivers about resuscitation decisions as early as possible (for example, when being admitted to the hospital); he or she may not be able to make these decisions later. Advance directives can ensure the patient's wishes are known ahead of time.

These issues are important to discuss whether a patient is being cared for at home, in a hospital, nursing home, or hospice, or elsewhere.

Part Three

Clinical Trials and Cancer Research Updates

Chapter 14

Should You Take Part in a Clinical Trial?

Taking Part in a Clinical Trial

Only you can make the decision about whether or not to participate in a clinical trial. Before you make your decision, you should:

- Learn as much as possible about your disease and the trials that are available to you.

- Then, talk about this information and how you feel about it with your doctor and/or nurse, family members and friends to help you determine what is right for you.

What are the potential risks and benefits of clinical trials?

Potential benefits include the following:

- Health care provided by leading physicians in the field of cancer research

- Access to new drugs and interventions before they are widely available

- Close monitoring of your health care and any side effects

This chapter includes text from "Should I Take Part In a Clinical Trial?" National Cancer Institute (NCI), August 30, 2001; "How Is a Clinical Trial Planned and Carried Out?" NCI, February 1, 2006; "How Do I Take Part in a Clinical Trial?" NCI, January 26, 2005; and "Clinical Trials: Questions and Answers," NCI, May 19, 2006.

- A more active role in your own health care
- If the approach being studied is found to be helpful, you may be among the first to benefit
- An opportunity to make a valuable contribution to cancer research

Potential risks include the following:

- New drugs and procedures may have side effects or risks unknown to the doctors
- New drugs and procedures may be ineffective, or less effective, than current approaches
- Even if a new approach has benefits, it may not work for you

Could I receive a placebo?

In treatment trials involving people who have cancer, placebos ("dummy" pills that contain no active ingredient) are very rarely used. Many treatment trials are designed to compare a new treatment with a standard treatment, which is the best treatment currently known for a cancer based on results of past research. In these studies, patients are randomly assigned to one group or another. When no standard treatment exists for a cancer, a study may compare a new treatment with a placebo. However, you will be told about this possibility during informed consent, before you decide whether or not to take part in the study.

How Clinical Trials Are Planned and Carried Out

Where do the ideas for trials come from?

The ideas for clinical trials often originate in the laboratory. Researchers develop a clinical trial protocol (the plan for a trial) after laboratory studies indicate the promise of a new drug or procedure. The first trials of a particular drug or procedure are focused on safety (phase I), and later trials focus on whether the drug or procedure is effective (phase II or phase III).

What is a protocol?

Every trial has a person in charge, usually a doctor, who is called the protocol chair or principal investigator. Phase I and phase II studies generally refer to the person in charge as the principal investigator. Phase

III studies generally have a protocol chair, under whose direction multiple principal investigators carry out the protocol in participating sites. The protocol chair or principal investigator prepares a plan for the study, called a protocol. The protocol explains what the study will do, how it will be carried out, and why each part of the study is necessary. For example, the protocol includes the following types of information:

- The reason for doing the study
- How many people will be in the study
- Who is eligible to participate in the study
- What study drugs participants will take, if any
- What medical tests they will have, if any, and how often
- What information will be gathered

Every doctor or research center that takes part in the trial uses the same protocol. This ensures that patients are treated identically no matter where or if they are receiving treatment, and that information from all the participating centers (if there is more than one) can be combined and compared.

Who sponsors clinical trials?

Clinical trials are sponsored by organizations or individuals who are seeking better treatments for cancer or better ways to prevent or detect cancer.

Individual physicians at cancer centers and other medical institutions can sponsor clinical trials themselves.

Drug companies or companies that make diagnostic equipment (like x-ray machines) sponsor trials of their products, hoping to demonstrate that their products are safe and effective. The U.S. Food and Drug Administration (FDA) will only permit companies to sell a product after it has been proven safe and effective in clinical trials.

What happens when a clinical trial is over?

After a phase I or phase II trial is completed, the researchers look carefully at the data collected during the trial and decide whether to:

- Move on to the next trial with the treatment, or
- Stop testing the treatment because it is not safe or effective.

When a phase III trial comes to an end, the researchers must look at the data and decide if the results have medical importance. When the analysis of a phase I, phase II, or phase III trial is complete, the researchers will inform the medical community and the public of the study results.

In most cases, the results of trials are published in scientific or medical journals. However, before that most medical and scientific journals have in place a process of peer review, in which experts critique the report before it is published, to make sure that the analysis and conclusions are sound. Particularly important results are likely to be featured by the print or electronic media, and widely discussed at scientific meetings and by patient advocacy groups. Once an intervention is proven safe and effective in a clinical trial, it may become the new standard of practice. In this way the development of better interventions for prevention, for treatment, or for detection and diagnosis is an ongoing, continuous process that builds progressively on itself to improve the quality of cancer care and prevention available to us all.

Considering Participation in a Clinical Trial?

Once you've decided that participating in a clinical trial could prove beneficial to you, there are other factors to consider that might affect your participation.

Who is eligible to participate in a clinical trial?

Each study has its own guidelines for who can participate, called eligibility criteria. To ensure the strongest results, researchers want study participants to be alike in key ways. Examples of eligibility criteria for a treatment trial might be a particular type and stage of cancer, age, gender, or previous treatments. The eligibility criteria are included in the study plan. To find out if you are eligible for a particular study, talk to your doctor or the doctor or nurse in charge of enrolling patients for the study.

Where are trials conducted?

If you were to participate in a clinical trial, you might do so at a large cancer center, a university hospital, or your local medical center or physician's office.

The trial may include participants at one or two highly specialized centers or it may involve hundreds of locations at the same time. You would participate in the trial under the guidance of a team including your physician and other health professionals, who would report your experience during the trial back to the center responsible for the trial's overall coordination. Experts then use the information from all of the participants to evaluate the intervention that the trial is testing.

Questions and Answers about Clinical Trials

What are the types of clinical trials?

There are several types of clinical trials:

- Prevention trials test new approaches, such as medications, vitamins, or other supplements, that doctors believe may lower the risk of developing a certain type of cancer. Most prevention trials are conducted with healthy people who have not had cancer. Some trials are conducted with people who have had cancer and want to prevent recurrence (return of cancer), or reduce the chance of developing a new type of cancer.

- Screening trials study ways to detect cancer earlier. They are often conducted to determine whether finding cancer before it causes symptoms decreases the chance of dying from the disease. These trials involve people who do not have any symptoms of cancer.

- Diagnostic trials study tests or procedures that could be used to identify cancer more accurately. Diagnostic trials usually include people who have signs or symptoms of cancer.

- Treatment trials are conducted with people who have cancer. They are designed to answer specific questions about, and evaluate the effectiveness of, a new treatment or a new way of using a standard treatment. These trials test many types of treatments, such as new drugs, vaccines, new approaches to surgery or radiation therapy, or new combinations of treatments.

- Quality-of-life (also called supportive care) trials explore ways to improve the comfort and quality of life of cancer patients and cancer survivors. These trials may study ways to help people who are experiencing nausea, vomiting, sleep disorders, depression, or other effects from cancer or its treatment.

- Genetics studies are sometimes part of another cancer clinical trial. The genetics component of the trial may focus on how genetic makeup can affect detection, diagnosis, or response to cancer treatment.

- Population-based and family-based genetic research studies differ from traditional cancer clinical trials. In these studies, researchers look at tissue or blood samples, generally from families or large groups of people, to find genetic changes that are associated with cancer. People who participate in genetics studies may or may not have cancer, depending on the study. The goal of these studies is to help understand the role of genes in the development of cancer.

How are participants protected?

Research with people is conducted according to strict scientific and ethical principles. Every clinical trial has a protocol, or action plan, which acts like a "recipe" for conducting the trial. The plan describes what will be done in the study, how it will be conducted, and why each part of the study is necessary. The same protocol is used by every doctor or research center taking part in the trial.

All clinical trials that are federally funded or that evaluate a new drug or medical device subject to Food and Drug Administration regulation must be reviewed and approved by an Institutional Review Board (IRB). Many institutions require that all clinical trials, regardless of funding, be reviewed and approved by a local IRB. The Board, which includes doctors, researchers, community leaders, and other members of the community, reviews the protocol to make sure the study is conducted fairly and participants are not likely to be harmed. The IRB also decides how often to review the trial once it has begun. Based on this information, the IRB decides whether the clinical trial should continue as initially planned and, if not, what changes should be made. An IRB can stop a clinical trial if the researcher is not following the protocol or if the trial appears to be causing unexpected harm to the participants. An IRB can also stop a clinical trial if there is clear evidence that the new intervention is effective, in order to make it widely available.

NIH-supported clinical trials require data and safety monitoring. Some clinical trials, especially phase III clinical trials, use a Data and Safety Monitoring Board (DSMB). A DSMB is an independent committee made up of statisticians, physicians, and patient advocates. The DSMB ensures that the risks of participation are as small as possible, makes sure the data are complete, and stops a trial if safety concerns arise or when the trial's objectives have been met.

What are eligibility criteria, and why are they important?

Each study's protocol has guidelines for who can or cannot participate in the study. These guidelines, called eligibility criteria, describe
characteristics that must be shared by all participants. The criteria
differ from study to study. They may include age, gender, medical history, and current health status. Eligibility criteria for treatment studies often require that patients have a particular type and stage of
cancer.

Enrolling participants with similar characteristics helps to ensure
that the results of the trial will be due to what is under study and not
other factors. In this way, eligibility criteria help researchers achieve
accurate and meaningful results. These criteria also minimize the risk
of a person's condition becoming worse by participating in the study.

What is informed consent?

Informed consent is a process by which people learn the important
facts about a clinical trial to help them decide whether to participate.
This information includes details about what is involved, such as the
purpose of the study, the tests and other procedures used in the study,
and the possible risks and benefits. In addition to talking with the
doctor or nurse, people receive a written consent form explaining the
study. People who agree to take part in the study are asked to sign
the informed consent form. However, signing the form does not mean
people must stay in the study. People can leave the study at any time—
either before the study starts or at any time during the study or the
follow-up period.

The informed consent process continues throughout the study. If
new benefits, risks, or side effects are discovered during the study, the
researchers must inform the participants. They may be asked to sign
new consent forms if they want to stay in the study.

How are clinical trials conducted?

Clinical trials are usually conducted in a series of steps, called
phases. Treatment clinical trials listed in PDQ®, the NCI's comprehensive cancer information database, are always assigned a phase.
However, screening, prevention, diagnostic, and quality-of-life studies do not always have a phase. Genetics clinical trials generally do
not have a phase.

Phase I trials are the first step in testing a new approach in people.
In these studies, researchers evaluate what dose is safe, how a new

agent should be given (by mouth, injected into a vein, or injected into the muscle), and how often. Researchers watch closely for any harmful side effects. Phase I trials usually enroll a small number of patients and take place at only a few locations. The dose of the new therapy or technique is increased a little at a time. The highest dose with an acceptable level of side effects is determined to be appropriate for further testing.

Phase II trials study the safety and effectiveness of an agent or intervention, and evaluate how it affects the human body. Phase II studies usually focus on a particular type of cancer, and include fewer than 100 patients.

Phase III trials compare a new agent or intervention (or new use of a standard one) with the current standard therapy. Participants are randomly assigned to the standard group or the new group, usually by computer. This method, called randomization, helps to avoid bias and ensures that human choices or other factors do not affect the study's results. In most cases, studies move into phase III testing only after they have shown promise in phases I and II. Phase III trials often include large numbers of people across the country.

Phase IV trials are conducted to further evaluate the long-term safety and effectiveness of a treatment. They usually take place after the treatment has been approved for standard use. Several hundred to several thousand people may take part in a phase IV study. These studies are less common than phase I, II, or III trials.

People who participate in a clinical trial work with a research team. Team members may include doctors, nurses, social workers, dietitians, and other health professionals. The health care team provides care, monitors participants' health, and offers specific instructions about the study. So that the trial results are as reliable as possible, it is important for participants to follow the research team's instructions. The instructions may include keeping logs or answering questionnaires. The research team may continue to contact participants after the trial ends.

Who pays for the patient care costs associated with a clinical trial?

Health insurance and managed care providers often do not cover the patient care costs associated with a clinical trial. What they cover varies by health plan and by study. Some health plans do not cover clinical trials if they consider the approach being studied "experimental" or "investigational." However, if enough data show that the approach is safe and effective, a health plan may consider the approach "established" and cover some or all of the costs. Participants may have difficulty obtaining coverage for costs associated with prevention and screening clinical trials; health plans are currently less likely to have review processes in place for these studies. It may, therefore, be more difficult to get coverage for the costs associated with them. In many cases, it helps to have someone from the research team talk about coverage with representatives of the health plan.

Health plans may specify other criteria a trial must meet to be covered. The trial might have to be sponsored by a specified organization, be judged "medically necessary" by the health plan, not be significantly more expensive than treatments the health plan considers standard, or focus on types of cancer for which no standard treatments are available. In addition, the facility and medical staff might have to meet the plan's qualifications for conducting certain procedures, such as bone marrow transplants. More information about insurance coverage can be found on the National Cancer Institute (NCI)'s Clinical Trials and Insurance Coverage: A Resource Guide webpage at http://www.cancer.gov/clinicaltrials/learning/insurance-coverage on the internet.

Federal programs that help pay the costs of care in a clinical trial include those listed below:

- Medicare reimburses patient care costs for its beneficiaries who participate in clinical trials designed to diagnose or treat cancer. Information about Medicare coverage of clinical trials is available at http://www.medicare.gov/ on the internet, or by calling Medicare's toll-free number for beneficiaries at 800-633-4227 (800-MEDICARE). The toll-free number for the hearing impaired is 877-486-2048.

- Beneficiaries of TRICARE, the Department of Defense's health program, can be reimbursed for the medical costs of participation in NCI-sponsored phase II and phase III cancer prevention (including screening and early detection) and treatment trials.

- The Department of Veterans Affairs (VA) allows eligible veterans to participate in NCI-sponsored prevention, diagnosis, and treatment studies nationwide. All phases and types of NCI-sponsored trials are included. The NCI fact sheet "The NCI/VA Agreement on Clinical Trials: Questions and Answers" has more information. It is available at http://www.cancer.gov/cancertopics/factsheet/NCI/VA-clinical-trials on the internet.

What are some questions people might ask their health care provider before entering a clinical trial?

It is important for people to ask questions before deciding to enter a clinical trial. Questions people might want to ask their doctor or nurse include the following:

The Study

- What is the purpose of the study?
- Why do the researchers think the approach being tested may be effective? Has it been tested before?
- Who is sponsoring the study?
- Who has reviewed and approved the study?
- What are the medical credentials and experience of the researchers and other study personnel?
- How are the study results and safety of participants being monitored?
- How long will the study last?
- How will the results be shared?

Possible Risks and Benefits

- What are the possible short-term benefits?
- What are the possible long-term benefits?
- What are the short-term risks, such as side effects?
- What are the possible long-term risks?
- What other treatment options are available?
- How do the possible risks and benefits of the trial compare with those of other options?

Participation and Care

- What kinds of treatment, medical tests, or procedures will the participants have during the study? How often will they receive the treatments, tests, or procedures?
- Will treatments, tests, or procedures be painful? If so, how can the pain be controlled?

- How do the tests in the study compare with what people might receive outside the study?
- Will participants be able to take their regular medications while in the clinical trial?
- Where will the participants receive their medical care? Will they be in a hospital? If so, for how long?
- Who will be in charge of the participants' care? Will they be able to see their own doctors?
- How long will participants need to stay in the study? Will there be follow-up visits after the study?

Personal Issues

- How could being in the study affect the participants' daily lives?
- What support is available for participants and their families?
- Can potential participants talk with people already enrolled in the study?

Cost Issues

- Will participants have to pay for any treatment, tests, or other charges? If so, what will the approximate charges be?
- What is health insurance likely to cover?
- Who can help answer questions from the insurance company or health plan?

Chapter 15

How to Find a Clinical Trial

This chapter will help you to look for a cancer treatment clinical trial that might benefit you. It is not intended to provide medical advice. You, your health care team, and your loved ones are in the best position to decide whether a clinical trial is right for you.

Before You Start: Steps 1–3

Step 1: Understand Clinical Trials

This guide assumes you already know what clinical trials are and why you might want to join one. If you need to, review your understanding of clinical trials before you continue the steps in this chapter.

Step 2: Talk with Your Doctor

When considering clinical trials, your best starting point is your doctor and other members of your health care team.

Your primary care physician, cancer doctor (oncologist), surgeon, or other health care provider might know about a clinical trial you should consider. He or she can help you determine whether a clinical trial might be a good option.

Excerpted from "How to Find a Cancer Treatment Trial," National Cancer Institute, March 21, 2005.

Note: In some cases, your doctor may be reluctant to discuss clinical trials as a treatment option for you. Some doctors are unfamiliar with clinical trials, cautious about turning your care over to another medical team, or wary of the extra time that joining a clinical trial might require of them and their staff. If so, you may wish to get a second opinion about your treatment options and clinical trials. Remember, you do not always need a referral from your doctor to join a clinical trial.

Step 3: Complete the Diagnosis Checklist

Before you begin looking for a clinical trial, you must know certain details about your cancer diagnosis. You will need to compare these details with the eligibility criteria of any trial in which you are interested. Eligibility criteria are the guidelines for who can and cannot participate in a particular study.

To help you gather the details of your diagnosis so you will know which trials you may be eligible to join, complete the following diagnosis checklist. Keep this checklist and your answers with you during your search for a clinical trial.

- What kind of cancer do you have?
- Where did the cancer first start?
- What is the cancer's cell type?
- If there's a solid tumor, what size is it?
- If there is a solid tumor, where is it located?
- What stage is the cancer?
- Have you had cancer before, different from the one you have now?
- What is your current performance status?
- If you have not yet had any treatment for cancer, what treatment(s) have been recommended to you?
- If you have had treatment for cancer, please list (for example: type of surgery; chemotherapy, immunotherapy, or radiation).
- Bone marrow function (blood tests that check whether your blood count is normal):
  - White blood cell count
  - Platelet count
  - Hemoglobin/hematocrit

- Liver function (blood tests that check whether your liver function is normal):

  - Bilirubin

  - Transaminases

- Renal function (blood test that checks whether your kidney function is normal):

  - Serum creatinine

To get the information you need for the form ask a nurse or social worker at your doctor's office for help. Explain to them that you are interested in looking for a clinical trial that may benefit you and that you need these details before starting to look. They will be able to review your medical records and help you fill out the form.

Searching for a Trial: Steps 4–6

Step 4: Search the PDQ® Clinical Trials Database

There are many nonprofit and for-profit resources in the United States that offer lists of cancer clinical trials. Unfortunately, no single list is complete. Clinical trials are run by many different organizations, so it is hard to collect information about all of them in one place.

However, the majority of trials listed in most resources are obtained from the Physician Data Query (PDQ) clinical trials database, which is maintained by the U.S. National Cancer Institute (NCI).

The NCI is the U.S. government's chief agency for cancer research and is part of the National Institutes of Health. The PDQ clinical trials database contains a list of more than 2,000 cancer clinical trials worldwide.

Steps 4 and 5 describe where to look for cancer clinical trials. Whichever resource you use, be sure to get a copy of the protocol summary for each trial you are interested in.

How to Search PDQ

- Search PDQ by telephone. Make a free telephone call—in English or Spanish—within the United States to the National Cancer Institute's Cancer Information Service (CIS) at 800-4-CANCER (800-422-6237). All calls to the CIS are strictly confidential.

- You can look for trials yourself using a PDQ search form on the NCI website. Remember to print out the protocol summaries for each trial you may be interested in.

Step 5: Search Other Resources

TrialCheck: TrialCheck is operated and maintained by the Coalition of National Cancer Cooperative Groups (CNCCG). The CNCCG is made up of groups of doctors and other health professionals that carry out many of the large cancer clinical trials in the United States funded by the National Cancer Institute. TrialCheck helps you search its list through an online form that "interviews" you about your cancer and the kind of treatment(s) you have received. You might prefer this kind of service. The Frequently Asked Questions (FAQs) page on the TrialCheck website provides helpful information about how to use TrialCheck.

Third-party clinical trial websites: There are a number of clinical trial websites that are not operated by funders, sponsors, or the organizations carrying out the trials. Some of these websites are operated by private companies—these may be funded through fees that industry sponsors pay to have their trials listed or according to how many participants the website refers to them.

Keep the following points in mind:

- They may include a few more trials than you'll find in the federal databases, but they may also include fewer.

- Unlike the federal databases, these sites may not regularly update their content or links.

- Unlike the federal databases, these sites might require you to register to search for trials or to obtain contact information about the trials that interest you.

Industry-sponsored cancer trials: Pharmaceutical and biotechnology companies sponsor many of the cancer clinical trials being carried out in the United States. Some of these trials are listed in the federal databases, but many are not.

Federal law requires that U.S. researchers submit to ClinicalTrials .gov all phase II, III, and IV trials of therapies for serious or life-threatening illnesses (including cancer) conducted as part of the approval process overseen by the U.S. Food and Drug Administration. However, this law is difficult to enforce and for business reasons, some drug companies have preferred to keep details about their clinical trials from the public.

If you are aware of an experimental cancer treatment and know the company that manufactures it, search the internet to find the website of the company. Find the company's customer service telephone number. When you call, ask to speak to the company's clinical trials department. Tell them you are looking for a trial that you might be eligible to join.

Cancer advocacy groups: Cancer advocacy groups work on behalf of people diagnosed with cancer and their loved ones. They provide education, support, financial assistance, and advocacy to help patients and families who are dealing with cancer. These organizations recognize that clinical trials are important to the cancer treatment process and, thus, work to educate and empower people to find information and access to treatment.

Because they work hard to know about the latest research advances in cancer treatment, these groups will sometimes have information about certain key government-sponsored trials, as well as some potentially significant trials sponsored by pharmaceutical companies or cancer care centers.

Contact the advocacy group for the type of cancer you are interested in and ask what they can tell you about ongoing clinical trials. The nonprofit Marti Nelson Cancer Foundation maintains a partial list of such groups on its CancerActionNow.org website.

Fee-based private search services: A number of private services will, for a fee, locate clinical trials for you. While having someone search for you may ease your stress, it is important to keep in mind that several of the resources mentioned earlier in this chapter provide elements of this kind of service for free. Also, be sure to ask the following questions:

- What list or lists of clinical trials does the service search? Are those lists likely to provide you with an unbiased and largely complete source of options?

- Does the service receive any money for directing patients to certain trials or for including certain trials in their list?

Step 6: Make a List of Potential Trials

Now it's time to take a closer look at the protocol summaries you have obtained for the trials you're interested in. You should remove from your list those trials you aren't actually able to join and come up with one or more top possibilities.

What follows are some key questions to consider about each trial. However, don't worry if you cannot answer all of these questions just yet. The idea is to narrow the list if you can, but don't give up on one that you're not sure of. Ideally, you should consult your doctor during this process, especially if you find the protocol summaries difficult to understand.

- **Trial objective:** What is the main purpose of the trial? Is it to improve your chances of a cure? To slow the rate at which your cancer may grow or return? To lessen the severity of treatment side effects? To establish whether a new treatment is safe and well tolerated? Read this information carefully to learn whether the trial's main objective matches your goals for treatment.

- **Eligibility criteria:** Do your diagnosis and current overall state of health match the eligibility criteria (sometimes referred to as enrollment or entry criteria)? This may tell you whether you could qualify for the trial. If you're not sure, keep the trial on your list for now.

- **Trial location:** Is the location of the clinical trial manageable for you? Some trials are available at more than one site. Look carefully at how often you will need to receive treatment during the course of the trial, and decide how far and how often you are willing to travel. You will also need to ask if the sponsoring organization will provide for some or all of your travel expenses.

- **Study duration:** How long will the study run? Not all protocol summaries list this information. If they do, consider the time commitment and whether it will work for you and your family.

If, after considering these questions, you are still interested in one or more of the clinical trials you have found, then you are ready for Step 7.

After Finding a Trial: Steps 7–10

Now that you have found one or more clinical trials for which you think you are eligible and that may be a good treatment option for you, it is time to make a telephone call to each trial's contact person so you can ask a few more crucial questions. Then, you will be ready to make a final treatment decision.

Step 7: Contact the Clinical Trial Team

There are several ways to contact the Clinical Trial Team.

- Contact the trial team directly. The protocol summary should include the name and telephone number of someone you can contact for more information. You do not need to talk to the lead researcher (called the "protocol chair" or "principal investigator") at this time, even if that is the name that is included with the telephone number. Instead, call the number and ask to speak with the "trial coordinator," the "referral coordinator," or the "protocol assistant." This person can answer questions from potential patients and their doctors. It is also this person's job to determine whether you are likely to be eligible to join the trial. (A final determination would be made only after you had gone in for a first appointment.)

- Ask your doctor or other health care team member to contact the trial team for you. Because the clinical trial coordinator will ask questions related to your diagnosis, you may want to ask your doctor or someone else on your health care team to contact the clinical trial team for you.

- The trial team may contact you. If you have used some a third-party website and identified a trial that interests you, you may have provided your name, phone number, and e-mail address so that the clinical trial team can contact you.

Step 8: Ask Questions about the Trial

Whether you or someone from your health care team calls the clinical trial coordinator, this is the time to get answers to questions that will help you decide whether or not to join this particular clinical trial.

It will be helpful if you can talk about your diagnosis in a manner that is brief and to the point. Before you make the call, rehearse with a family member or friend how you will present the key details of your diagnosis (the diagnosis checklist listed before). This will make you more comfortable when you are talking with the clinical trial coordinator and will enable you to answer his or her questions smoothly.

Questions to Ask the Trial Coordinator

- Is the trial still open?
- Am I eligible for this trial?
- Why do researchers think the new treatment might be effective?
- What are the risks and benefits associated with the treatments I may receive?

- Who will monitor my care and safety?

- May I get a copy of the protocol document?

- May I get a copy of the informed consent document?

- Is there a chance I will receive a placebo?

- Is the trial randomized?

- What is the treatment dose and schedule in each arm of the trial?

- What costs will I be responsible for?

- If I have to travel, who will pay for travel and lodging?

- Will participation in this trial require more time than if I had elected to receive standard care? Will participation require a hospital stay?

- How will participating in the clinical trial affect my everyday life?

Step 9: Discuss Your Options with Your Doctor

To make a final decision, you will want to know the possible risks and benefits of all the various treatment options open to you. You may decide that joining a trial for which you are eligible is your best option, or you may decide not to join a trial. It is your choice.

Step 10: If You Want to Join a Trial, Schedule an Appointment

If you decide to participate in a clinical trial for which you are eligible, schedule an appointment with the trial coordinator.

You might also want your doctor to contact the study's principal investigator to further discuss your medical history and overall current state of your health. The principal investigator's name should be listed in the protocol summary.

Your doctor might disagree with your decision to participate in a clinical trial. If so, be sure you understand his or her concerns. You also may wish to seek a second opinion about your treatment options at this time. Ultimately, it is up to you to decide what treatment is in your best interest.

Chapter 16

Access to Investigational Drugs

What is an investigational drug?

An investigational drug is one that is under study but does not have permission from the U.S. Food and Drug Administration (FDA) to be legally marketed and sold in the United States.

FDA approval is the final step in the process of drug development. The first step is for the new drug to be tested in the laboratory. If the results are promising, the drug company or sponsor must apply for FDA approval to test the drug on people. This is called an Investigational New Drug (IND) Application. Once the IND is approved, clinical trials can begin. Clinical trials are research studies to determine the safety and measure the effectiveness of the drug in people. Once clinical trials are completed, the sponsor submits the study results in a New Drug Application (NDA) or Biologics License Application (BLA) to the FDA. This application is carefully reviewed and, if the drug is found to be reasonably safe and effective, it is approved.

How do patients get investigational drugs?

By far, the most common way that patients get investigational drugs is by taking part in a clinical trial sponsored under an IND. A patient's doctor may suggest a clinical trial as one treatment option.

"Access to Investigational Drugs: Questions and Answers," a National Cancer Institute (NCI) FactSheet, reviewed November 19, 2004. For additional information, visit the NCI website at http://www.cancer.gov.

Or a patient or family member can ask the doctor about clinical trials or new drugs available for cancer treatment.

Another way patients and their families can learn about new drugs being tested in clinical trials is through the National Cancer Institute's (NCI) PDQ® database. This database contains information on a large number of ongoing studies. Individuals can search this database at http://www.cancer.gov/clinicaltrials, or they can call the NCI's Cancer Information Service at 800-4-CANCER (800-422-6237). Information specialists can search the database and provide a list of trials for individuals to discuss with their doctor.

Are there other ways to get investigational drugs?

Less common ways that patients can receive investigational drugs include mechanisms such as an expanded access protocol or as special or compassionate exception. The sponsor must agree to provide the drug for this use.

Investigational drugs given under these mechanisms must meet the following criteria:

- There must be substantial clinical evidence that the drug may benefit persons with particular types of cancer.

- The drug must be able to be given safely outside a clinical trial.

- The drug must be in sufficient supply for ongoing and planned clinical trials.

Expanded access: The purpose of an expanded access protocol is to make investigational drugs that have significant activity against specific cancers available to patients before the FDA approval process has been completed. Expanded access protocols allow a larger group of people to be treated with the drug.

The sponsor must apply to the FDA to make the drug available through an expanded access protocol. There must be enough evidence from studies already completed to show that the drug is likely to be effective against a specific type of cancer and that it does not have unreasonable risks. The FDA generally approves expanded access only if there are no other satisfactory treatments available for the disease.

The NCI's Treatment Referral Center (TRC) protocols are one type of expanded access protocol. The NCI establishes a TRC protocol when clinical evidence suggests that an investigational drug should be made more widely available to patients, even though the

FDA approval process has not been completed. The TRC protocol is made available at NCI-designated cancer centers and other institutions selected to provide wide geographic availability of the drug to patients.

Special Exception/Compassionate Exemption: Patients who do not meet the eligibility criteria for a clinical trial of an investigational drug may be eligible to receive the drug under a mechanism known as a special exception or a compassionate exemption to the policy of administering investigational drugs only in a clinical trial. The patient's doctor contacts the sponsor of the investigational agent and provides the patient's medical information and treatment history. The sponsor (the drug company or NCI) evaluates the requests on a case-by-case basis. There should be reasonable expectation that the drug will prolong survival or improve quality of life.

In some cases, even patients who qualify for treatment with an investigational drug on a compassionate basis might not be able to obtain the drug if the supply is limited and the demand is high.

Are all investigational drugs available through an expanded access or special exception mechanism?

No. The sponsor decides whether to provide an investigational drug outside a clinical trial. Availability may be limited in part by drug supply, patient demand, or other factors.

What is the NCI's role in providing access to investigational drugs?

The NCI acts as the sponsor for many, but not all, investigational drugs. When acting as sponsor, the NCI provides the investigational drug to the physicians who are participating in clinical trials or TRC protocols. A physician who wishes to treat a patient with the investigational drug as a special exception must request the drug from the NCI. These requests are reviewed on a case-by-case basis.

Who can provide access to investigational drugs being developed by pharmaceutical companies?

In the case of investigational drugs sponsored by a drug company, the drug company in collaboration with the FDA provides access to the drug. The process is similar to that described above.

The patient's physician must submit a request to the drug company and to the FDA. The drug company can provide the name of the appropriate reviewing division at the FDA. (FDA reviewing divisions are prohibited from divulging proprietary information such as whether a sponsor has filed an IND or the status of an IND.)

Are there specific criteria used to determine whether patients can receive an investigational drug outside a clinical trial?

To be considered for treatment with an investigational drug outside a clinical trial, generally patients must meet the following criteria:

- Have undergone standard treatment that has not been successful
- Be ineligible for any ongoing clinical trials of this drug
- Have no acceptable treatment alternatives
- Have a cancer diagnosis for which the investigational drug has demonstrated activity
- Be likely to experience benefits that outweigh the risks involved

What should patients do if they are interested in receiving an investigational drug through a special exception or expanded access mechanism?

Patients interested in gaining access to investigational drugs should talk to their physician about available options. Physicians can make requests for special exceptions by contacting the study sponsor. Physicians will be required to follow strict guidelines, including gaining approval from their Institutional Review Board and obtaining informed consent from the patient. Informed consent is a process that includes a document to be signed by the patient which outlines the known risks and benefits of the treatment, as well as the rights and responsibilities of the patient.

What are the costs involved in receiving an investigational drug?

In general, the drug is provided free of charge. However, there may be other costs associated with the treatment. Before beginning treatment, patients should check with their insurer about coverage of these costs.

What are some of the potential drawbacks to receiving an investigational drug?

It is not known whether an investigational drug is better than standard therapy for treating a disease, and a patient may not receive any benefit. Side effects (both long-term and short-term) from the drug may not be fully understood, especially if the drug is in early phases of testing. Finally, a patient's health insurance company may not pay expenses associated with receiving the investigational drug.

How can patients find out more information about a specific investigational drug?

Patients can find out more about a specific drug by contacting the drug company that is developing the drug. Information may also be available from the NCI's Cancer Information Service at 800-4-CANCER (800-422-6237).

What other resources are available on this topic?

The following list of resources may be helpful:

- The NCI's website has a feature titled "Understanding the Approval Process for New Cancer Treatments: Special Needs," which can be found at http://www.cancer.gov/clinicaltrials/learning/approval-process-for-cancer-drugs/page4 on the internet.

- Another NCI website titled "Developing Cancer Therapies" can be found at http://ctep.cancer.gov on the internet.

- The FDA's Center for Drug Evaluation and Research website has "Oncology Tools," which contains a variety of information related to cancer, including a section on access to unapproved drugs. This resource is at http://www.fda.gov/cder/cancer/index.htm on the internet.

Chapter 17

Cancer Vaccines: An Emerging Therapy

For many years, the treatment of cancer was focused primarily on surgery, chemotherapy, and radiation. However, as researchers learn more about how the body fights cancer on its own, therapies are being developed that harness the potential of the body's defense system in this fight, including efforts to prevent some forms of cancer.

The body's defense system—called the immune system—consists of a network of specialized cells and tissues that fight infection and disease. Therapies that use the immune system to fight or prevent cancer are called biological therapies.

Cancer vaccines represent an emerging type of biological therapy that is still mostly experimental. Many clinical trials are underway to test vaccines as potential treatments for a wide variety of cancer types. The U.S. Food and Drug Administration (FDA) has not approved any cancer vaccine as a standard treatment for any type of cancer. This means that cancer-fighting vaccines are only available to those who enroll in clinical trials.

The FDA has, however, approved two vaccines that can help prevent cancer. One of these vaccines prevents infection with the human papillomavirus (HPV), which causes almost all cervical cancers. The other vaccine prevents infection with the hepatitis B virus, which can cause liver cancer. Other vaccines that may prevent or reduce the risk of cancer are also being tested in ongoing clinical trials.

"Treating and Preventing Cancer with Vaccines," a National Cancer Institute (NCI) Fact Sheet, updated June 12, 2006. For additional information, visit the NCI website at http://www.cancer.gov.

171

About Vaccines

A vaccine is a substance designed to stimulate the immune system to launch an immune response. This response is directed against specific targets, or antigens, that are part of the vaccine. An antigen is any substance that the immune system recognizes as foreign.

The flu vaccine, for example, contains copies of the flu virus that cannot cause the flu. Antigens on the viruses in the vaccine stimulate the immune system to produce cells that can fight the flu virus if it shows up in your nose or throat.

The flu vaccine only works if it is given at least two weeks before exposure to infectious flu virus. The immune system needs those two weeks to produce immune cells that can attack the flu virus.

Because the flu virus changes from year to year, a new flu vaccine is needed every year. Your immune system, however, still protects you against last year's flu type. This type of vaccine is called a preventive vaccine—it stimulates a long-lasting immunity that helps protect you from getting sick for years or even for a lifetime.

Cancer Vaccines

Cancer vaccines are intended either to treat existing cancer or to prevent the development of cancer. Cancer treatment vaccines are designed to strengthen the body's natural defenses against a cancer that has already developed. These vaccines may stop an existing tumor from growing, stop a tumor from coming back after it has been treated, or eliminate cancer cells not killed by previous treatments.

Cancer preventive vaccines are given to healthy people and are designed to target infectious agents that can cause cancer. The HPV vaccine is an example of a cancer preventive vaccine. It is used to help prevent cervical cancer.

Substances Used to Make Vaccines

Vaccines can be made using specific types of molecules from viruses or cells, including molecules from bacterial cells or human cells. These molecules may contain a single antigen or several different antigens. Carbohydrates (sugars), proteins, and peptides (pieces of proteins) are among the types of molecules that have been used to make vaccines. Molecules of DNA or RNA that contain genetic instructions for one or more antigens can also be used as vaccines.

In addition, whole viruses or cells, or parts of viruses or cells that contain different types of molecules, can be used to make vaccines.

The flu vaccine, for example, is made using inactive whole flu viruses. If whole human cells are used as vaccines, they are usually treated with enough radiation to keep them from dividing (growing and multiplying) or enough to kill them.

Immune System Basics

The immune system is made up, in part, of a network of immune cells that form in the bone marrow from a very basic type of cell called a stem cell. Many different types of immune cells can be made from stem cells.

Immune cells circulate in the blood or in a network of channels similar to blood vessels called the lymphatic system. They also congregate in special areas of the lymphatic system called lymph nodes.

Some immune cells have very specific functions. Others have general or non-specific functions. T lymphocytes (T cells) and B lymphocytes (B cells) are examples of specific immune cells.

Each T cell and B cell recognizes and is activated by a single substance. This single substance is called the T cell's or B cell's antigen. When a T cell or a B cell recognizes its antigen and is activated, it makes many identical copies of itself. Each copy recognizes the same antigen as the original T cell or B cell.

T Cells, B Cells, and APCs

There are two main types of T cells. Cytotoxic T cells identify and kill cells that contain the antigen they recognize. Helper T cells release chemical messengers called cytokines that recruit other immune cells to the site of attack. Helper T cells also help cytotoxic T cells do their job.

B cells make antibodies. Each B cell makes only one type of antibody, which is directed against its specific antigen. Just as helper T cells help cytotoxic T cells do their job, helper T cells help stimulate B cells to make antibodies. Antibodies specific for an antigen on a cancer cell can attach to the antigen and, by several indirect mechanisms, cause the cancer cell's death.

The immune system also contains antigen-presenting cells (APCs). APCs sample their surrounding environment, eating whatever they come across, and then they display little bits of what they have eaten on their surface. Macrophages and dendritic cells are examples of APCs.

Macrophages patrol the body, eating dead cells, debris, viruses, and bacteria. Dendritic cells are more stationary, monitoring the surrounding environment from one spot, such as the skin. Lymphocytes (T cells or B cells) that "meet" an APC can look at the APC cell surface and see if their specific antigen is present. If their antigen is present, the lymphocytes become activated.

Both T cells and B cells can be activated in immune responses against cancer treatment or cancer preventive vaccines. With preventive vaccines against infectious agents that cause cancer, the activated B cells may produce antibodies that bind to the agents and interfere with their ability to infect cells. Because the agents must infect cells to make them cancerous, this lowers chances that cancer will occur.

Cancer Vaccine Strategies

Researchers used to think that the immune system prevented cancer from growing and spreading by constantly looking to see if cancer cells are present and killing them once they are found. It was thought that the growth and spread of cancer resulted from a breakdown of the immune system. In a broken-down immune system, effective anti-cancer immune responses could not occur.

However, this theory of immune system control over cancer growth has now been shown to be only partially correct. Researchers now know that strong immune responses against cancer cells are hard to generate, and they are studying ways to strengthen the ability of the immune system to fight cancer.

Part of the problem is that the immune system has the job of knowing the difference between normal cells and cancer cells. To keep us healthy, the immune system must be able to ignore or "tolerate" normal cells and recognize and attack abnormal ones.

To the immune system, cancer cells differ from normal cells in very small, subtle ways. Therefore, the immune system largely tolerates cancer cells rather than attacking them. Although tolerance is essential to keep the immune system from attacking normal cells, tolerance of cancer cells is a problem. Therapeutic cancer vaccines must not only provoke an immune response but stimulate the immune system strongly enough to overcome its usual tolerance of cancer cells.

Another reason cancer cells may not stimulate a strong immune response is that they have developed ways to evade the immune system. Scientists now understand some of the ways in which cancer cells do this. For example, they may shed certain types of molecules that inhibit the ability of the body to attack cancer cells. As a result, cancers become less "visible" to the immune system.

Researchers are now using these advances in knowledge in their efforts to design more effective cancer vaccines. They have developed several strategies for stimulating immune responses against cancers, including the following:

- Identify unusual or unique cancer-related molecules that are rarely present on normal cells and use these so-called "tumor antigens" as vaccines.

- Intervene to make tumor antigens more visible to the immune system. This can be done in several ways:

  - Alter the structure of a tumor antigen slightly (that is, make it look more foreign) and give the altered antigen as a vaccine. One way to alter an antigen is modify the gene needed to make it. This can be done in the laboratory.

  - Put the gene for a tumor antigen into a viral vector (a harmless virus) and use the virus as a vehicle to deliver the gene to cancer cells or to normal cells. Cells infected with the viral vector will make much more tumor antigen than uninfected cancer cells and may be more visible to the immune system. Cells can also be infected with the viral vector in the laboratory and then given to patients as a vaccine. In addition, patients can be infected (that is, vaccinated) with the viral vector as another way to get virus-infected cells inside the body.

  - Put genes for other molecules that normally help stimulate the immune system into a viral vector along with a tumor antigen gene.

- Use "primed" dendritic cells or other APCs as a vaccine. There are three ways to prime a dendritic cell.

  - APCs can be fed tumor antigens in the laboratory and then injected into a patient. The injected cells are primed to activate T cells.

  - Alternatively, APCs can be infected with a viral vector that contains the gene for a tumor antigen.

  - A third way to make primed APCs is to feed the cells DNA or RNA that contains genetic instructions for the antigen. The APCs will then make the tumor antigen and present it on their surface.

- Use antibodies that have antigen-binding sites that mimic, or look like, a tumor antigen. These antibodies are called anti-idiotype antibodies. They can stimulate B cells to make to make antibodies against tumor antigens. Anti-idiotype antibodies present tumor antigens in a different way to the immune system.

Making Cancer Treatment Vaccines

Cancer treatment vaccines can be made using a patient's own tumor antigens or cells, or someone else's. Most tumors of a given type share many antigens. When a patient's own tumor antigens or cells are used, the vaccine is called an autologous vaccine. When someone else's tumor antigens or cells are used, the vaccine is called an allogeneic vaccine.

Added Ingredients

Cancer vaccines often have added ingredients, called adjuvants, that help boost the immune response. These substances may also be given separately to increase a vaccine's effectiveness. Many different kinds of substances have been used as adjuvants, including cytokines, proteins, bacteria, viruses, and certain chemicals.

Deciding about Cancer Vaccine Trials

Only you can make decisions about what treatment you should have. You should always discuss any treatment option thoroughly with your doctor and possibly your loved ones. The following questions and answers may help you to think about whether taking part in a cancer vaccine trial might be an appropriate option for you.

Is a standard treatment available for my cancer?

If a standard treatment exists for your cancer, you should not choose an experimental vaccine therapy over the standard treatment. The FDA has not yet approved any cancer vaccine for use as a standard treatment. A vaccine may be appropriate addition to standard therapy but not a replacement for it. Currently, many therapeutic cancer vaccines are being used after the patient finishes standard treatment.

Some cancer vaccine trials test a standard treatment with or without the vaccine. A few test the standard therapy against the vaccine. Some cancer vaccine trials test the cancer vaccine against a placebo vaccine or test the cancer vaccine in combination with various adjuvants. In these cases, the patient has already received standard therapy.

Is the main goal of treatment to prevent my cancer from coming back or to shrink existing tumors?

In studies using laboratory animals, cancer vaccines show the most promise at preventing cancer from coming back after the primary tumor has been eliminated by surgery, radiation, or chemotherapy. When the immune system has to detect and fight a smaller number of cancer cells, it is more likely to be successful. In contrast, shrinking existing tumors using vaccine therapy is more difficult. When the immune system is matched against a large number of cancer cells, it is more likely to be overwhelmed and ineffective—an out-numbered army.

It may be appropriate to consider experimental cancer vaccines for advanced cancers once all other therapies have been exhausted, when standard therapy is no longer effective, or in combination with other therapies. For example, in some patients with melanoma and renal cell cancers, treatment with the cytokine called interleukin-2 (IL-2) has caused large tumors to shrink. Many current cancer vaccine clinical trials are testing vaccines in combination with other therapies such as IL-2. It is also possible that newer and more potent vaccine strategies could cause advanced cancers to shrink.

Present and Future of Cancer Vaccines

In studies conducted in laboratory animals, cancer vaccines that stimulate the immune system have caused cancers to recede. In humans, however, the situation is more complicated. As discussed in Cancer Vaccine Strategies, cancers have developed ways of evading the immune system. Researchers now have a better understanding of how cancer cells avoid detection by the immune system, and they have developed new strategies for stimulating a more powerful anti-cancer immune response.

Therapeutic cancer vaccines have shown promise in early-stage clinical trials against several types of cancer, for example:

- In one early-stage study, 18 of 20 patients who were vaccinated against non-Hodgkin lymphoma stayed in remission for an average of four years. The vaccine used in this study contained a protein specific to each patient's tumor cells (that is, each patient was given an autologous vaccine) as well as two other substances to help boost the immune response. A large, randomized, phase III trial of this vaccine is now under way.

- In a phase I/II study, three of 33 patients with advanced non-small cell lung cancer had a complete remission of disease and were still alive at least three years after vaccine therapy. To make the vaccine, researchers added the gene for the cytokine granulocyte-macrophage colony stimulating factor (GM-CSF) to each patient's tumor cells—that is, each patient was given an autologous vaccine.

- Another early-stage trial showed that, when administered along with a melanoma peptide vaccine, an antibody that blocks the activity of a key immune-system regulatory molecule caused tumors to shrink in patients with metastatic melanoma.

It is important to note that the promise of early-stage clinical trials, which usually enroll only a small number of patients, is not always sustained in larger trials. Early studies of another melanoma vaccine suggested that the vaccine might help prevent melanoma from coming back in patients who were at high risk for recurrence. However, in a subsequent large trial that included 774 patients who were at high risk for melanoma recurrence, high-dose interferon proved superior to the vaccine in preventing melanoma from coming back.

Researchers still have a lot of work to do to demonstrate clearly that cancer treatment vaccines can be effective. It is possible that vaccines will prove more effective when combined with other therapies and that multiple vaccinations may be necessary for a benefit to be seen.

Much work also remains to be done to develop vaccines that can reliably prevent cancers associated with infectious agents. Cervical cancer, for example, is almost always caused by infection with HPV. The FDA has approved a vaccine that prevents infections with two types of HPV that cause nearly 70 percent of all cervical cancers. Researchers must develop new vaccines that are able to prevent infections by all HPV types that can cause this disease.

Ongoing trials seek to find the most promising situations for the use of cancer vaccines and the best approaches for making such vaccines work. Only when rigorous trials provide evidence that a particular cancer vaccine is both safe and effective against a specific type of cancer will the FDA consider approving that vaccine as standard treatment.

Chapter 18

Angiogenesis Inhibitors: A Potential Anti-Cancer Tool

Angiogenesis means the formation of new blood vessels. It plays an important role in the growth and spread of cancer. New blood vessels "feed" the cancer cells with oxygen and nutrients, allowing these cells to grow, invade nearby tissues, spread to other parts of the body, and form new colonies of cancer cells.

Because cancer cannot grow or spread without the formation of new blood vessels, scientists are trying to find ways to stop angiogenesis. Whether angiogenesis inhibitors will be effective against cancer in humans is not yet known. The process of producing and testing angiogenesis inhibitors is likely to take several years.

Understanding Angiogenesis

Metastasis and How It Requires Angiogenesis

When patients are diagnosed with cancer, they want to know whether their disease is local or has spread to other locations. Cancer spreads by metastasis, the ability of cancer cells to penetrate into lymphatic and blood vessels, circulate through the bloodstream, and then invade and grow in normal tissues elsewhere.

In large measure, it is this ability to spread to other tissues and organs that makes cancer a potentially life-threatening disease, so there

---

This chapter begins with an excerpt from "Angiogenesis Inhibitors in the Treatment of Cancer," National Cancer Institute (NCI), May 20, 2002. Additional information is from "Understanding Cancer Series: Angiogenesis," NCI, January 28, 2005.

179

is great interest in understanding what makes metastasis possible for a cancerous tumor.

Cancer researchers studying the conditions necessary for cancer metastasis have discovered that one of the critical events required is the growth of a new network of blood vessels. This process of forming new blood vessels is called angiogenesis.

Tumor Angiogenesis

Tumor angiogenesis is the proliferation of a network of blood vessels that penetrates into cancerous growths, supplying nutrients and oxygen and removing waste products. Tumor angiogenesis actually starts with cancerous tumor cells releasing molecules that send signals to surrounding normal host tissue. This signaling activates certain genes in the host tissue that, in turn, make proteins to encourage growth of new blood vessels.

Angiogenesis is regulated by both activator and inhibitor molecules. Normally, the inhibitors predominate, blocking growth. Should a need for new blood vessels arise, angiogenesis activators increase in number and inhibitors decrease. This prompts the growth and division of vascular endothelial cells and, ultimately, the formation of new blood vessels.

Normal Angiogenesis

In addition to its role in tumors, angiogenesis occurs normally in the human body at specific times in development and growth. For example, a developing child in a mother's womb must create the vast network of arteries, veins, and capillaries that are found in the human body. A process called vasculogenesis creates the primary network of vascular endothelial cells that will become major blood vessels. Later on, angiogenesis remodels this network into the small new blood vessels or capillaries that complete the child's circulatory system.

Proliferation of new blood vessels also takes place in adults, although it is a relatively infrequent event. In women, angiogenesis is active a few days each month as new blood vessels form in the lining of the uterus during the menstrual cycle. Also, angiogenesis is necessary for the repair or regeneration of tissue during wound healing.

Angiogenesis and Cancer

Before the 1960s, cancer researchers believed that the blood supply reached tumors simply because pre-existing blood vessels dilated.

But later experiments showed that angiogenesis—the growth of the new blood vessels—is necessary for cancerous tumors to keep growing and spreading.

In early experiments, researchers asked whether cancer growth requires angiogenesis. Scientists removed a cancerous tumor from a laboratory animal and injected some of the cancer cells into a normal organ removed from the same strain of animal. The organ was then placed in a glass chamber and a nutrient solution was pumped into the organ to keep it alive for a week or two. Scientists found that the cancer cells grew into tiny tumors but failed to link up to the organ's blood vessels. As a result, tumor growth stopped at a diameter of about 1–2mm. Without angiogenesis, tumor growth stopped.

What Prompts Angiogenesis?

In an experiment designed to find out whether molecules from the cancer cells or from the surrounding host tissues are responsible for starting angiogenesis, scientists implanted cancer cells in a chamber bounded by a membrane with pores too small for the cells to exit. Under these conditions, angiogenesis still began in the region surrounding the implant. Small activator molecules produced by the cancer cells must have passed out of the chamber and signaled angiogenesis in the surrounding tissue.

Once researchers knew that cancer cells could release molecules to activate the process of angiogenesis, the challenge became to find and study these angiogenesis-stimulating molecules in animal and human tumors.

From such studies more than a dozen different proteins, as well as several smaller molecules, have been identified as "angiogenic," meaning that they are released by tumors as signals for angiogenesis. Among these molecules, two proteins appear to be the most important for sustaining tumor growth: vascular endothelial growth factor (VEGF) and basic fibroblast growth factor (bFGF). VEGF and bFGF are produced by many kinds of cancer cells and by certain types of normal cells, too.

The Angiogenesis Signaling Cascade

VEGF and bFGF are first synthesized inside tumor cells and then secreted into the surrounding tissue. When they encounter endothelial cells, they bind to specific proteins, called receptors, sitting on the outer surface of the cells. The binding of either VEGF or bFGF to its appropriate receptor activates a series of relay proteins that transmits a signal into the nucleus of the endothelial cells. The nuclear signal ultimately prompts a group of genes to make products needed for new endothelial cell growth.

The activation of endothelial cells by VEGF or bFGF sets in motion a series of steps toward the creation of new blood vessels. First, the activated endothelial cells produce matrix metalloproteinases (MMPs), a special class of degradative enzymes. These enzymes are then released from the endothelial cells into the surrounding tissue. The MMPs break down the extracellular matrix—support material that fills the spaces between cells and is made of proteins and polysaccharides. Breakdown of this matrix permits the migration of endothelial cells. As they migrate into the surrounding tissues, activated endothelial cells begin to divide. Soon they organize into hollow tubes that evolve gradually into a mature network of blood vessels.

The Possibility of Inhibitors of Angiogenesis

The discovery of angiogenesis inhibitors raises the question of whether such molecules might therapeutically halt or restrain cancer's growth. Researchers have addressed this question in numerous experiments involving animals. In one striking study, mice with several different kinds of cancer were treated with injections of endostatin. After a few cycles of treatment, the initial (primary) tumor formed at the site of the injected cancer cells almost disappeared, and the animals did not develop resistance to the effects of endostatin after repeated usage.

The discovery that angiogenesis inhibitors such as endostatin can restrain the growth of primary tumors raises the possibility that such inhibitors might also be able to slow tumor metastasis.

To test this hypothesis, researchers injected several kinds of mouse cancer cells beneath the animals' skin and allowed the cells to grow for about two weeks. The primary tumors were then removed, and the animals checked for several weeks. Typically, mice developed about 50 visible tumors from individual cancer cells that had spread to the lungs prior to removal of the primary tumor. But mice treated with angiostatin developed an average of only 2–3 tumors in their lungs. Inhibition of angiogenesis by angiostatin had reduced the rate of spread (metastasis) by about 20-fold.

It has been known for many years that cancer cells originating in a primary tumor can spread to another organ and form tiny, microscopic tumor masses (metastases) that can remain dormant for years. A likely explanation for this tumor dormancy is that no angiogenesis occurred, so the small tumor lacked the new blood vessels needed for continued growth.

One possible reason for tumor dormancy may be that some primary tumors secrete the inhibitor angiostatin into the bloodstream, which then circulates throughout the body and inhibits blood vessel growth at other sites. This could prevent microscopic metastases from growing into visible tumors.

Additional support for the idea that interfering with the process of angiogenesis can restrain tumor growth has come from genetic studies of mice. Scientists have recently created strains of mice that lack two genes, called Id1 and Id3, whose absence hinders angiogenesis. When mouse breast cancer cells are injected into such angiogenesis-deficient mutant mice, there is a small period of tumor growth, but the tumors regress completely after a few weeks, and the mice remain healthy with no signs of cancer. In contrast, normal mice injected with the same breast cancer cells die of cancer within a few weeks.

When lung cancer cells are injected into the same strain of angiogenesis-deficient mutant mice, the results are slightly different. The lung cancer cells do develop into tumors in the mutant, but the tumors grow more slowly than in normal mice and fail to spread (metastasize) to other organs. As a result, the mutant mice live much longer than normal mice injected with the same kinds of lung cancer cells.

Angiogenesis Inhibitors in the Treatment of Human Cancer

Researchers are now asking if inhibiting angiogenesis can slow down or prevent the growth and spread of cancer cells in humans.

To answer this question, almost two dozen angiogenesis inhibitors are currently being tested in cancer patients. The inhibitors being tested fall into several different categories, depending on their mechanism of action. Some inhibit endothelial cells directly, while others inhibit the angiogenesis signaling cascade or block the ability of endothelial cells to break down the extracellular matrix.

One class of angiogenesis inhibitors being tested in cancer patients are molecules that directly inhibit the growth of endothelial cells. Included in this category is endostatin, the naturally occurring protein known to inhibit tumor growth in animals. Another drug, combretastatin A4, causes growing endothelial cells to commit suicide (apoptosis). Other drugs, which interact with a molecule called integrin, also can promote the destruction of proliferating endothelial cells.

Another interesting drug is thalidomide, a sedative used in the 1950s that was subsequently taken off the market because it caused birth defects when taken by pregnant women. Although this drug clearly would not be suitable for pregnant women, its ability to prevent endothelial cells from forming new blood vessels might make it useful in treating non-pregnant cancer patients.

A second group of angiogenesis inhibitors being tested in human clinical trials are molecules that interfere with steps in the angiogenesis signaling cascade. Included in this category are anti-VEGF antibodies that block the VEGF receptor from binding growth factor. Bevacizumab (Avastin), a monoclonal antibody, is the first of these anti-VEGF antibodies to be FDA-approved. This new drug has been proven to delay tumor growth and more importantly, to extend the lives of patients. Another agent, interferon-alpha, is a naturally occurring protein that inhibits the production of bFGF and VEGF, preventing these growth factors from starting the signaling cascade.

Also, several synthetic drugs capable of interfering with endothelial cell receptors are being tested in cancer patients.

A third group of angiogenesis inhibitors are directed against one of the initial products made by growing endothelial cells, namely, the MMPs, enzymes that catalyze the breakdown of the extracellular matrix. Because breakdown of the matrix is required before endothelial cells can migrate into surrounding tissues and proliferate into new blood vessels, drugs that target MMPs also can inhibit angiogenesis.

Several synthetic and naturally occurring molecules that inhibit the activity of MMPs are currently being tested to see if interfering with this stage in the process of angiogenesis will prolong the survival of cancer patients.

A miscellaneous group of drugs, whose ability to inhibit angiogenesis involves mechanisms that are either nonspecific or are not clearly understood, is also being tested in cancer patients. One example, a drug called CAI, exerts its effects by inhibiting the influx of calcium ions into cells. While this inhibition of calcium uptake suppresses the growth of endothelial cells, such a general mechanism may affect many other cellular processes.

On to Clinical Trials

Researchers have answered many questions about angiogenesis, but many questions still remain. Scientists do not know whether using angiogenesis inhibitors to treat cancer will trigger unknown side effects, how long treatment will need to last, or whether tumor cells will find alternative routes to vascularization. To answer such questions, human clinical trials are currently under way.

Chapter 19

Studying Hyperthermia as a Cancer Treatment

What is hyperthermia?

Hyperthermia (also called thermal therapy or thermotherapy) is a type of cancer treatment in which body tissue is exposed to high temperatures (up to 113° F). Research has shown that high temperatures can damage and kill cancer cells, usually with minimal injury to normal tissues.[1] By killing cancer cells and damaging proteins and structures within cells,[2] hyperthermia may shrink tumors.

Hyperthermia is under study in clinical trials (research studies with people) and is not widely available (this topic is addressed later in another question).

How is hyperthermia used to treat cancer?

Hyperthermia is almost always used with other forms of cancer therapy, such as radiation therapy and chemotherapy.[1, 3] Hyperthermia may make some cancer cells more sensitive to radiation or harm other cancer cells that radiation cannot damage. When hyperthermia and radiation therapy are combined, they are often given within an hour of each other. Hyperthermia can also enhance the effects of certain anticancer drugs.

"Hyperthermia in Cancer Treatment: Questions and Answers," a National Cancer Institute (NCI) FactSheet reviewed August 12, 2004. For additional information, visit the NCI website at http://www.cancer.gov.

185

Numerous clinical trials have studied hyperthermia in combination with radiation therapy and chemotherapy. These studies have focused on the treatment of many types of cancer, including sarcoma, melanoma, and cancers of the head and neck, brain, lung, esophagus, breast, bladder, rectum, liver, appendix, cervix, and peritoneal lining (mesothelioma).[1, 3, 4, 5, 6, 7] Many of these studies, but not all, have shown a significant reduction in tumor size when hyperthermia is combined with other treatments.[1, 3, 6, 7] However, not all of these studies have shown increased survival in patients receiving the combined treatments.[3, 5, 7]

What are the different methods of hyperthermia?

Several methods of hyperthermia are currently under study, including local, regional, and whole-body hyperthermia.[1, 3, 4, 5, 6, 7, 8, 9]

- In local hyperthermia, heat is applied to a small area, such as a tumor, using various techniques that deliver energy to heat the tumor. Different types of energy may be used to apply heat, including microwave, radiofrequency, and ultrasound. Depending on the tumor location, there are several approaches to local hyperthermia:

  - External approaches are used to treat tumors that are in or just below the skin. External applicators are positioned around or near the appropriate region, and energy is focused on the tumor to raise its temperature.

  - Intraluminal or endocavitary methods may be used to treat tumors within or near body cavities, such as the esophagus or rectum. Probes are placed inside the cavity and inserted into the tumor to deliver energy and heat the area directly.

  - Interstitial techniques are used to treat tumors deep within the body, such as brain tumors. This technique allows the tumor to be heated to higher temperatures than external techniques. Under anesthesia, probes or needles are inserted into the tumor. Imaging techniques, such as ultrasound, may be used to make sure the probe is properly positioned within the tumor. The heat source is then inserted into the probe. Radiofrequency ablation (RFA) is a type of interstitial hyperthermia that uses radio waves to heat and kill cancer cells.

- In regional hyperthermia, various approaches may be used to heat large areas of tissue, such as a body cavity, organ, or limb.

- Deep tissue approaches may be used to treat cancers within the body, such as cervical or bladder cancer. External applicators are positioned around the body cavity or organ to be treated, and microwave or radiofrequency energy is focused on the area to raise its temperature.

- Regional perfusion techniques can be used to treat cancers in the arms and legs, such as melanoma, or cancer in some organs, such as the liver or lung. In this procedure, some of the patient's blood is removed, heated, and then pumped (perfused) back into the limb or organ. Anticancer drugs are commonly given during this treatment.

- Continuous hyperthermic peritoneal perfusion (CHPP) is a technique used to treat cancers within the peritoneal cavity (the space within the abdomen that contains the intestines, stomach, and liver), including primary peritoneal mesothelioma and stomach cancer. During surgery, heated anticancer drugs flow from a warming device through the peritoneal cavity. The peritoneal cavity temperature reaches 106–108° F.

- Whole-body hyperthermia is used to treat metastatic cancer that has spread throughout the body. This can be accomplished by several techniques that raise the body temperature to 107–108° F, including the use of thermal chambers (similar to large incubators) or hot water blankets.

The effectiveness of hyperthermia treatment is related to the temperature achieved during the treatment, as well as the length of treatment and cell and tissue characteristics.[1, 2] To ensure that the desired temperature is reached, but not exceeded, the temperature of the tumor and surrounding tissue is monitored throughout hyperthermia treatment.[3, 5, 7] Using local anesthesia, the doctor inserts small needles or tubes with tiny thermometers into the treatment area to monitor the temperature. Imaging techniques, such as CT (computed tomography), may be used to make sure the probes are properly positioned.[5]

Does hyperthermia have any complications or side effects?

Most normal tissues are not damaged during hyperthermia if the temperature remains under 111° F. However, due to regional differences in tissue characteristics, higher temperatures may occur in various spots. This can result in burns, blisters, discomfort, or pain.[1, 5, 7]

Perfusion techniques can cause tissue swelling, blood clots, bleeding, and other damage to the normal tissues in the perfused area; however, most of these side effects are temporary. Whole-body hyperthermia can cause more serious side effects, including cardiac and vascular disorders, but these effects are uncommon.[1, 3, 7] Diarrhea, nausea, and vomiting are commonly observed after whole-body hyperthermia.[7]

What does the future hold for hyperthermia?

A number of challenges must be overcome before hyperthermia can be considered a standard treatment for cancer.[1, 3, 6, 7] Many clinical trials are being conducted to evaluate the effectiveness of hyperthermia. Some trials continue to research hyperthermia in combination with other therapies for the treatment of different cancers. Other studies focus on improving hyperthermia techniques.

To learn more about clinical trials, call the National Cancer Institute's (NCI) Cancer Information Service at the telephone number listed below or visit the clinical trials page of the NCI's website at http://www.cancer.gov/clinical_trials/ on the internet.

Selected References

1. van der Zee J. Heating the patient: A promising approach? *Annals of Oncology* 2002; 13:1173–1184.

2. Hildebrandt B, Wust P, Ahlers O, et al. The cellular and molecular basis of hyperthermia. *Critical Reviews in Oncology/Hematology* 2002; 43:33–56.

3. Wust P, Hildebrandt B, Sreenivasa G, et al. Hyperthermia in combined treatment of cancer. *The Lancet Oncology* 2002; 3:487–497.

4. Alexander HR. Isolation perfusion. In: DeVita VT Jr., Hellman S, Rosenberg SA, editors. *Cancer: Principles and Practice of Oncology*. Vol. 1 and 2. 6th ed. Philadelphia: Lippincott Williams and Wilkins, 2001.

5. Falk MH, Issels RD. Hyperthermia in oncology. *International Journal of Hyperthermia* 2001; 17(1):1–18.

6. Dewhirst MW, Gibbs FA Jr, Roemer RB, Samulski TV. Hyperthermia. In: Gunderson LL, Tepper JE, editors. *Clinical Radiation Oncology*. 1st ed. New York, NY: Churchill Livingstone, 2000.

7. Kapp DS, Hahn GM, Carlson RW. Principles of Hyperthermia. In: Bast RC Jr., Kufe DW, Pollock RE, et al., editors. *Cancer Medicine* e.5. 5th ed. Hamilton, Ontario: B.C. Decker Inc., 2000.

8. Feldman AL, Libutti SK, Pingpank JF, et al. Analysis of factors associated with outcome in patients with malignant peritoneal mesothelioma undergoing surgical debulking and intraperitoneal chemotherapy. *Journal of Clinical Oncology* 2003; 21(24): 4560–4567.

9. Chang E, Alexander HR, Libutti SK, et al. Laparoscopic continuous hyperthermic peritoneal perfusion. *Journal of the American College of Surgeons* 2001; 193(2):225–229.

Chapter 20

Cancer Genomics

The Human Genome

The complete supply of DNA—all the genes and spaces in between—in all the chromosomes of a species is called its genome. Except for red blood cells, which have no nucleus, the human genome is located in the nucleus of every cell in the body. There it is organized into 46 very large molecules called chromosomes; 44 are called autosomes and 2 are called the sex chromosomes. There are about 25,000 genes present.

Genes: Keepers of the Code

The 25,000 genes scattered throughout the human chromosomes comprise only about 3 percent of the total genome. These genes hold information critical to all human life. While all the component bases in a gene are copied as information leaves the nucleus, not all this information is kept. This is because within a gene there are both coding and noncoding stretches of bases. For example, in split genes, coding sections called exons supply the genetic instructions that are copied to direct protein building. These sections are preserved, but other noncoding sections within the gene, called introns, are rapidly removed and degraded.

Close to each gene is a "regulatory" sequence of DNA, which is able to turn the gene "on" or "off." Farther away, there are enhancer regions, which can speed up a gene's activity.

Excerpted from "Understanding Cancer Series: Cancer Genomics," National Cancer Institute, January 28, 2005.

The massive DNA molecules known as chromosomes also have many noncoding regions located outside the genes. These contain large stretches of repetitive sequences. Some of the sequences in these locations are involved in the regulation of gene expression, and others simply act as spacers. Still other regions have functions as yet undiscovered.

Genes to mRNA to Proteins

When a gene "switches on," it eventually makes a protein, but it does not do so directly. First, the gene codes an intermediary molecule called mRNA. To transfer a gene's information from DNA to mRNA, base pairing is used. However, there is one change: An adenine base (A) in the DNA matches with a new base called uracil (U) in the mRNA. This difference helps to distinguish mRNA from DNA.

mRNA travels from the nucleus into the cytoplasm to cell organelles called ribosomes. There it directs the assembly of amino acids that fold into a unique protein.

Before mRNA leaves the nucleus, it undergoes further processing. The regions not involved in building proteins, called introns, are cut out of the message. The mature RNA that arrives at a ribosome contains only exons that will be used to build a protein in a process called translation.

Triplet Code

The translation of base sequences from DNA to protein is dependent on the nucleotide triplet in mRNA. Each mRNA triplet of nucleotides, called a codon, codes for a single amino acid, and, ultimately, a string of amino acids makes up a protein. Since the complementary DNA that specifies a particular mRNA has only four nucleotide bases in a gene, 64 (4X4X4) possible combinations of codons are available to code for 20 amino acids. So there is great redundancy. There are 60 mRNA triplets for 19 amino acids, 3 triplets for "stop," and 1 triplet to call for methionine, the 20th amino acid that signals "start." Most amino acids are coded for by more than one triplet codon. However, each triplet is linked to only one amino acid.

Mutations

All mutations are changes in the normal base sequence of DNA. These changes may occur in either coding or noncoding regions. Mutations may be silent and have no effect on the resulting protein. This is especially true if they occur in noncoding regions of the DNA. But even base pair changes in the coding region may be silent because of the redundancy of the code. For example, a mutation within a codon may occur, yet still call for the same amino acid as was called for earlier.

Most cancers arise from several genetic mutations that accumulate in cells of the body over a person's lifespan. These are called somatic mutations, and the genes involved are usually located on autosomes (non-sex chromosomes). Cancer may also have a germline mutation component, meaning that they occur in germ cells, better known as the ovum or sperm. Germline mutations may occur de novo (for the first time) or be inherited from parents' germ cells. An example of germline mutations linked to cancer are the ones that occur in cancer susceptibility genes, increasing a person's risk for the disease.

Each cell, when it divides, generates two identical new ones. So, when a cell acquires a mutation, it passes that mutation on to its progeny during cell growth and division. Because cells with cancer-linked mutations tend to proliferate more than normal cells, cellular candidates for additional mutations grow in number. Mutations continue to accumulate and are copied to descendant cells. If one cell finally acquires enough mutations to become cancerous, subsequent cancer cells will be derived from that one single transformed cell. So all tumors are clonal, which means that they originate from a single parent cell, whether that first mutant cell was of germline or somatic origin.

Mitosis and Somatic Mutations

The majority of human cancers result from an accumulation of somatic mutations. Somatic mutations are not passed on to the next generation. An 80-year cancer-free lifespan is no small accomplishment. It requires as many as 10 million billion body cells to copy themselves correctly. It is easy to see how random errors can occur. These changes are acquired during a person's lifetime from exposures to carcinogens and other mutagens, or from random unrepaired errors that occur during routine cell growth and division. Occasionally, one of these somatic mutations alters the function of some critical genes, providing a growth advantage to the cell in which it has occurred. A clone then arises from that single cell.

Normal human cells with a nucleus having 23 pairs of chromosomes are called diploid or 2N to indicate these homolog pairs. During the cell growth cycle for body (somatic) cells, the DNA of all 23 pairs—46 chromosomes—copies itself (4N). When the cell next divides by a process called mitosis, each daughter cell ends up with 23 pairs or 2N, a complete set of chromosomes. If a mutation occurs during the process of mitosis, only the offspring of the mutated somatic cell will have the alteration present.

Meiosis and Germline Mutations

Unlike other human body cells, maturing germ cells, like ova or sperm, must cut their chromosome number from 46 to 23, from 2N to N. They do this through two specialized cell divisions in a process called meiosis. After meiosis is complete, each germ cell has only one-half of the 44 original body chromosomes (or autosomes) plus either an X or a Y sex chromosome.

De Novo Mutations

Inherited mutations had to start somewhere, and that somewhere is a de novo mutation. A de novo mutation is a new mutation that occurs in a germ cell and is then passed on to an offspring. All germline mutations started as a de novo mutation in some ancestor. De novo mutations are common in a few inherited cancer susceptibility syndromes.

Point Mutations

Point mutations, single base changes in DNA sequences, are the most common type of alteration in DNA. They can have varying effects on the resulting protein.

A missense point mutation substitutes one nucleotide for a different one, but leaves the rest of the code intact. The impact of these point mutations depends on the specific amino acid that is changed and the protein sequence that results. If the change is critical to the protein's catalytic site or to its folding, damage may be severe.

Frameshift Mutations

Another type of mutation that can occur is a frameshift mutation. When a gene is copied, the action begins in the nucleus. There an mRNA strand copies the DNA strand exactly. It codes for a protein precisely, leaving no gaps or spaces separating the triplets. This set of connected triplets is called the reading frame. A frameshift mutation is caused by the addition or loss of a nucleotide, or nucleotides. This alters the content of every triplet codon that follows in a reading frame. Frameshift mutations usually result in a shortened abnormal or nonfunctional protein, and they can create an early STOP codon downstream. If the number of added or missing base pairs is a multiple of three, the resulting protein may be drastically altered, and its function will depend on the extent of these alterations.

Splice-Site Mutations

Splice-site mutations occur within genes in the noncoding regions (introns) just next to the coding regions (exons). They can have profound effects on the resulting protein, which may lead to disease. Before mRNA leaves the nucleus, the introns are removed and the exons are joined together. This process is called splicing. Splicing is controlled by specific intron sequences, called splice-donor and splice-acceptor sequences, which flank the exons. Mutations in these sequences may lead to retention of large segments of intronic DNA by the mRNA, or to entire exons being spliced out of the mRNA. These changes could result in production of a nonfunctional protein.

Regulatory Mutations

Although mutations in the noncoding region are generally silent, that is not always the case. Some of the most important regulatory regions are in the 5' noncoding flanking region of the gene. Promoter sequences that regulate the gene are located there. Also, enhancer sequences that regulate the rate of gene activity are in noncoding regions a considerable distance from the gene. And gene repressor regions, which negatively regulate gene activity, also exist. Mutations in any of these regions can change the rate of protein production.

Large Deletions or Insertions

Large deletions or insertions in a chromosome also may lead to cancer. These may occur during mitosis or during recombination in meiosis. Translocations occur when segments of one chromosome break off and fuse to a different chromosome, without any loss of genetic material. Many of these have been found to enable tumor development. Inversions are mutations that arise when two breaks occur in a chromosome and the piece is reinserted in reversed order. Other chromosomal abnormalities include nondisjunction, the failure of the homologs (chromosome pairs) to separate as new cells divide.

Cancer-Associated Mutations

Cancer-associated mutations, whether somatic or germline, whether point mutations or large deletions, alter key proteins and their functions in the human biosystem. A wide variety of mutations seems to be involved. Even mutations in noncoding regions, such as in promoters, enhancers, or negative regulatory regions, can result in under or over expression of proteins needed for normalcy. Other mutations may cause production of important checkpoint proteins to malfunction. Collectively, these mutations conspire to change a genome from normal to cancerous.

Genotypes and Phenotypes

Cancer may start as a new genotype, that is, as a change in the genetic makeup of a person, but it ultimately produces a new phenotype as well. A phenotype is the physical manifestation of a genotype in the form of a trait or disease. Cancer is known for its ever-changing genotypes and phenotypes.

All genotypes are not created equal in their influence on phenotype. Genes come in many varieties called alleles, and some are more dominant than others. In a pair of alleles, the effect of a dominant allele prevails over the effect of a recessive allele. And the effects of a recessive allele become apparent only if the dominant allele becomes inactivated or lost.

Many cancer susceptibility syndromes are genetically heterogeneous (a mixture), which means that different mutations (genotypes) can be expressed as the same phenotype. These different mutations may be located within the same gene but at different locations (locus heterogeneity) or on different genes altogether (allelic heterogeneity). For example, hereditary breast and ovarian cancer susceptibility has both locus and allelic heterogeneity. More than 500 different mutations have been identified that can occur in the BRCA1 gene on chromosome 17 and increase a woman's risk for breast cancer. And more than 300 mutations scattered throughout the BRCA2 gene on chromosome 13 are associated with hereditary breast and ovarian cancer susceptibility.

Penetrance

Sometimes one person with a dominant allele will express a trait, yet that same genotype in another person will remain silent. This is an example of differences in penetrance. In classic Mendelian genetics, if an individual carries a dominant allele, the trait will be expressed. However, if all carriers of a certain dominant allele in a population do not express the trait (same genotypes/different phenotypes), the gene is said to have incomplete penetrance.

Modifier genes affect the expression of some alleles, which may increase or decrease the penetrance of a germline mutation such as an altered cancer susceptibility allele. Penetrance may also be affected by mutations in DNA damage response genes, whose normal function is to recognize and repair genetic damage. If repair malfunctions, mutations may accumulate in other genes, increasing the likelihood that a given cell will progress to cancer.

Age-related penetrance: Penetrance is usually age related, meaning that the trait is not expressed in most carriers at birth but occurs with increased frequency as the carriers get older. For example, germline mutations in mismatch repair genes associated with hereditary nonpolyposis colorectal cancer (HNPCC) are incompletely penetrant. So not all individuals who carry these mutations will get colorectal cancer, but the risk increases as individuals age. About 20 percent of carriers will never develop colorectal cancer.

Epigenetic factors and penetrance: Epigenetic factors are mechanisms outside the gene such as a cell's exposure to carcinogens or hormones, or genetic variations that modify a gene or its protein by methylation, demethylation, phosphorylation, or dephosphorylation. These factors can alter what is ultimately expressed; they can change a phenotype. For example, hormone and reproductive factors may influence the penetrance of certain cancer-linked mutations. Breast and ovarian cancer are more likely to occur in women with early menarche, late menopause, and a first child after age 30 (or no children at all). These factors are believed to be linked to a woman's exposure to estrogen and progesterone and their effects on cell differentiation in the breast that occur during pregnancy.

In cancer, both the genotype and the phenotype change over time. Epigenetic factors play a key role in these changes.

Carrier Frequency

Carrier frequency describes the prevalence in a given population of germline mutations in a specific gene. A mutation carrier is sometimes called a heterozygote because two different alleles are present at a given locus—one with a germline mutation and one normal allele. Here, two out of 10 individuals carry a mutated allele at a particular gene locus, so the carrier frequency is 20 percent.

Autosomal Dominant Inheritance

Most hereditary cancer syndromes are inherited in autosomal dominant fashion.

Dominant inheritance occurs when only one copy of an allele is required for a particular trait to be expressed (phenotype). In autosomal dominant inheritance, multiple generations express the traits, with no skipped generations (assuming complete penetrance).

Hereditary cancer syndromes are relatively uncommon, accounting for only about 5 to 10 percent of all cancers. Nevertheless, as many as 50,000 cancers newly diagnosed in the U.S. each year are associated with a hereditary syndrome.

Cancer Susceptibility: Incomplete Penetrance and Phenocopies

Individuals who inherit cancer susceptibility mutations inherit a predisposition to cancer, not cancer itself. Some mutation carriers inherit their predisposing genotypes in an autosomal dominant fashion, yet they do not develop cancer, indicating that their altered genes are incompletely penetrant. A somatic mutation in a second allele is required for cancer to develop.

Further confusing the situation is the fact that sporadic forms of cancer may also occur in families along with a hereditary cancer syndrome. These cases of sporadic cancer are called phenocopies because their phenotype is similar to that of the affected mutation carriers, but their genotype is different. Genetic testing may determine if the cancer is hereditary or sporadic in nature.

Autosomal Recessive Inheritance

In autosomal recessive inheritance, two copies of the allele are required for the trait to be expressed. Carriers of one disease allele will not develop the illness, and several generations may be unaffected, leading to the appearance of skipped generations. Males and females are equally affected. If both parents carry one copy of the recessive allele, one in four offspring, on average, will express the trait.

In X-linked inheritance, the gene of interest is on the X chromosome, not on an autosome. Because females have two X chromosomes, they must inherit two copies of the disease allele to express the disease phenotype. Females with only one mutated allele are carriers.

Males are more frequently affected because they only have one X chromosome and need only one allele mutated to express a disease phenotype. All males who inherit a copy of the abnormal X chromosome are affected by the disease (assuming 100 percent penetrance).

Other Genetic Conditions Linked to Increased Cancer Risk

Hereditary susceptibility to breast cancer occurs in several other rare genetic conditions. Breast cancer is the most common adult manifestation of Li-Fraumeni syndrome, a multiple cancer syndrome caused by germline mutations in the TP53 gene. Breast cancer also is the most frequent malignancy diagnosed in Cowden syndrome, a condition with germline mutations in the PTEN gene. Both benign and malignant breast tumors occur in Muir-Torre syndrome, a condition related to hereditary nonpolyposis colon cancer (HNPCC), characterized by germline mutations in the DNA mismatch repair genes MSH2 and MLH1. Patients with Peutz-Jeghers syndrome display abnormal pigmentation, gastrointestinal polyps, and, if they are women, they are at increased risk for breast cancer and they experience early onset bilateral disease.

Abnormal Cell Growth: Oncogenes

In normal cells, tumor suppressor genes act as braking signals during G1 to stop or slow the cell cycle before S phase. DNA repair genes are active throughout the cell cycle, particularly during G2 after DNA replication and before the chromosomes prepare for mitosis.

Most cancers have mutations in protooncogenes, the normal genes involved in the regulation of controlled cell growth. These genes encode proteins that function as growth factors, growth factor receptors, signal-relaying molecules, and nuclear transcription factors (proteins that bind to genes to start transcription). When the proto-oncogene is mutated or overregulated, it is called an oncogene and results in unregulated cell growth and transformation. At the cellular level, only one mutation in a single allele is enough to trigger an oncogenic role in cancer development. The chance that such a mutation will occur increases as a person ages.

Tumor Suppressor Genes

Most cancer susceptibility genes are tumor suppressor genes. Tumor suppressor genes are just one type of the many genes malfunctioning in cancer. These genes, under normal circumstances, suppress cell growth. Some do so by encoding transcription factors for other genes needed to slow growth. For example, the protein product of the suppressor gene TP53 is called p53 protein. It binds directly to DNA and leads to the expression of genes that inhibit cell growth or trigger cell death. Other tumor suppressor genes code for proteins that help control the cell cycle.

Mutations in Tumor Suppressor Genes

Both copies of a tumor suppressor gene must be lost or mutated for cancer to occur. A person who carries a germline mutation in a tumor suppressor gene has only one functional copy of the gene in all cells. For this person, loss or mutation of the second copy of the gene in any of these cells can lead to cancer.

Loss of Heterozygosity

In hereditary cancer syndromes, individuals are called heterozygous (having one or more dissimilar gene pairs) because they start life with a germline mutation in one of the alleles linked to cancer susceptibility, but it is balanced by a normal counterpart. These individuals are predisposed to cancer because all their cells have already sustained the first hit to cancer-linked genes. If the critically needed normal suppressor gene that balances this germline mutation is lost at some time during an individual's life, a condition called loss of heterozygosity (LOH) occurs.

There are several ways a cell can suffer loss of heterozygosity. An entire chromosome containing a normal allele may be lost due to failure of the chromosomes to segregate properly at mitosis (nondisjunction). Alternatively, an unbalanced exchange of genetic material can occur in a process called translocation, resulting in loss of a chromosomal region containing the normal gene. Sometimes when a normal gene is lost, a reduplication of the remaining chromosome with an abnormal gene occurs, leaving the cell with two abnormal gene copies. Normal genes may also be lost during normal mitotic recombination events or as a consequence of a point mutation in the second allele, leading to inactivation of the normal counterpart.

Repair Failure

Some mutations linked to cancer appear to involve a failure of one or many of the cell's repair systems. One example of such error involves DNA mismatch repair. After DNA copies itself, proteins from mismatch repair genes act as proofreaders to identify and correct mismatches. If a loss or mutation occurs in the mismatch repair genes, sporadic mutations will more likely accumulate. Other errors in repair may involve incorrect cutting out of bases—or whole nucleotides—as repair proteins try to fix DNA after bulky molecules, such as the carcinogens in cigarettes, have attached. This is faulty excision repair. Sometimes both strands of DNA suffer breaks at the same time, and faulty recombinational repair occurs. Any of these mistakes may enable mutations to persist, get copied, and eventually contribute to cancer's development.

Epigenetic Changes: Much Still Unknown

Much remains unknown about the role of epigenetic factors and cancer. Epigenetic changes are reversible modifications to genes or proteins that occur in the tumor and its microenvironment. Epigenetic modifier molecules have been observed making tumor-friendly, nonmutational changes in an already confused biosystem. For example, by heavily methylating genes or promoter regions, gene activity critical to counteract a tumor's drive toward metastasis gets turned off. Or noncoding ribonucleic acids meddle in epigenetic fashion, interfering with a cell's regulation of growth or attempt to repair damage.

In addition to oncogenes and tumor suppressor genes, most cancers acquire several other key mutations that enable cancer to progress. While researchers don't yet know all the mutations involved, they have organized them in terms of their activities in support of tumor growth and metastasis. In addition to the contributions of oncogenes and mutated suppressor genes, additional genomic mutations enable the invasion of neighboring tissue, evasion of immune system detection, recruitment of a new blood supply, dissemination and targeting of new sites, and the penetration and reinvasion through new blood and tissue layers. Over time, successful metastasis occurs.

A Daunting Challenge

A comprehensive analysis of the cancer genome remains a daunting challenge. There is no single technology at present that will detect all the types of abnormality implicated in cancer. Microarrays and gene chip analysis, however, are beginning to unveil some key genomic drivers.

Many clinical trials now include genomic profiles of cancer patients as prognostic and diagnostic indicators. Genomic profiles are even used to monitor where and how the cancer genome has been hit during molecularly targeted therapies. Mining and sharing all this data should eventually help oncologists to better integrate the genotypic and phenotypic changes that occur in a biosystem during cancer's progression. This knowledge will be used to bring earlier and better interventions to cancer patients.

Chapter 21

Gene Therapy

What is gene therapy and how does it work?

In the center of every cell in your body is a region called the nucleus. The nucleus contains your DNA (deoxyribose nucleic acid), which is the genetic code you inherited from each of your parents. The DNA is ribbon-like in structure, but normally exists in a condensed form called chromosomes. You have 46 chromosomes, which are in turn comprised of thousands of genes. These genes carry specific instructions that tell cells how to work, control our growth and development, and determine what we look like and how our bodies work. They also play a role in the repair of damaged cells and tissues. Each person has more than 30,000 genes, which are made up of DNA. You have two copies of every gene, one inherited from your mother and one from your father.

So, now that we know what genes are, how can they be used to help fight cancer? If a gene becomes damaged, this damage is called a mutation. This can lead to a gene not functioning properly and a cell growing uncontrollably. This can eventually lead to cancer formation. (Keep in mind that developing a cancer is not quite as simple as this, but probably requires a complex series of multiple mutations.) These mutations may be caused by things like smoking or the environment, or they may be inherited. It makes sense that if we could repair these mutations, we could potentially stop a cancer from starting. The question is, how do we do this?

Researchers are testing several ways of applying gene therapy to the treatment of cancer:

- Replace missing or non-functioning genes. For example, p53 is a gene called a tumor suppressor gene. Its job is just that: to suppress tumors from forming. Cells that are missing this gene or have a non-functioning copy due to a mutation may be "fixed" by adding functioning copies of p53 to the cell.

- Oncogenes are mutated genes that are capable of causing either development of a new cancer, or the spread of an existing cancer (metastasis). By stopping the function of these genes, the cancer or spread of cancer may be stopped.

- Use the body's own immune system by inserting genes into cancer cells that then trigger the body to attack the cancer cells as foreign invaders.

- Insert genes into cancer cells to make them more susceptible to or prevent resistance to chemotherapy, radiation therapy, or hormone therapies.

- Create "suicide genes" that can enter cancer cells and cause them to self-destruct.

- Cancers require a blood supply to grow and survive, and they form their own blood vessels to accomplish this. Genes can be used to prevent these blood vessels from forming, thus starving the tumor to death (also called angiogenesis).

- Use genes to protect healthy cells from the side effects of therapy, allowing higher doses of chemotherapy and radiation to be given.

How is gene therapy given?

You can imagine it would be hard to actually inject these genes into the tiny cells, so a carrier, or a "vector", is used to accomplish this. Typically, viruses are used as the vectors. These viruses are like those that cause the common cold, only they are "deactivated" so that they will not cause the patient to actually get the cold. In some cases, some cells are taken from the patient and the virus is exposed to the cells in the laboratory. The virus with the desired gene attached finds its way into the cells. These cells are allowed to grow in the laboratory, and are then given back to the patient by intravenous (IV) infusion or are injected into a body cavity (that is the lung) or a tumor. In other cases, the vector with the attached gene is directly inserted into the patient by intravenous infusion or is injected into a body cavity or a tumor. Gene therapy is still experimental, so the means by which it is given may change as the technology develops.

What are the side effects of gene therapy?

Given that gene therapy is so new, we do not know what side effects it may have, particularly long-term side effects that may occur years after receiving this therapy. After initially receiving a type of gene therapy, the patient's immune system may react to the foreign vector, causing fever, severe chills (rigors), drop in blood pressure, nausea, vomiting, and headache. These symptoms typically resolve within 24–48 hours of the infusion. Other side effects are dependent upon the type of vector used and how it is given. If the gene is given into a patient's lung, the side effects may affect the lung.

Some side effects are theoretical, meaning that it is feasible that they could happen, yet they have not actually occurred in clinical trials to date. There is a fear that the genes could enter healthy cells, causing damage to them, which could then lead to another disease or another cancer. If genes enter reproductive cells, they could potentially cause damage to sperm or eggs. It is feared that this damage could then be passed on to future generations. At this time, researchers are particularly careful to monitor for these unwanted complications, and perform tests in animal studies before any particular therapy is given to humans.

How do I know if gene therapy is working for me?

At this time, gene therapy on its own is not thought to cure any cancer. It is generally given in conjunction with other therapies with more reliable track records, such as chemotherapy.

That being said, the real answer varies, depending on the type of cancer being treated. Many patients will have radiology studies (computed tomography scans, magnetic resonance imaging scans, positron emission tomography scans) periodically to assess the tumor's status (shrunk, stayed the same, or grown). Some types of tumors can be followed using tumor markers. Tumor markers are substances that are either produced by the tumor or by the body in response to the tumor, and can be measured by a blood test. If the chemotherapy is working, one would expect the tumor marker to decrease. In some cases, a decrease in a patient's symptoms may be able to signal if the medications are shrinking the tumor or not. Talk with your doctor or nurse about how your response will be measured.

Chapter 22

The Challenges and Promise of Proteomics Research

What is proteomics?

The term 'proteome' was first coined in 1994 and refers to all the proteins in a cell, tissue, or organism. Proteomics refers to the study of the proteome. Because proteins are involved in almost all biological activities, the proteome is a rich source of biological information.

Protein scientists have diverse interests. These include determining the function and amino acid sequence of proteins; their three-dimensional structure; how the addition of sugar, phosphate, or fat affects protein function; and how proteins interact with other molecules, including other proteins. Some researchers are focused on the proteins present in particular parts of the cell such as the outer cell membrane, the nucleus, the cytoplasm (the region of the cell outside the nucleus), or the nuclear membrane; others are analyzing protein-protein interactions in a particular cell or organism; some are studying the differences between the proteins present in diseased vs. healthy cells.[1]

How does studying the proteome compare to studying the genome? What are some of the challenges in proteomics research?

The total number of proteins in human cells is estimated to be between 250,000 to 500,000, and only a small percentage have been

Excerpted from "Questions and Answers: Proteomics and Cancer," National Cancer Institute (NCI), September 29, 2005. The complete text of this document can be accessed online through the NCI website (www.cancer.gov).

sequenced or identified. The complete proteome has not been characterized for any organism. In contrast, the genome or the entire set of genes for several organisms has been sequenced, including humans. The human genome is estimated to contain about 35,000 protein-encoding genes.

Besides the difference in quantity, another important difference between the genome and proteome is that the genome is static and relatively unchanged from day to day. Cellular proteins, on the other hand, are continually moving and undergoing changes such as binding to a cell membrane, partnering with other proteins, gaining or losing a chemical group (such as a sugar, fat, or phosphate), or breaking into two or more pieces. Proteins play a central role in the complex communication network within and between cells and are constantly responding to the needs of the organism.

Several other properties of proteins add to their complexity:

- Proteins and/or modified proteins may vary among individuals, between cell types, and even within the same cell under different stimuli or different disease-states.

- One gene can produce more than one protein and one protein can be modified in multiple ways, which may change its behavior. This can happen when the cell uses a single gene DNA template to produce several different messenger RNAs, which are then used as templates to make different proteins, or it may happen when a protein is modified by cellular processes after it is created. The result is that instead of one gene producing one protein, one gene can produce as many as 1,000 different proteins. On average, however, a gene produces five to ten different proteins from its messenger RNAs.[2]

- The quantity of different proteins can vary greatly. For example, in human blood, the concentration of the protein albumin is more than a billion times greater than another protein, interleukin-6.

- There is no laboratory amplification technique for proteins like there is for amplifying genes. This means that it is not possible to make copies of proteins that are present in very small amounts.

What are the approaches used in the development of clinical proteomics?

The goal of clinical proteomics is to develop proteomics technology for the benefit of patient care. This new research technology is now being used in clinical research studies ranging from cancer to cardiovascular disease and organ transplants.[3] Researchers are searching for proteins that can be used as early biomarkers of disease, or that may predict response to therapy or the likelihood of relapse after treatment in blood, urine, or diseased tissue.[4, 5]

Ovarian cancer: Ovarian cancer is a major focus of early biomarker discovery because it is usually diagnosed at an advanced stage with a five-year survival rate of about 20 percent. To evaluate the potential use of proteomics as a diagnostic tool, a group of researchers from the National Cancer Institute (NCI) in Bethesda, Maryland, collected serum from 50 ovarian cancer patients and 50 controls and used a computer algorithm to search for the protein patterns that distinguished cancer from non-cancer. When they tested this pattern with a set of blinded serum samples, the test pattern correctly identified all 50 patients with cancer, and was able to discriminate them from 63 out of 66 patients who were unaffected or had benign disease.[6] Using the same approach, two other groups reported similar results.[5,6]

Prostate cancer: A similar proteomic analysis of prostate cancer patients vs. healthy controls was carried out by looking for differences in protein patterns between the two groups. Using blood samples from 167 prostate cancer patients, 77 patients with benign prostate hyperplasia and 82 healthy men, the computer was able to develop a classification system that correctly classified 96 percent of the samples as either prostate cancer or non-cancer (benign prostate hyperplasia/healthy men).[9] Another proteomic approach is to determine whether the changes in specific phosphoproteins (proteins with phosphate groups attached) believed to be important in cellular signaling events and cancer progression in prostate cancer patients can serve as a biomarker of early disease.[10]

Breast cancer: A combination of three candidate proteins in the blood were found to be useful in discriminating between 169 patients at various stages of breast cancer compared to women with benign breast disease and healthy controls.[11] In three other studies, nipple aspirate fluid was used to identify tumor marker candidates.[12–14] Nipple aspirate fluid has a higher concentration of breast specific proteins than blood. Mammary ducts are thin tubes that lead to the nipples and are where 70 percent to 80 percent of breast cancers originate.

Lung and bladder: Several laboratories have successfully analyzed tumor tissue from patients with lung and bladder cancer and discovered protein patterns that could discriminate diseased from healthy tissue.[15] Likewise, preliminary results using a proteomic approach to detect bladder cancer have been promising.[16]

Future use: At this point, none of the above described proteomics analyses is mature enough to be used in the clinic as a screening tool. However, these exploratory studies point to the promise of proteomics as a diagnostic marker. Validation in clinical trials in large groups of patients is necessary before proteomics patterns can be used routinely in the clinic as biomarkers for early disease.

What are some of the technologies used in proteomics research?

Traditionally, proteomics experiments have been done using two-dimensional gel electrophoresis (2DE), a process by which large mixtures of proteins are separated by electrical charge and size. In the first dimension, the proteins migrate through a gel-like substance until they are separated by their charge; for the second dimension, they are transferred to a second semi-solid gel and are separated by size. The advantage of this method is that a large number (3,000 to 10,000) proteins can be visually separated. The drawback is that certain kinds of proteins such as membrane proteins, proteins present in very small amounts, or very large or very small proteins are difficult or impossible to visualize by 2DE.

In the last ten years or so, mass spectrometry (MS) has increasingly become the method of choice for analyses of complex protein samples. Mass spectrometry is a technique that measures two properties: the mass-to-charge ratio (m/z) of a mixture of ions (particles with an electric charge) in the gas phase under vacuum; and the number of ions present at each m/z value. The end product is a mass spectrum or chart with a series of spiked peaks, each representing the ion or charged protein fragment present in a given sample. The height of the peak is related to the abundance of the protein fragment. The size of the peaks and the distance between them are a fingerprint of the sample and provide a clue to its identity.[26]

The mass spectrometer consists of an ionization source, a mass analyzer, and a detector:

- The ionization source ionizes the proteins or protein fragments present in the sample. Ionizing means removing electrons from protein fragments resulting in positively charged particles.

- The mass analyzer measures the mass-to-charge ratio of the ionized protein fragments in the sample.

- The detector registers the number of ions at each m/z value. The end product is a mass spectrum described in the previous paragraph.

Ionization sources: Two ionization techniques, MALDI and ESI, have had a major impact on protein biochemistry because they are able to produce ions in the gas phase without fragmenting the proteins too extensively, a problem with older methods. MALDI (matrix-assisted laser desorption ionization) produces ions by sublimating (transforming a solid to a gas) and ionizing the proteins out of a dry, crystalline stage. ESI (electrospray ionization) ionizes the protein mixtures out of a liquid. MALDI is normally used to analyze relatively simple peptide mixtures while ESI is preferred for more complex samples. However, a variant of MALDI, where the surface of the MALDI target has been modified, is used with more complex mixtures. Known as surface-enhanced laser-desorption ionization (SELDI) MS, this technique is widely used in cancer proteomics. Only a small fraction of protein fragments in the sample bind to the SELDI surface because they have an affinity for the substances on the surface.[26]

Mass analyzer and detector: Once the ions are produced, the mass analyzer/detector separates them by the mass-to-charge ratio and produces a mass spectrum, or a series of spiked peaks, which are used to identify the proteins. The mass of the protein peaks increases from left to right; the height of each peak is proportional to the number of ions at that particular mass-to-charge ratio. Four types of mass analyzers are commonly used: ion trap, time of flight (TOF), quadrupole, and Fourier transform ion cyclotron (FT-MS).[26]

Ionizers, analyzers, and detectors: The ionization method, MALDI, is commonly coupled to TOF mass analyzers, while ESI is most often coupled to ion-trap or quadrupole spectrometers. Most serum protein mass spectrum data have been generated by using the Ciphergen Biosystems (Fremont, California) ProteinChip array surface-enhanced laser-desorption ionization-time-of-flight (SELDI-TOF) MS system. In this system, specific substances are applied to the surface of the SELDI chip array to capture peptides in the sample. Once captured, the proteins are detected by TOF MS.

What are some of the advantages of using mass spectrometry techniques in clinical research?

The great advantage of mass spectrometry (MS) over other technologies for detecting and monitoring subtle changes in substances in the body is the ability to measure rapidly and inexpensively thousands of elements in a few drops of blood. Unlike 2DE, MS patterns generated from the thousands of proteins present in blood are difficult to analyze visually. However, the powerful computational ability of today's computers makes it possible to analyze MS spectra rapidly and distinguish subtle differences in patterns between diseased and healthy people.

Mass spectrometry-based proteomics analysis is extremely rapid. The entire process, from collecting blood to analyzing the MS spectrum, can occur in less than one minute. In addition, hundreds of samples can be analyzed sequentially, and extremely small amounts of protein can be detected.

References

1. Patterson SD & Aebersold RH. Proteomics: the first decade and beyond. *Nature Genetics Supplement* 2003;33:311–32.

2. Ullrich B, Ushkaryov YA, and Sudhof TC. Cartography of neurexins: more than 1,000 isoforms generated by alternative splicing and expressed in distinct subsets of neurons. *Neuron* 1995:14:497–507.

3. Petricoin EF, Rajapaske V, Herman EH, Arekani AM, Ross S, Johann D, Knapton,A, Zhang J, Hitt BA, Conrads TP, Veenstra TD, Liotta LA, and Sistare FD. Toxicoproteomics: Serum Proteomic Pattern Diagnostics for Early Detection of Drug Induced Cardiac Toxicities and Cardioprotection. *Journal of Toxicologic Pathology* 2004;32 (S1):1–9.

4. Clarke W, Zhang Zhen, Chan DW. The application of clinical proteomics to cancer and other diseases. *Clin Chem Lab Med* 2003;41(12):1562–1570.

5. Liotta LA, Espina V, Mehta AI, Calvert V, Rosenblatt K, Geho D, Munson PJ, Young L, Wulfkuhle J, Petricoin EF. Protein microarrays: Meeting analytical challenges for clinical applications. *Cancer Cell* 2003; Apr;3(4):317–25.

6. Petricoin EF, Ardekani AM, Hitt BA, Levine PF, Fusara VA, Steinberg SM, et al. Use of proteomic patterns in serum to identify ovarian cancer. *Lancet* 2002;369:572–7.

7. Sorace JM, Zhan M. A data review and re-assessment of ovarian cancer serum proteomic profiling. *BMC Bioinformatics* 2003;4:24.

8. Zhu W, Wang X, Ma Y, Rao M, Glimm J, Kovach JS. Detection of cancer-specific markers amid massive mass spectral data. *Proceedings of the National Academy of Sciences* 2003;100: 14666–14671.

9. Adam B-L, Qu Y, Davis JW, Ward MD, Clements MA, Cazares LH, et al. Serum Protein Fingerprinting couple with a pattern-matching algorithm distinguishes prostate cancer from benign prostate hyperplasia and healthy men. *Cancer Research* 2003; 62:3609–3614.

10. Grubb RL, Calvert VS, Wulkuhle JD, Paweletz CP, Linehan WM, Phillips JL, et al. Signal pathway profiling of prostate cancer using reverse phase protein array. *Proteomics* 2003;3:2142–2146.

11. Li J, Zhang Z, Rosenzweig J, Wang YY, Chan DW. Proteomics and bioinformatics approaches for identification of serum bio-markers to detect breast cancer. *Clinical Chemistry* 2002;48: 1296–1304.

12. Sauter ER, Zhu W, Fan XJ, Wassell RP, Chervoneva I, Du Bois GC. Proteomic analysis of nipple aspirate fluid to detect biologic markers of breast cancer. *Br J Cancer* 2002; 86:1440–3.

13. Pawaletz CP, Trock B, Pennanen M, Tsangaris T, Magnant C, Liotta LA, et al. Proteomic patterns of nipple aspirate fluids obtained by SELDI-TOF: potential for new biomarkers to aid in the diagnosis of breast cancer. *Disease Markers* 2001;17:301–7.

14. Varnum SM, Covington CC, Woodbury RL, Petritis K, Kangas LJ, Abdullah MS, et al. Proteomic characterization of nipple aspirate fluid: identification of potential biomarkers of breast cancer. *Breast Cancer Research and Treatment* 2003;80:87–97.

15. Celis JE and Gromov. Proteomics in translational cancer research: Toward an integrated approach. *Cancer Cell* 2003 Jan;3:9–15.

16. Vlahou A, Schellhammer PF, Mendrinos S et al. Development of a novel proteomic approach for the detection of transitional cell carcinoma of the bladder in urine. *American Journal of Pathology* 2001;158:1491–1502.

17. Conrads TP, Fusaro VA, Ross S, Johann D, Rajapakse Vinodh, Hitt BA, et al. High-resolution serum proteomic features for ovarian cancer detection. Accepted for publication in *Endocrine-related Cancer*, June 2004.

18. Alexe G, Alexe S, Liotta LA, Petricoin E, Reiss M, Hammer PL. Ovarian cancer detection by logical analysis of proteomic data. *Proteomics* 2004;4:766.

19. Petricoin EF 3rd, Liotta LA. Serum Proteomic Patterns for Detection of Prostate Cancer 2003. *Journal of the National Cancer Institute* 2003;95(6):490–1.

20. Hingorani SR, Petricoin EF, Maitra A, Rajapakse V, King C, Jacobetz MA, Ross S, Conrads TP, Veenstra TD, Hitt BA, Kawaguchi Y, Johann D, Liotta LA, Crawford HC, Putt ME, Jacks T, Wright CV, Hruban RH, Lowy AM, Tuveson DA. Pre-invasive and invasive ductal pancreatic cancer and its early detection in the mouse. *Cancer Cell* 2004;5(1):103.

21. Wulfkuhle JD, Aquino JA, Calvert VS, Fishman DA, Coukos G, Liotta LA, and Petricoin EF. Signal pathway profiling of ovarian cancer from human tissue specimens using reverse-phase micro-arrays. *Proteomics* 2003 Nov;3(11):2085–90.

22. Liotta LA, Ferrari M, Petricoin EP. Written in Blood. *Nature* Oct 2003;425:905.

23. Tirumalai RS, Chan KC, Prieto DA, Issaq HJ, Conrads TP, Veenstra TD. Characterization of the low molecular weight human serum proteome. *Molecular and Cellular Proteomics* 2003;2(10):1096–103.

24. Mehta AI, Ross S, Lowenthal MS, Fusaro V, Fishman DA, Petricoin EF, Liotta LA. Biomarker amplification by serum carrier protein binding. *Disease Markers* 2003-2004; 19:1–10.

25. Petricoin EF, Fishman, DA, Conrads TP, Veenstra TD, and Liotta, LA. Proteomic Pattern Diagnostics: Producers and Consumers in the Era of Correlative Science. *BMC*

Bioinformatics, Posted March 12, 2004 (http://www.biomedcentral.com/1471-2105/4/24/comments).

26. Aebersold R and Mann M. Mass spectrometry-based proteomics. *Nature* 2003;422:198–207.

27. Wulfkuhle JD, Aquino JA, Calvert VS, Fishman DA, Coukos G, Liotta LA, and Petricoin EF. Signal pathway profiling of ovarian cancer from human tissue specimens using reverse-phase microarrays. *Proteomics* 2003 Nov;3(11):208–590.

28. Liotta LA, Ferrari M, Petricoin EP. Written in Blood. *Nature* Oct 2003;425:905.

29. Tirumalai RS, Chan KC, Prieto DA, Issaq HJ, Conrads TP, Veenstra TD. Characterization of the low molecular weight human serum proteome. *Molecular and Cellular Proteomics* 2003;2(10):1096–103.

30. Mehta AI, Ross S, Lowenthal MS, Fusaro V, Fishman DA, Petricoin EF, Liotta LA. Biomarker amplification by serum carrier protein binding. *Disease Markers* 2003-2004; 19:1–10.

31. Petricoin EF, Fishman,DA, Conrads TP, Veenstra TD, and Liotta, LA. Proteomic Pattern Diagnostics: Producers and Consumers in the Era of Correlative Science. *BMC Bioinformatics*, Posted March 12, 2004 (http://www.biomedcentral.com/1471-2105/4/24/comments).

32. Aebersold R and Mann M. Mass spectrometry-based proteomics. *Nature* 2003;422:198–207.

Chapter 23

Nanotechnology in Cancer Research

For several years, the National Cancer Institute (NCI) has supported exploratory work integrating nanotechnology into cancer research. The NCI is moving the science of nanotechnology into the clinic to change the way we diagnose, treat and prevent cancer.

Today, nanodevices are used in detecting cancer at its earliest stages, pinpointing its location within the body, delivering anticancer drugs specifically to malignant cells, and determining if these drugs are killing malignant cells. As research continues and nanodevices are evaluated for safety and efficacy, nanotechnology will result in significant advances in early detection, molecular imaging, assessment and therapeutic efficacy, targeted and multifunctional therapeutics, and the prevention and control of cancer.

Over the next five years, the NCI will fund $144.3 million in research and development through the NCI Alliance for Nanotechnology in Cancer. This Alliance will direct research efforts and facilitate partnerships across the scientific and research communities and the public and private sectors. These efforts capitalize on the multidisciplinary nature of nanotechnology development and will hasten its application to the elimination of suffering and death due to cancer.

"Nanotechnology in Cancer: Tools to Relieve Human Suffering," a National Cancer Institute (NCI) Technology Backgrounder, July 2004. For additional information, visit the NCI website at http://www.cancer.gov.

What Is Nanotechnology?

Nanotechnology is the development and engineering of devices so small that they are measured on a molecular scale. This emerging field involves scientists from many different disciplines, including physicists, chemists, engineers, information technologists, and material scientists, as well as biologists. Nanotechnology is being applied to almost every field imaginable, including electronics, magnetics, optics, information technology, materials development, and biomedicine.

The Size of Things

Nanoscale devices are one hundred to ten thousand times smaller than human cells. They are similar in size to large biological molecules ("biomolecules") such as enzymes and receptors. As an example, hemoglobin, the molecule that carries oxygen in red blood cells, is approximately five nanometers in diameter. Nanoscale devices smaller than 50 nanometers can easily enter most cells, while those smaller than 20 nanometers can move out of blood vessels as they circulate through the body.

Because of their small size, nanoscale devices can readily interact with biomolecules on both the surface and inside cells. By gaining access to so many areas of the body, they have the potential to detect disease and deliver treatment in ways unimagined before now.

Nanotechnology in Cancer Diagnosis and Therapy

Biological processes, including events that lead to cancer, occur at the nanoscale. Nanotechnology offers unprecedented access to the interior of living cells, and therefore provides researchers with the opportunity to study and interact with normal and cancer cells in real time, at the molecular and cellular scales, and during the earliest stages of the cancer process.

Nanodevices can provide rapid and sensitive detection of cancer-related molecules by enabling scientists to detect molecular changes even when they occur only in a small percentage of cells. They also have the potential to radically change cancer therapy for the better and to dramatically increase the number of highly effective therapeutic agents. Nanoscale constructs can serve as customizable, targeted drug delivery vehicles capable of ferrying large doses of chemotherapeutic agents or therapeutic genes into malignant cells while sparing healthy cells, greatly reducing or eliminating the side effects that accompany many current cancer therapies.

Examples of Nanotechnologies

Nanowires

Nano-sized sensing wires lay across a microfluidic channel. These nanowires by nature have incredible properties of selectivity and specificity. As particles flow through the microfluidic channel, the nanowire sensors pick up the molecular signatures of these particles and can immediately relay this information through a connection of electrodes to the outside world.

These nanodevices are man-made constructs made with carbon, silicon and other materials that have the capability to monitor the complexity of biological phenomenon and relay the information, as it is monitored, to the medical care provider. They can detect the presence of altered genes associated with cancer and may help researchers pinpoint the exact location of those changes.

Cantilevers

Nanoscale cantilevers—microscopic, flexible beams resembling a row of diving boards—are built using semiconductor lithographic techniques and coated with molecules capable of binding to the biomarkers of cancer.

As a cancer cell secretes its molecular products, the antibodies coated on the cantilever fingers selectively bind to these secreted proteins, changing the physical properties of the cantilever and signaling the presence of cancer. Researchers can read this change in real time and provide not only information about the presence and the absence but also the concentration of different molecular expressions.

Nanoscale cantilevers, constructed as part of a larger diagnostic device, can provide rapid and sensitive detection of cancer-related molecules.

Nanoshells

Nanoshells have a core of silica and a metallic outer layer. Scientists can link the nanoshells to antibodies that recognize tumor cells. Once the cancer cells take them up, scientists apply near-infrared light that is absorbed by the nanoshells, creating an intense heat that selectively kills the tumor cells and not neighboring healthy cells.

The result is greater efficacy of the therapeutic treatment and a significantly reduced set of side effects.

Nanoparticles

Nanoparticles can be engineered to target cancer cells for use in the molecular imaging of a malignant lesion. Large numbers of nanoparticles are safely injected into the body and preferentially bind to the cancer cell, defining the anatomical contour of the lesion and making it visible.

These nanoparticles give us the ability to see cells and molecules that we otherwise cannot detect through conventional imaging. The ability to pick up what happens in the cell—to monitor therapeutic intervention and to see when a cancer cell is mortally wounded or is actually activated—is critical to the successful diagnosis and treatment of the disease.

Nanoparticulate technology can prove to be very useful in cancer therapy allowing for effective and targeted drug delivery by overcoming the many biological, biophysical and biomedical barriers that the body stages against a standard intervention such as the administration of drugs or contrast agents.

Strategic Implementation: The Cancer Nanotechnology Plan

The Cancer Nanotechnology Plan (CNPlan) is a focused strategy to capitalize on past NCI investments in nanotechnology and direct those and new efforts on the immediate mission of the NCI. The plan carries an aggressive timeline and specific milestones to achieve the NCI goals. The projects initiated under the CNPlan will be integrated, milestone driven, and product oriented. The efforts will include targeted objectives and goals, and will use a project-management approach to help capitalize on today's opportunities to create the tools that both cancer researchers and clinicians need.

Based on the input NCI solicited from researchers and clinicians, the cancer community will be extremely involved in the implementation of the plan. NCI will continue to utilize traditional funding mechanisms to further promising research, and will supplement these efforts with a targeted approach that stresses interdisciplinary team efforts involving partners from across the cancer research and nanotechnology development communities.

The NCI Alliance for Nanotechnology in Cancer is a comprehensive, systematized initiative encompassing the public and private sectors, designed to accelerate the application of the best capabilities of nanotechnology to cancer. The Alliance is one of the first steps in implementing the CNPlan and focuses on applying research and translating it into clinical products in six key programmatic areas:

- **Molecular imaging and early detection:** diagnostics to detect cancer in the earliest, most easily treatable, pre-symptomatic stage

- **In vivo imaging:** targeted contrast agents that improve the resolution of cancer and address the diversity of tumors at the single cell level

- **Reporters of efficacy:** systems to provide real-time assessments of therapeutic and surgical efficacy

- **Multifunctional therapeutics:** multifunctional targeted devices to deliver multiple therapeutic agents directly to cancer cells

- **Prevention and control:** agents to monitor predictive molecular changes and prevent precancerous cells from becoming malignant

- **Research enablers:** research tools to identify new biological targets, opening new pathways for research

Part Four

Coping with Side Effects and Complications of Cancer Treatment

Chapter 24

Nausea and Vomiting

Nausea is an unpleasant wavelike feeling in the back of the throat and stomach that may or may not result in vomiting. Vomiting is the forceful elimination of the contents of the stomach through the mouth. Retching is the movement of the stomach and esophagus without vomiting and is also called dry heaves. Although treatments have improved, nausea and vomiting continue to be worrisome side effects of cancer therapy. Nausea may be even more distressing for patients than vomiting.

It is very important to prevent and control nausea and vomiting in patients with cancer. Uncontrolled nausea and vomiting can interfere with the patient's ability to receive cancer treatment and care for himself or herself by causing chemical changes in the body, loss of appetite, physical and mental difficulties, a torn esophagus, broken bones, and the reopening of surgical wounds.

Nausea and vomiting that are caused by cancer therapy are classified as follows:

Anticipatory nausea and vomiting: If a patient has had nausea and vomiting after the previous three or four chemotherapy treatments, he or she may experience anticipatory nausea and vomiting. The smells, sights, and sounds of the treatment room may remind the patient of previous episodes and may trigger nausea and vomiting before a new cycle of chemotherapy (or radiation therapy) has even begun.

PDQ® Cancer Information Summary. National Cancer Institute; Bethesda, MD. Nausea and Vomiting (PDQ®): Supportive Care - Patient. Updated 11/2005. Available at http://cancer.gov. Accessed November 10, 2006.

Acute nausea and vomiting: Usually occurs within 24 hours after beginning chemotherapy.

Delayed nausea and vomiting: Occurs more than 24 hours after chemotherapy. Also called late nausea and vomiting.

Chronic nausea and vomiting: May affect people who have advanced cancer. It is not well understood.

Causes

Nausea is controlled by a part of the central nervous system that controls involuntary bodily functions. Vomiting is a reflex controlled by a vomiting center in the brain. Vomiting can be stimulated by various triggers, such as smell, taste, anxiety, pain, motion, poor blood flow, irritation, or changes in the body caused by inflammation.

The most common causes of nausea and vomiting are chemotherapy drugs and radiation therapy directed at the gastrointestinal (GI) tract, liver, or brain.

Nausea and vomiting are more likely to occur if these characteristics are associated with the patient:

- Experienced severe episodes of nausea and vomiting after past chemotherapy sessions
- Is female
- Is younger than 50 years
- Has a fluid or electrolyte imbalance (hypercalcemia, dehydration, or an excess of fluid in the body's tissues)
- Has a tumor in the GI tract, liver, or brain
- Has constipation
- Is receiving certain drugs
- Has an infection or blood poisoning
- Has kidney disease
- Experiences anxiety

Anticipatory Nausea and Vomiting

Anticipatory nausea and vomiting occur after the patient has undergone several cancer treatments. It occurs in response to triggers, such as odors in the therapy room. For example, a person who begins chemotherapy and smells an alcohol swab at the same time may later experience nausea and vomiting at the smell of alcohol alone. Patients usually do not experience nausea or vomiting before or during chemotherapy until after they have received several courses of treatment. The following factors may help predict which patients are more likely to experience anticipatory nausea and vomiting:

- Being younger than 50 years

- Being female

- The severity of nausea and vomiting after the last chemotherapy session

- Feeling warm or hot after the last chemotherapy session

- A history of motion sickness

- Feeling dizzy or lightheaded after chemotherapy

- Sweating after the last chemotherapy session

- Experiencing weakness after the last chemotherapy session

- Having a high level of anxiety

- The type of chemotherapy (some are more likely to cause nausea and vomiting)

- Having morning sickness during pregnancy

Acute Nausea and Vomiting

Chemotherapy is the most common treatment-related cause of nausea and vomiting. The drug, dose, schedule of administration, route, and factors that are unique to the patient all determine how often nausea occurs and how severe it will be. Usually, these symptoms can be prevented or controlled.

Acute nausea and vomiting are more likely to occur in patients with these characteristics:

- Have experienced nausea and vomiting after previous chemotherapy sessions

- Are female

- Drink little or no alcohol

- Are young

Delayed Nausea and Vomiting

Delayed nausea and vomiting occurs more than 24 hours after chemotherapy. It is more likely to occur in patients with these characteristics:

- Are receiving high-dose chemotherapy regimens
- Have experienced acute nausea and vomiting with chemotherapy
- Are female
- Drink little or no alcohol
- Are young

Drugs to prevent nausea and vomiting may be given alone or in combinations to patients who are receiving chemotherapy.

Nausea and Vomiting in Advanced Cancer

Patients who have advanced cancer commonly experience chronic nausea and vomiting, which can significantly impair quality of life. Nausea and vomiting related to advanced cancer may be caused by the following:

- Use of opioids, antidepressants, and other pain medications
- Constipation (a common side effect of opioid use)
- Brain and colon tumors
- Abnormal levels of certain substances in the blood
- Dehydration
- Stomach ulcers

Radiation Therapy and Nausea and Vomiting

Radiation therapy may also cause nausea and vomiting, especially in patients who are undergoing radiation to the GI tract (particularly the small intestine and stomach) or brain. The risk for nausea and vomiting increases as the dose of radiation and area being irradiated increase. Nausea and vomiting associated with radiation therapy usually occurs one-half hour to several hours after treatment. Symptoms may improve on days the patient does not undergo radiation therapy.

Treatment

Anticipatory Nausea and Vomiting

Treatment of anticipatory nausea and vomiting is more likely to be successful when symptoms are recognized and treated early. Although antinausea drugs do not seem to be effective, the following may reduce symptoms:

- Guided imagery
- Hypnosis
- Relaxation
- Behavioral modification techniques
- Distraction (such as playing video games)

Acute/Delayed Nausea and Vomiting

Acute and delayed nausea and vomiting are most commonly treated with antinausea drugs. Some drugs last only a short time in the body, and need to be given more often; others last a long time and are given less frequently. Blood levels of the drug(s) must be kept constant to control nausea and vomiting effectively.

The following drugs are commonly given alone or in combinations to treat nausea and vomiting:

- Prochlorperazine
- Droperidol, haloperidol
- Metoclopramide
- Ondansetron, granisetron, dolasetron, palonosetron
- Aprepitant
- Dexamethasone, methylprednisolone
- Dronabinol
- Lorazepam, midazolam, alprazolam
- Olanzapine

Nausea and Vomiting Related to Constipation and Bowel Obstruction in Advanced Cancer

In patients with advanced cancer, constipation is one of the most common causes of nausea. To prevent constipation and decrease the risk for nausea and vomiting, it is important that a regular bowel routine be followed, even if the patient isn't eating. High-fiber diets and bulk-forming laxatives with psyllium or cellulose require large amounts of fluid, however, and are not well tolerated by patients with advanced cancer. Laxatives that soften the stool or stimulate the bowel may be prescribed to prevent constipation, especially if the patient is being treated with opioids for cancer pain. The use of enemas and rectal suppositories is limited to short-term, severe episodes of constipation. Patients who have a loss of bowel function because of nerve damage (such as a tumor pressing on the spinal cord) may require suppositories for regular bowel emptying. Enemas and rectal suppositories should not be used in patients who have damage to the bowel wall. Severe constipation may result in bowel obstruction.

Malignant bowel obstruction: Patients who have advanced cancer may develop a bowel obstruction that cannot be removed with surgery. The doctor may insert a nasogastric tube through the nose and esophagus into the stomach to temporarily relieve a partial obstruction. If the obstruction completely blocks the bowel, the doctor may insert a gastrostomy tube through the wall of the abdomen directly into the stomach to relieve fluid and air build-up. A gastrostomy tube also allows medications and liquids to be given directly into the stomach by pouring them down the tube. Sometimes, the doctor may create an ileostomy or colostomy by bringing part of the small intestine or colon through the abdominal wall to form an opening; or an expandable metal tube called a stent may be inserted into the bowel to open the blocked area. Injections or infusions of medications may be prescribed to relieve pain, nausea, and vomiting.

Alternative Therapies for Nausea and Vomiting

Nausea and vomiting may be controlled without using drugs. The following may be helpful in relieving symptoms, especially for anticipatory nausea and vomiting, and may improve the effectiveness of antinausea drugs:

- Nutrition
- Hypnosis
- Acupuncture
- Acupressure
- Guided imagery

Chapter 25

Appetite Loss
and Nutrition Therapy

Appetite Loss

Appetite changes are common with cancer and cancer treatment. Individuals with poor appetite or appetite loss may eat less than usual, not feel hungry at all, or feel full (satiated) after eating only a small amount. Ongoing appetite loss can lead to weight loss, malnutrition, and loss of muscle mass and strength. The combination of weight loss and loss of muscle mass, also called wasting, is referred to as cachexia.

Causes

Appetite loss is common in people with cancer. Certain types of cancer, including ovarian, pancreatic, and stomach cancers, can cause a loss of appetite, usually by affecting a person's metabolism. Cancer-related weight loss is not like starvation, and eating enough food doesn't solve the problem—unlike starvation. Weight loss associated with cancer results in a loss of muscle mass.

Appetite loss also occurs in 80% to 90% of people with advanced cancer for various reasons, including changes in metabolism, early satiety

---

This chapter begins with "Appetite Loss," reprinted with permission from the American Society of Clinical Oncology. © 2005. All rights reserved. Text under the heading "Nutrition Therapy Overview" is excerpted from PDQ® Cancer Information Summary. National Cancer Institute; Bethesda, MD. Nutrition in Cancer Care (PDQ®): Supportive Care - Patient. Updated 04/2006. Available at http://cancer.gov. Accessed June 26, 2006.

(feeling of fullness) from ascites (accumulation of fluid in the abdomen), and other symptoms of cancer.

Other causes of appetite loss include chemotherapy, immunotherapy, and sedative medications (drugs that cause feelings of calm or sleepiness). In addition, radiation treatment or surgery to any part of the gastrointestinal system, such as the stomach or intestines, can also cause appetite loss.

Several of the side effects commonly experienced with chemotherapy and radiation treatment may also cause appetite loss, including the following:

- Nausea and vomiting
- Mouth sores and mouth pain
- Dry mouth
- Swallowing difficulties
- Chewing difficulties
- Changes in taste and smell
- Pain
- Fatigue
- Depression

Management

If possible, the first step in treating appetite loss is to treat the underlying cause. Treatment for conditions such as mouth sores, dry mouth, pain, or depression should help improve appetite. Additional treatment for appetite loss and associated weight loss may include appetite-stimulating medications, medications that help food move through the intestine, nutritional supplement drinks, and tube feeding (often a nasogastric tube that passes through the nose into the stomach).

Although you may not feel like eating, it is important to remember that good nutrition and maintaining a healthy weight are important parts of overall cancer care and recovery. Eating well can also help a person better cope physically and emotionally with the effects of cancer and cancer treatment. The following tips may be helpful in maintaining proper nutrition when your appetite is poor.

- Eat five to six small meals a day and snack whenever you are hungry.

- Determine what times of day you are hungry, make sure to eat at those times, and do not limit how much you eat.

- Eat nutritious snacks that are high in calories and protein (for example, dried fruits, nuts, yogurt, cheeses, eggs, milkshakes, ice cream, cereal, pudding, and granola bars).

- Keep favorite foods on hand for snacking.

- Add calories and protein to foods by adding sauces, gravy, butter, cheese, peanut butter, cream, and nuts.

- Drink fluids between meals rather than with meals. Drinking during a meal can make you feel full too quickly.

- Choose nutritious drinks, such as milk, milkshakes, and juices.

- Ask family members or friends to prepare foods when you are too tired to cook. Ask them to shop for groceries or buy precooked meals.

- Try to eat in pleasant surroundings and eat meals with family or friends.

- Eat food that is cold or at room temperature to decrease its odor and reduce its taste.

- Ask your doctor about ways to relieve other gastrointestinal symptoms, such as nausea, vomiting, and constipation.

- If your sense of taste is diminished, try adding spices and condiments to foods to make them more appealing.

- Try light exercise, such as a 20 minute walk, about an hour before meals to stimulate your appetite. (Consult your doctor before starting an exercise program.) Exercise also helps maintain muscle mass.

- Drink a glass of sherry or wine before a meal to help increase appetite.

- Meet with a registered dietitian (RD) for additional advice on meal planning.

Nutrition Therapy Overview

Nutrition Screening and Assessment

Early nutrition screening and assessment can identify problems that affect the success of anticancer therapy. Patients who are underweight or malnourished may not respond well to cancer treatments. Malnutrition may be caused by the cancer or made worse as the cancer progresses. Finding and treating nutrition problems early may help the patient gain or maintain weight, improve the patient's response to therapy, and reduce complications of treatment.

Because the ability to tolerate treatment is better for the well-nourished patient, screening and assessment are done before beginning anticancer therapy. Appropriate nutrition management is begun early, and nutritional status is checked often during treatment.

Screening is used to identify patients who may be at nutritional risk. Assessment determines the complete nutritional status of the patient and identifies if nutrition therapy is needed. The patient or caregiver may be asked for the following information:

- Weight changes over the past six months
- Changes in the amount and type of food eaten compared to what is usual for the patient
- Problems that have affected eating, such as nausea, vomiting, diarrhea, constipation, dry mouth, changes in taste and smell, mouth sores, pain, or loss of appetite
- Ability to walk and perform the activities of daily living

A physical exam is part of the assessment. The physical exam will check the body for general health and signs of disease, such as lumps or growths. The physician will look for loss of weight, fat and muscle, and fluid buildup in the body.

A nutrition support team will monitor the patient's nutritional status during cancer treatment and recovery. The team may include the following specialists:

- Physician
- Nurse
- Registered dietitian
- Social worker
- Psychologist

Goals of Nutrition Therapy

The goals of nutrition therapy for cancer patients in active treatment and recovery are designed to restore nutrient shortages, maintain nutritional health, and prevent complications. The goals of nutrition therapy for patients in active treatment and recovery are to do the following:

- Prevent or correct malnutrition
- Prevent wasting of muscle, bone, blood, organs, and other lean body mass
- Help the patient tolerate treatment
- Reduce nutrition-related side effects and complications
- Maintain strength and energy
- Protect ability to fight infection
- Help recovery and healing
- Maintain or improve quality of life

A patient whose religion forbids eating certain foods may consider speaking with a religious leader about waiving the restriction during cancer treatment and recovery.

Good nutrition continues to be important for patients who are in remission or whose cancer has been cured.

The goals of nutrition therapy for patients who have advanced cancer are designed to improve the quality of life. The goals of nutrition therapy for patients who have advanced cancer are to do the following:

- Reduce side effects
- Reduce risk of infection
- Maintain strength and energy
- Improve quality of life

Methods of Nutrition Care

Nutrition support provides nutrition to patients who cannot eat normally. Eating by mouth is the preferred method and should be used whenever possible, but some patients may not be able to take any or enough food by mouth due to complications from cancer or cancer treatment. This may include patients with cancer of the head, neck, esophagus, or stomach. A patient may be fed using enteral nutrition (through a tube inserted into the stomach or intestine) or parenteral nutrition infused into the bloodstream directly). The nutrients are delivered in formulas, liquids that contain water, protein, fats, carbohydrates, vitamins, or minerals. The content of the formula depends on the needs of the patient and the method of feeding.

Nutritional support can improve a patient's quality of life during cancer, but there are risks and disadvantages that should be considered before making the decision to use it. The effect of nutritional support on tumor growth is not known. Also, each form of nutrition therapy has its own benefits and disadvantages. For example, enteral nutrition keeps the stomach and intestines working normally and has fewer complications than parenteral nutrition; nutrients are used more easily by the body in enteral feeding. These and other issues should be discussed with the patient's health care providers so that an informed decision can be made.

Patients with certain conditions are most appropriate for treatment with nutrition support. Nutrition support may be helpful for patients who have one or more of the following characteristics:

- Low body weight
- Inability to absorb nutrients
- Holes or draining abscesses in the esophagus or stomach
- Inability to eat or drink by mouth for more than five days
- Moderate or high nutritional risk
- Ability, along with the caregiver, to handle tube feedings at home

Enteral Nutrition

Enteral nutrition is also called tube feeding. Enteral nutrition is food (in liquid form) given to the patient through a tube that is inserted into the stomach or the small intestine. The following types of tube feeding may be used:

- A tube inserted through the nose and throat down into the stomach or small intestine. This kind of tube is usually used for short-term use.

- A tube inserted into the stomach or small intestine through a stoma (an opening made on the outside of the abdomen). This kind of tube is usually chosen for long-term use or for patients who cannot tolerate a tube in the nose and throat.

If the tube is placed in the stomach, food may be given through the tube continuously or in batches several times a day. If the tube is placed in the small intestine, the food is delivered continuously. Different formulas are available. Some provide complete nutrition and others provide certain nutrients. Formulas that meet the patient's specific needs are selected. Formulas are available for patients who have other health conditions, such as diabetes.

Enteral nutrition is sometimes used when the patient is able to eat small amounts by mouth but cannot obtain enough food that way. The patient may continue to eat or drink as able, and the tube feeding provides the balance of calories and nutrients that are needed.

Enteral nutrition may be appropriate for patients whose gastrointestinal tract is still working. Enteral nutrition continues to use the stomach and intestines to digest food. Enteral nutrition may be used for patients who have cancer of the head, neck, or digestive system and whose treatment with chemotherapy and radiation therapy causes side effects that limit eating or drinking.

Enteral nutrition is not appropriate for the following patients:

- Patients whose stomach and intestines are not working, or have been removed

- Patients who have a blockage in the bowel

- Patients who have severe nausea, vomiting, or diarrhea

- Patients whose platelet count is low. Platelets are blood cells that help prevent bleeding by causing blood clots to form.

- Patients who have low levels of all blood cells (white blood cells, red blood cells, and platelets)

Enteral nutrition may continue after a patient leaves the hospital. If enteral nutrition is to be part of the patient's care after leaving the hospital, the patient and caregiver will be trained in use of the tube and pump, and in care of the patient. The home must be clean and the patient must be monitored often by the nutrition support team.

Parenteral Nutrition

Parenteral nutrition provides the patient with nutrients delivered into the blood stream. Parenteral nutrition is used when the patient cannot take food by mouth or by enteral feeding. Parenteral feeding bypasses the normal digestive system. Nutrients are delivered to the patient directly into the blood, through a catheter (thin tube) inserted into a vein. Patients with the following problems may benefit from parenteral nutrition:

- Stomach and intestines that are not working or have been removed

- Severe nausea, diarrhea, or vomiting
- Severe sores in the mouth or esophagus
- A fistula (hole) in the stomach or esophagus
- Loss of body weight and muscle with enteral nutrition

A central venous catheter is placed beneath the skin and into a large vein in the upper chest. Placement of a central venous catheter is done by a surgeon.

A peripheral venous catheter is placed into a vein in the arm. Placement of a peripheral venous catheter is done by trained medical staff. This site may be used for short-term parenteral feeding.

The patient is checked often for infection or bleeding at the site (place) where the catheter enters the body.

Some drugs should not be given with parenteral formulas. Many drugs and other substances do not mix safely with the formulas used for parenteral feeding. A pharmacist or doctor should be consulted before adding anything to the formula or using the catheter for another substance.

Trained medical staff should manage the use of parenteral nutrition. The techniques and formulas involved in parenteral nutrition support are precise and require management by trained medical staff or a nutrition support team. Some of the serious complications that may occur with parenteral feeding include the following:

- Placement of the tip of the catheter into the wrong place
- Blood clots
- A collapsed lung
- A high or low sugar level in the blood
- A low potassium level in the blood
- Elevated liver enzymes

If parenteral nutrition is to be part of the patient's care after leaving the hospital, the patient and caregiver will be trained in the procedures and in care of the patient. The home must be clean and the patient must be monitored often by the nutrition support team.

Experienced medical staff should manage the patient's removal from parenteral nutrition support. Going off parenteral nutrition support needs to be done gradually and under medical supervision. The parenteral feedings are reduced by small amounts over time as the patient is changed to enteral or oral feeding.

Chapter 26

Weight Gain

Although it is more common to lose weight during cancer treatment, some people with cancer gain weight. Slight increases in weight during cancer treatment are generally not problematic. However, significant weight gain may affect a person's health and the ability to tolerate treatments.

Weight gain is an especially important health issue for people living with breast cancer, as over half of women experience weight gain during treatment. Reports have shown that weight gain is linked to a poorer prognosis (chance of recovery). Being overweight before treatment begins also increases the risk of serious health conditions, such as high blood pressure, diabetes, and cardiovascular disease.

Causes

The following cancer treatments may produce symptoms that lead to weight gain:

Chemotherapy: Some chemotherapy causes the body to retain (hold on) to excess fluid in cells and tissues, called edema.

- A decrease in physical activity, usually from fatigue, can cause people to exercise less and leads to weight gain.

- Chemotherapy can increase hunger (especially for high-fat foods) and can trigger intense food cravings.

- Chemotherapy has been shown to decrease metabolism (the rate that energy is used), which can cause weight gain.

- Chemotherapy can cause menopause in some women, which is associated with changes in metabolism that can increase the likelihood of weight gain.

Steroid medications: Steroids are hormonal substances that are used in cancer treatment. They can cause an increase in fatty issue, resulting in a big belly and fullness in the neck or face. Steroids can also cause peripheral wasting (the loss of muscle mass). A noticeable increase in weight usually only happens when people have been taking steroids continuously for many weeks.

Hormone therapy: Hormone therapy for the treatment of breast, uterine, prostate, and testicular cancers involves medications that decrease the amount of estrogen or progesterone in women and testosterone in men. Hormone therapy can increase body mass from fat, decrease body mass from muscle, and change how food is metabolized, resulting in weight gain.

Managing Weight Gain

If gaining weight becomes a concern, consult a doctor or registered dietitian (RD) before starting a diet or changing eating habits. They can help discover the possible cause of the weight gain and find the best way to manage it. In addition, an RD can provide nutritional guidelines or a customized diet plan.

Ways to manage diet and physical activity include the following:

- Eat plenty of fruits, vegetables, breads, and cereals.

- Limit fats, simple sugars, and refined flour.

- Drink plenty of water.

- Evaluate everyday eating habits and try to identify behavior patterns that lead to overeating and inactivity.

- Check with a doctor about increasing the amount of exercise.

- Do strength-building exercises for the arms and shoulders if muscle mass has been lost.

Signs of Fluid Retention

It is important to immediately call a doctor if there are any of the following signs of fluid retention:

- Skin that feels stiff (small indentations left on the skin after pressing on the swollen area)
- Swelling around ankles and wrists
- Rings, wristwatches, bracelets, or shoes that fit tighter than usual
- Decreased flexibility in hands, elbows, wrists, fingers, or legs

The following tips can help a person manage fluid retention:

- Ask a doctor about prescribing a diuretic medication to rid the body of excess water.
- Lower the amount of salt in the diet.
- Avoid standing for long periods and elevate feet as often as possible.
- Avoid crossing the legs, which restricts blood flow.
- Monitor body weight daily.
- Avoid tight clothing.

Chapter 27

Gastrointestinal Complications of Cancer Treatment

Constipation

In persons with cancer, constipation may be a symptom of cancer, a result of a growing tumor, or a result of cancer treatment. Constipation may also be a side effect of medications for cancer or cancer pain and may be a result of other changes in the body (organ failure, decreased ability to move, and depression). Other causes of constipation include dehydration and not eating enough. Cancer, cancer treatment, aging, and declining health can contribute to causing constipation.

More specific causes of constipation that can result in bowel impaction include the following:

Diet

- Not including enough high-fiber foods in the diet
- Not drinking enough water or other fluids

Changed Bowel Habits

- Repeatedly ignoring the urge to pass stool
- Using too many laxatives and enemas

Excerpted from PDQ® Cancer Information Summary. National Cancer Institute; Bethesda, MD. Gastrointestinal Complications (PDQ®): Supportive Care - Patient. Updated 01/2006. Available at http://cancer.gov. Accessed April 30, 2006.

Immobility and Lack of Exercise

- Spinal cord injury, spinal cord compression, bone fractures, fatigue, weakness, long periods of bed rest
- Inability to tolerate movement and exercise due to respiratory or cardiac problems

Medications

- Chemotherapy treatments
- Pain medications
- Medications for anxiety and depression
- Stomach antacids
- Diuretics
- Vitamin supplements such as iron and calcium
- Sleep medications
- General anesthesia

Bowel Disorders

- Irritable colon
- Diverticulitis
- Tumor

Muscle and Nerve Disorders (nerve damage can lead to loss of muscle tone in the bowel)

- Brain tumors
- Spinal cord compression from a tumor or other spinal cord injury
- Stroke or other disorders that cause muscle weakness or movement
- Weakness of the diaphragm or abdominal muscles making it difficult to take a deep breath and push to have a bowel movement

Body Metabolism Disorders

- Under-secretion of the thyroid gland

- Increased level of calcium in the blood
- Low levels of potassium or sodium in the blood
- Diabetes with nerve dysfunction

Environmental Factors

- Needing assistance to go to the bathroom
- Being in unfamiliar surroundings or a hurried atmosphere
- Living in extreme heat leading to dehydration
- Needing to use a bedpan or bedside commode
- Lack of privacy

Assessment of Constipation

A medical history and physical examination can identify the causes of constipation. The examination may include a digital rectal exam (the doctor inserts a gloved, lubricated finger into the rectum to check for stool impaction) or a test for blood in the stool. If cancer is suspected, a thorough examination of the rectum and colon may be done with a lighted tube inserted through the anus and into the colon.

Treatment

Treatment of constipation includes prevention (if possible), elimination of possible causes, and limited use of laxatives. Suggestions for the patient's treatment plan may include the following:

- Keep a record of all bowel movements.
- Increase the fluid intake by drinking eight 8-ounce glasses of fluid each day (patients who have kidney or heart disease may need to limit fluid intake).
- Exercise regularly, including abdominal exercises in bed or moving from the bed to chair if the patient cannot walk.
- Increase the amount of dietary fiber by eating more fruits (raisins, prunes, peaches, and apples), vegetables (squash, broccoli, carrots, and celery), and whole grain cereals, breads, and bran. Patients must drink more fluids when increasing dietary fiber or they may become constipated. Patients who have had a bowel

obstruction or have undergone bowel surgery (for example, a colostomy) should not eat a high-fiber diet.

- Drink a warm or hot drink about one half-hour before the patient's usual time for a bowel movement.

- Provide privacy and quiet time when the patient needs to have a bowel movement.

- Help the patient to the toilet or provide a bedside commode instead of a bedpan.

- Take only medications prescribed by the doctor.

- Do not use suppositories or enemas unless ordered by the doctor. In some cancer patients, these treatments may lead to bleeding, infection, or other harmful side effects.

Impaction

Five major factors can cause impaction:

1. Opioid pain medications

2. Inactivity over a long period

3. Changes in diet

4. Mental illness

5. Long-term use of laxatives

Regular use of laxatives for constipation contributes most to the development of constipation and impaction. Repeated use of laxatives in higher and higher doses makes the colon less able to signal the need to have a bowel movement. (Refer to the Constipation section for causes of constipation that can result in impaction.)

Patients with impaction may have symptoms similar to patients with constipation, or they may have back pain (the impaction presses on sacral nerves) or bladder problems (the impaction presses on the ureters, bladder, or urethra). The patient's abdomen may become enlarged causing difficulty breathing, rapid heartbeat, dizziness, and low blood pressure. Other symptoms can include explosive diarrhea (as stool moves around the impaction), leaking stool when coughing, nausea, vomiting, abdominal pain, and dehydration. Patients who have an impaction may become very confused and disoriented with rapid heartbeat, sweating, fever, and high or low blood pressure.

Assessment of Impaction

The doctor will ask questions concerning bowel movement and do a physical examination to find out if the patient has an impaction. The examination may also include x-rays of the abdomen or chest, blood tests, and an electrocardiogram (a test that shows the activity of the heart).

Treatment of Impaction

Impactions are usually treated by moistening and softening the stool with an enema. Enemas must be given very carefully as prescribed by the doctor since too many enemas can damage the bowel. Some patients may need to have stool manually removed from the rectum after it is softened. Glycerin suppositories may also be prescribed. Laxatives that stimulate the bowel and cause cramping must be avoided since they can damage the bowel even more.

Bowel Obstruction

A bowel obstruction may be caused by a narrowing of the intestine from inflammation or damage to the bowel, tumors, scar tissue, hernias, twisting of the bowel, or pressure on the bowel from outside the intestinal tract. It can also be caused by factors that interfere with the function of muscles, nerves, and blood flow to the bowel. Most bowel obstructions occur in the small intestine and are usually caused by scar tissue or hernias. The rest occur in the colon (large intestine) and are usually caused by tumors, twisting of the bowel, or diverticulitis. Symptoms will vary depending on whether the small or large intestine is involved.

The most common cancers that cause bowel obstructions are cancers of the colon, stomach, and ovary. Other cancers, such as lung and breast cancers, and melanoma, can spread to the abdomen and cause bowel obstruction. Patients who have had abdominal surgery or radiation are at a higher risk of developing a bowel obstruction. Bowel obstructions are most common during the advanced stages of cancer.

Assessment of Bowel Obstruction

The doctor will do a physical examination to find out whether the patient has abdominal pain, vomiting, or any movement of gas or stool in the bowel. Blood and urine tests may be done to detect any fluid and blood chemistry imbalances or infection. Abdominal x-rays and a barium enema may also be done to find the location of the bowel obstruction.

Treatment of Acute Bowel Obstruction

Patients who have abdominal symptoms that continue to become worse must be monitored frequently to prevent or detect early signs and symptoms of shock and constricting obstruction of the bowel. Medical treatment is necessary to prevent fluid and blood chemistry imbalances and shock.

A nasogastric tube may be inserted through the nose and esophagus into the stomach, or a colorectal tube may be inserted through the rectum into the colon to relieve pressure from a partial bowel obstruction. The nasogastric tube or colorectal tube may decrease swelling, remove fluid and gas build-up, or decrease the need for multiple surgical procedures; however, surgery may be necessary if the obstruction completely obstructs the bowel.

Treatment of Chronic, Malignant Bowel Obstruction

Patients who have advanced cancer may have chronic, worsening bowel obstruction that cannot be removed with surgery. Sometimes, the doctor may be able to insert an expandable metal tube called a stent into the bowel to open the area that is blocked.

When neither surgery nor a stent placement is possible, the doctor may insert a gastrostomy tube through the wall of the abdomen directly into the stomach by a very simple procedure. The gastrostomy tube can relieve fluid and air build-up in the stomach and allow medications and liquids to be given directly into the stomach by pouring them down the tube. A drainage bag with a valve may also be attached to the gastrostomy tube. When the valve is open, the patient may be able to eat or drink by mouth without any discomfort because the food drains directly into the bag. This gives the patient the experience of tasting the food and keeping the mouth moist. Solid food should be avoided because it may block the tubing to the drainage bag.

If the patient's comfort is not improved with a stent or gastrostomy tube, and the patient cannot take anything by mouth, the doctor may prescribe injections or infusions of medications for pain, nausea, or vomiting.

Diarrhea

In cancer patients, the most common cause of diarrhea is cancer treatment (chemotherapy, radiation therapy, bone marrow transplantation, or surgery). Other causes of diarrhea include antibiotic therapy, stress and anxiety related to being diagnosed with cancer and undergoing cancer treatment; and infection. Infection may be caused by viruses, bacteria, fungi, or other harmful microorganisms. Antibiotic therapy can cause inflammation of the lining of the bowel, resulting in diarrhea that often does not respond to treatment. Other causes of diarrhea in cancer patients include the following:

- The cancer itself
- Physical reactions to diet
- Medical problems and diseases other than cancer
- The laxative regimen
- Bowel impaction with leakage of stool around the blockage

Undergoing surgery to the stomach or intestines can affect normal bowel function and cause diarrhea. Some chemotherapy drugs cause diarrhea by affecting how nutrients are broken down and absorbed in the small bowel. Radiation therapy to the abdomen and pelvis can cause inflammation of the bowel. Patients may have problems digesting food, and experience gas, bloating, cramping, and diarrhea. These symptoms may last up to 8 to 12 weeks after therapy or may not develop for months or years. Treatment may include diet changes, medications, or surgery. Patients who are undergoing radiation therapy while receiving chemotherapy often experience severe diarrhea. Hospitalization may not be required, since an outpatient clinic or special home care nursing may give the care and support needed. Each patient's symptoms should be evaluated to determine if intravenous fluids or special medication should be prescribed.

Patients who undergo donor bone marrow transplantation may develop graft-versus-host disease (GVHD). Stomach and intestinal symptoms of GVHD include nausea and vomiting, severe abdominal pain and cramping, and watery, green diarrhea. Symptoms may occur one week to three months after transplantation. Some patients may require long-term treatment and diet management.

Assessment

Because diarrhea can be life-threatening, it is important to identify the cause so treatment can begin as soon as possible. The doctor may ask the following questions:

- How often have you had bowel movements in the past 24 hours?
- When was your last bowel movement? What was it like (how much, how hard or soft, what color)? Was there any blood?

- Have you been dizzy, extremely drowsy, or had any cramping, abdominal pain, nausea, vomiting, fever, or rectal bleeding?
- What have you eaten? What and how much have you had to drink in the past 24 hours?
- Have you lost weight recently? How much?
- How often have you urinated in the past 24 hours?
- What medicine are you taking? How much and how often?
- Have you traveled recently?

The doctor will also do a physical examination that should include checking blood pressure, pulse, and respirations; evaluation of the skin and tissue lining the inside of the mouth to check for blood circulation and amount of fluid in the tissue; examination of the abdomen for pain, tenderness, and bowel sounds; and a rectal exam to check for stool impaction and collect stool to test for blood.

Stool may be tested in the laboratory to check for bacterial, fungal, or viral infections. Blood and urine tests may be done to detect fluid and blood chemistry imbalances or infection.

In some cases, abdominal x-rays may also be done to identify bowel obstruction or other abnormalities. In rare cases, a thorough examination of the rectum and colon may be done with a lighted tube inserted through the anus and into the colon.

Treatment

Diarrhea is treated by identifying and treating the problems causing diarrhea. For example, diarrhea may be caused by stool impaction and medications to prevent constipation. The doctor may make changes in medications, diet, and fluids. Diet changes that may help decrease diarrhea include eating small frequent meals and avoiding some of the following foods:

- Milk and dairy products
- Spicy foods
- Alcohol
- Caffeine-containing foods and drinks
- Some fruit juices
- Gas-forming foods and drinks
- High-fiber foods
- High-fat foods

For mild diarrhea, a diet of bananas, rice, apples, and toast (the BRAT diet) may decrease the frequency of stools. Patients should be encouraged to drink up to three quarts of clear fluids per day including water, sports drinks, broth, weak decaffeinated tea, caffeine-free soft drinks, clear juices, and gelatin. For severe diarrhea, the patient may need intravenous fluids or other forms of intravenous nutrition.

To manage diarrhea caused by graft-versus-host disease (GVHD), the doctor may recommend a special 5-phase diet. During phase 1, the patient receives intravenous fluids and nothing by mouth to rest the bowel until the diarrhea slows down. In phase 2, the patient may begin drinking fluids. If the patient is able to drink fluids and the diarrhea improves, he or she may begin phase 3, eating solid foods that are low-fiber, low-fat, low-acid, and do not irritate the stomach. In phase 4, the patient is gradually allowed to eat regular foods. If the patient is able to eat regular foods without any episodes of diarrhea, he or she may begin phase 5, eating their regular diet. Many patients may continue to have problems digesting milk and dairy products.

Depending on the cause of the diarrhea, the doctor may change the laxative therapy regimen or may prescribe medications that slow down bowel activity, decrease bowel fluid secretions, and allow nutrients to be absorbed by the bowel.

Radiation Enteritis

Radiation therapy stops the growth of rapidly dividing cells, such as cancer cells. Since normal cells in the lining of the bowel also divide rapidly, radiation treatment can stop those cells from growing, making it difficult for bowel tissue to repair itself. As bowel cells die and are not replaced, gastrointestinal problems develop over the next few days and weeks.

Patients with acute enteritis may have the following symptoms:

- Nausea
- Vomiting
- Abdominal cramps
- Frequent urges to have a bowel movement
- Rectal pain, bleeding, or mucus-like discharge
- Watery diarrhea

With diarrhea, the gastrointestinal tract does not function normally, and nutrients such as fat, lactose, bile salts, and vitamin B_{12} are not well absorbed.

251

Symptoms of acute enteritis usually gets better two to three weeks after treatment ends.

Patients with chronic enteritis may have the following symptoms:

- Wave-like abdominal pain
- Bloody diarrhea
- Frequent urges to have a bowel movement
- Greasy and fatty stools
- Weight loss
- Nausea
- Vomiting

Less common symptoms of chronic enteritis are bowel obstruction, holes in the bowel, and heavy rectal bleeding.

Symptoms usually appear six to 18 months after radiation therapy ends. Before determining that chronic radiation enteritis is causing these symptoms, recurrent tumors need to be ruled out. The radiation history of the patient is important in making the correct diagnosis.

Assessment of Radiation Enteritis

Patients will be given a physical exam and be asked questions about the following:

- Usual pattern of bowel movements
- Pattern of diarrhea, including when it started; how long it has lasted; frequency, amount, and type of stools; and other symptoms (such as gas, cramping, bloating, urgency, bleeding, and rectal soreness).
- Nutritional health of the patient, including height and weight, usual eating habits, any change in eating habits, amount of fiber in the diet, and signs of dehydration (such as poor skin tone, increased weakness, or feeling very tired)
- Current level of stress, ability to cope, and changes in lifestyle caused by the enteritis

Treatment of Acute Radiation Enteritis

Treatment of acute enteritis includes treating the diarrhea, loss of fluids, poor absorption, and stomach or rectal pain. These symptoms usually get better with medications, changes in diet, and rest. If symptoms become worse even with this treatment, then cancer treatment may have to be stopped, at least temporarily.

Medications that may be prescribed include antidiarrheals to stop diarrhea, opioids to relieve pain, and steroid foams to relieve rectal inflammation and irritation. If patients with pancreatic cancer have diarrhea during radiation therapy, they may need pancreatic enzyme replacement, because not having enough of these enzymes can cause diarrhea.

Nutrition: Nutrition also plays a role in acute enteritis. Intestines damaged by radiation therapy may not make enough or any of certain enzymes needed for digestion, especially lactase. Lactase is needed for the digestion of milk and milk products. A lactose-free, low-fat, and low-fiber diet may help to control symptoms of acute enteritis.

Foods to avoid include the following:

- Milk and milk products, except buttermilk and yogurt. Processed cheese may not cause problems because the lactose is removed during processing. Lactose-free milkshake supplements, such as Ensure, may also be used.
- Whole-bran bread and cereal
- Nuts, seeds, and coconut
- Fried, greasy, or fatty foods
- Fresh and dried fruit and some fruit juices (such as prune juice)
- Raw vegetables
- Rich pastries
- Popcorn, potato chips, and pretzels
- Strong spices and herbs
- Chocolate, coffee, tea, and soft drinks with caffeine
- Alcohol and tobacco

The following are examples of foods to choose:

- Fish, poultry, and meat that are cooked, broiled, or roasted
- Bananas, applesauce, peeled apples, and apple and grape juices
- White bread and toast
- Macaroni and noodles
- Baked, boiled, or mashed potatoes

- Cooked vegetables that are mild, such as asparagus tips, green and waxed beans, carrots, spinach, and squash
- Mild processed cheese, eggs, smooth peanut butter, buttermilk, and yogurt

Here are some helpful hints:

- Eat food at room temperature.
- Drink three liters (about 12 eight-ounce glasses) of fluid a day.
- Allow carbonated beverages to lose their fizz before drinking them.
- Add nutmeg to food to help decrease movement of the gastrointestinal tract.
- Start a low-fiber diet on the first day of radiation therapy.

Treatment of Chronic Radiation Enteritis

Treatment of the symptoms of chronic radiation enteritis is the same as treatment of acute radiation enteritis. Surgery is used to treat severe damage. Fewer than 2% of affected patients will need surgery to control their symptoms.

Two types of surgery may be used:

- Intestinal bypass, a procedure in which the doctor creates a new pathway for the flow of bowel contents.
- Complete removal of the diseased intestines.

The patient's general health and the amount of damaged tissue are considered before surgery is attempted, however, because wound healing is often slow and long-term tube-feeding may be needed. Even after surgery, many patients still have symptoms.

To lower the risk that chronic radiation enteritis will occur, different treatment methods are used to reduce the area that is exposed to radiation. Patients may be positioned to protect as much of the small bowel as possible from the radiation treatment, or may be asked to have a full bladder during treatment to help push the small bowel out of the way. The amount of radiation may be adjusted to deliver lower amounts more evenly or higher amounts to specific areas. If a patient has surgery, clips may be placed at the tumor site to help show the area to be irradiated.

Chapter 28

Oral Complications of Cancer Treatment

Oral complications are common in patients receiving chemotherapy or undergoing radiation therapy to the head and neck. The oral cavity is at high risk of side effects from chemotherapy and radiation therapy for a number of reasons.

- Chemotherapy and radiation therapy stop the growth of rapidly dividing cells, such as cancer cells. Since normal cells in the lining of the mouth also divide rapidly, anticancer treatment can prevent cells in the mouth from reproducing, making it difficult for oral tissue to repair itself.

- The mouth contains hundreds of different bacteria, some helpful and some harmful. Chemotherapy and radiation therapy can cause changes in the lining of the mouth and production of saliva and upset the healthy balance of bacteria. These changes may lead to mouth sores, infections, and tooth decay.

- Wear and tear occurs from normal use of the mouth, teeth, and jaws, making healing more difficult.

Oral complications associated with chemotherapy and radiation therapy may be caused directly by the treatment or may result indirectly from side effects of the treatment. Radiation therapy may directly

Excerpted from PDQ® Cancer Information Summary. National Cancer Institute; Bethesda, MD. Oral Complications of Chemotherapy and Head/Neck Radiation (PDQ®): Supportive Care - Patient. Updated 09/2005. Available at http://cancer.gov. Accessed April 30, 2006.

damage oral tissue, salivary glands, and bone. Areas treated may scar or waste away.

Slow healing and infection are indirect complications of cancer treatment. Both chemotherapy and radiation therapy can affect the ability of cells to reproduce, which slows the healing process in the mouth. Chemotherapy may reduce the number of white blood cells and weaken the immune system (the organs and cells that defend the body against infection and disease), making it easier for the patient to develop an infection.

Complications can be acute or chronic. Acute complications are those that occur during therapy. Chemotherapy usually causes acute complications that heal after treatment ends.

Chronic complications are those that continue or develop months to years after therapy ends. Radiation can cause acute complications but may also cause permanent tissue damage that puts the patient at a lifelong risk of oral complications. The following chronic complications commonly continue after radiation therapy to the head or neck has ended:

- Dry mouth
- Tooth decay
- Infections
- Taste changes
- Problems using the mouth and jaw due to tissue and bone loss or the growth of benign tumors in the skin and muscle

Prevention and Treatment before Chemotherapy and Radiation Therapy Begins

Oral complications in patients undergoing treatment for head and neck cancer may be reduced by aggressive prevention measures taken before treatment begins. This will get the mouth and teeth in the best possible condition to withstand treatment.

Preventive measures include the following:

- Eating a well-balanced diet. Proper nutrition can help the body tolerate the stress of cancer treatment, maintain energy, fight infection, and rebuild tissue.

- Learning how to care for the mouth and teeth during and after anticancer therapy. Good dental hygiene helps prevent cavities, mouth sores, and infections.

- Having a complete oral health exam by a dentist familiar with the oral side effects of anticancer treatments.

The cancer care team should include the patient's dentist. It is important to choose a dentist familiar with the oral side effects of chemotherapy and radiation therapy. An evaluation of the patient's oral health at least a month before treatment begins usually provides enough time for the mouth to heal after dental work. The dentist will identify and treat teeth at risk for infection or decay, so the patient may avoid having invasive dental treatment during anticancer therapy. The dentist may also provide appropriate preventive care to lessen the severity of dry mouth, a common complication of radiation therapy to the head and neck.

The goal of the oral care plan is to find and treat oral disease that may produce complications during treatment and to continue oral care throughout treatment and recovery. Different oral complications may occur during the different phases of transplantation. Steps can be taken ahead of time to prevent or lessen the severity of these side effects.

Ongoing oral care during radiation therapy will depend on the specific needs of the patient; the dose, locations, and duration of the radiation treatment; and the specific complications that occur.

Management during and after Chemotherapy and Radiation Therapy

Routine Oral Care

Continuing good dental hygiene during and after cancer treatment can reduce complications such as cavities, mouth sores, and infections. It is important to clean the mouth after eating. The following are helpful hints for everyday oral care during chemotherapy and radiation therapy:

- Rinse the toothbrush in hot water every 15 to 30 seconds to soften the bristles, if needed.

- Choose toothpaste with care:
  - Use a mild-tasting toothpaste; flavoring may irritate the mouth.
  - If toothpaste irritates the mouth, brush with a solution of 1 teaspoon of salt added to 4 cups (1 quart) of water.
  - Use a fluoride toothpaste.

- One of the following rinses made with salt or baking soda may be used:
  - 1 teaspoon of salt in 4 cups of water.
  - 1 teaspoon of baking soda in 1 cup (8 ounces) of water.
  - ½ teaspoon salt and 2 tablespoons baking soda in 4 cups of water.

Oral Mucositis

Mucositis is an inflammation of mucous membranes in the mouth. The terms "oral mucositis" and "stomatitis" are often used in place of each other, but their meanings are different.

- Mucositis is an inflammation of mucous membranes in the mouth. It usually appears as red, burn-like sores or as ulcer-like sores throughout the mouth.

- Stomatitis is an inflammation of tissues in the mouth, such as the gums, tongue, roof and floor of the mouth, and tissues inside the lips and cheeks. It includes infections of mucous membranes.

Mucositis may be caused by either radiation therapy or chemotherapy. In patients receiving chemotherapy, mucositis will heal by itself, usually in two to four weeks when there is no infection. Mucositis caused by radiation therapy usually lasts six to eight weeks, depending on the duration of treatment.

The following problems may occur:

- Pain
- Infection
- Bleeding, in patients receiving chemotherapy. Patients undergoing radiation therapy usually do not have a bleeding risk.
- Inability to breathe and eat normally

Swishing ice chips in the mouth for 30 minutes may help prevent mucositis from developing in patients who are given fluorouracil. Medication may be given to help prevent mucositis or keep it from lasting as long in patients who undergo high-dose chemotherapy and bone marrow transplant.

Treatment of mucositis caused by either radiation therapy or chemotherapy is generally the same. After mucositis has developed, proper treatment depends on its severity and the patient's white blood cell count. The following are guidelines for treating mucositis during chemotherapy, stem cell transplantation, and radiation therapy:

Cleaning the Mouth

- Use water-soluble lubricating jelly to moisturize the mouth.

- Use bland rinses or plain sterile water. Frequent rinsing removes particles and bacteria from the mouth, prevents crusting of sores, and moistens and soothes sore gums and the lining of the mouth. The following rinse may be used to neutralize acid and dissolve thick saliva:

  - ½ teaspoon salt and 2 tablespoons baking soda in 4 cups of water.

- If crusting of sores occurs, the following rinse may be used:

  - Equal parts hydrogen peroxide and water or saltwater (1 teaspoon of salt in 4 cups of water). This should not be used for more than two days because it will keep mucositis from healing.

Relieving Pain

- Try topical medications for pain. Rinse the mouth before applying the medication onto the gums or lining of the mouth. Wipe mouth and teeth gently with wet gauze dipped in saltwater to remove particles.

- Painkillers may provide relief when topical medications do not. Nonsteroidal anti-inflammatory drugs (NSAIDs, aspirin-type painkillers) should not be used by patients receiving chemotherapy because these patients have a bleeding risk.

- Capsaicin, the active ingredient in hot peppers, may be used to increase a person's ability to tolerate pain. When capsaicin is put on inflamed tissues in the mouth, mucositis pain may decrease as the burning feeling from the capsaicin decreases. The side effects of capsaicin are not known.

Infection

Oral mucositis breaks down the lining of the mouth, allowing germs and viruses to get into the bloodstream. When the immune system is weakened by chemotherapy, even good bacteria in the mouth can cause infections, as can disease-causing organisms picked up from the hospital or other sources. As the white blood cell count gets lower, infections may occur more often and become more serious. Patients who have low white blood cell counts for a long time are more at risk of developing serious infections. Dry mouth, common during radiation therapy to the head and neck, may also raise the risk of infections in the mouth. Preventive dental care during chemotherapy and radiation therapy can reduce the risk of mouth, tooth, and gum infections. The following types of infections may occur:

Bacterial infections: Treatment of bacterial infections in patients who have gum disease and receive high-dose chemotherapy may include the following:

- Medicated and peroxide mouth rinses
- Brushing and flossing
- Wearing dentures as little as possible

Bacterial infections in patients undergoing radiation therapy are usually treated with antibiotics.

Fungal infections: The mouth normally contains fungi that can exist on or in the body without causing any problems. An overgrowth of fungi, however, can be serious and requires treatment.

Antibiotics and steroid drugs are often used when a patient receiving chemotherapy has a low white blood cell count. These drugs change the balance of bacteria in the mouth, making it easier for a fungal overgrowth to occur. Fungal infections are common in patients treated with radiation therapy.

Drugs may be given to prevent fungal infections from occurring. Treatment of surface fungal infections in the mouth only may include mouthwashes and lozenges that contain antifungal drugs. These are used after removing dentures, brushing the teeth, and cleaning the mouth. An antibacterial rinse should be used on dentures and dental appliances and to rinse the mouth.

Deeper fungal infections, such as those in the esophagus or intestines, are treated with drugs taken by mouth or injection.

Viral infections: Patients receiving chemotherapy, especially those with weakened immune systems, are at risk of mild to serious viral infections. Finding and treating the infections early is important. Drugs may be used to prevent or treat viral infections.

Herpesvirus infections may recur in radiation therapy patients who have these infections.

Bleeding

Bleeding may occur during chemotherapy when anticancer drugs affect the ability of blood to clot. Areas of gum disease may bleed on their own or when irritated by eating, brushing, or flossing. Bleeding may be mild (small red spots on the lips, soft palate, or bottom of the mouth) or severe, especially at the gumline and from ulcers in the mouth. When blood counts drop below certain levels, blood may ooze from the gums.

With close monitoring, most patients can safely brush and floss throughout the entire time of decreased blood counts. Continuing regular oral care will help prevent infections that may further complicate bleeding problems. The dentist or doctor can provide guidance on how to treat bleeding and safely keep the mouth clean when blood counts are low.

Treatment for bleeding during chemotherapy may include the following:

- Medications to reduce blood flow and help clots form

- Topical products that cover and seal bleeding areas

- Rinsing with a mixture of one part 3% hydrogen peroxide to 2 or 3 parts saltwater solution (1 teaspoon of salt in 4 cups of water) to help clean oral wounds. Rinsing must be done carefully so clots are not disturbed.

Dry Mouth

Dry mouth (xerostomia) occurs when the salivary glands produce too little saliva. Saliva is needed for taste, swallowing, and speech. It helps prevent infection and tooth decay by neutralizing acid and cleaning the teeth and gums. Chemotherapy and radiation therapy can damage salivary glands, causing them to produce too little saliva. The mouth is less able to clean itself. Acid in the mouth is not neutralized, and minerals are lost from the teeth. Tooth decay and gum disease are more likely to develop. Symptoms of dry mouth include the following:

- Thick, stringy saliva

261

- Increased thirst
- Changes in taste, swallowing, and speech
- A sore or burning feeling (especially on the tongue)
- Cuts or cracks in the lips or at the corners of the mouth
- Changes in the surface of the tongue
- Difficulty wearing dentures

Dry mouth during chemotherapy is usually temporary. The salivary glands often recover two to eight weeks after chemotherapy ends.

Saliva production drops within one week after starting radiation therapy to the head or neck and continues to decrease as treatment continues. The severity of dry mouth depends on the dose of radiation and the number of glands irradiated. The salivary glands in the upper cheeks near the ears are more affected than other salivary glands.

Partial recovery of salivary glands may occur in the first year after radiation therapy, but recovery is usually not complete, especially if the salivary glands were directly irradiated. Salivary glands that were not irradiated may become more active to offset the loss of saliva from the destroyed glands.

Careful oral hygiene can help prevent mouth sores, gum disease, and tooth decay caused by dry mouth. The following are guidelines for managing dry mouth:

- Use a fluoride toothpaste when brushing
- Apply fluoride gel once a day at bedtime, after cleaning the teeth
- Rinse 4 to 6 times a day with a solution of salt and baking soda (mix ½ teaspoon salt and ½ teaspoon baking soda in 1 cup of warm water). Avoid foods and liquids that contain a lot of sugar. Sip water to relieve mouth dryness.

Tooth Decay

Dry mouth and changes in the balance of oral bacteria increase the risk of tooth decay. Meticulous oral hygiene and regular care by a dentist can help prevent cavities.

Taste Changes

Change in the sense of taste (dysgeusia) is a common side effect of both chemotherapy and head or neck radiation therapy. Foods may have no taste or may not taste as they did before therapy. These taste changes are caused by damage to the taste buds, dry mouth, infection, or dental problems. Chemotherapy patients may experience unpleasant taste related to the spread of the drug within the mouth. Radiation may cause a change in sweet, sour, bitter, and salty tastes.

In most patients receiving chemotherapy and in some patients undergoing radiation therapy, taste returns to normal a few months after therapy ends. For many radiation therapy patients, however, the change is permanent. In others, the taste buds may recover six to eight weeks, or later, after radiation therapy ends. Zinc sulfate supplements may help with the recovery for some patients.

Unpleasant changes in the taste of food can cause a patient with cancer to lose the desire to eat. The patient's quality of life and nutritional well-being may be affected by loss of appetite. The following suggestions may help patients with cancer manage taste changes and meet nutritional needs:

- Change the texture of food. Serving food chopped, ground, or blended can reduce the amount of time it needs to stay in the mouth before being swallowed.
- Eat between-meal snacks to add calories and nutrients.
- Choose foods high in calories and protein.
- Take supplements that provide vitamins, minerals, and calories.

Pain

If an anticancer drug is causing the pain, stopping the drug usually stops the pain. Because there may be many causes of oral pain during cancer treatment, a careful diagnosis is important. This may include obtaining a medical history, performing physical and dental exams, and taking x-rays of the teeth.

Tooth sensitivity may occur in some patients weeks or months after chemotherapy has ended. Fluoride treatments or toothpaste for sensitive teeth may relieve the discomfort.

Pain in the teeth or jaw muscles may occur in patients who grind their teeth or clench their jaws, often because of stress or the inability to sleep. Treatment may include the following:

- Muscle relaxers
- Drugs to treat anxiety
- Physical therapy (moist heat, massage, and stretching)
- Mouthguards to wear while sleeping

Jaw Stiffness

A long-term complication of radiation therapy is the growth of benign tumors in the skin and muscles. These tumors may make it difficult for the patient to move the mouth and jaw normally. Oral surgery may also affect jaw mobility. Management of jaw stiffness may include the following:

- Physical therapy
- Oral appliances
- Pain treatments
- Medication

Tissue and Bone Loss

Radiation therapy can cause tissue and bone in the treated area to waste away. When tissue death occurs, ulcers may form in the soft tissues of the mouth, grow in size, and cause pain or loss of feeling. Infection becomes a risk. As bone tissue is lost, fractures can occur. Preventive care can lessen the severity of tissue and bone loss. Treatment of tissue and bone loss may include the following:

- Eating a well-balanced diet
- Wearing removable dentures or appliances as little as possible
- Not smoking
- Not drinking alcohol
- Using topical antibiotics
- Using painkillers
- Undergoing surgery to remove dead bone or to reconstruct bones of the mouth and jaw
- Receiving hyperbaric oxygen therapy, a method of delivering oxygen under pressure to the surface of a wound to help it heal

Management of Oral Complications of High-Dose Chemotherapy and Stem Cell Transplant

Graft-versus-host disease (GVHD) is a reaction of donated bone marrow or stem cells against the patient's tissue. Symptoms of oral GVHD include the following:

- Sores that appear in the mouth two to three weeks after the transplant
- Dry mouth
- Pain from spices, alcohol, or flavoring (such as mint in toothpaste)

Biopsies taken from the lining of the mouth and salivary glands may be needed to diagnose oral GVHD. Treatment of oral GVHD may include the following:

- Topical rinses, gels, creams, or powders
- Antifungal drugs taken by mouth or injection
- Psoralen (a drug used with ultraviolet light to treat skin disease)
- Drugs that promote the production of saliva
- Fluoride treatments
- Treatments to replace minerals lost from teeth by acids in the mouth

The following are guidelines for the care and use of dentures, braces, and other oral appliances during high-dose chemotherapy or stem cell transplant:

- Remove brackets, wires, and retainers before high-dose chemotherapy begins.
- Wear dentures only when eating during the first three to four weeks after the transplant.
- Brush dentures twice a day and rinse them well.
- Soak dentures in an antibacterial solution when they are not being worn.
- Clean denture soaking cups and change denture soaking solution every day.
- Remove appliances or dentures when cleaning the mouth.
- If mouth sores are present, avoid wearing removable appliances until the mouth is healed.

Routine dental treatments, including scaling and polishing, should be delayed until the transplant patient's immune system returns to normal. Caution is advised for at least a year after the transplant.

Relapse and Second Cancers

Cancer survivors who received chemotherapy or a transplant or who underwent radiation therapy are at risk of developing a second cancer later in life. Oral squamous cell cancer is the most common second cancer occurring in transplant patients. The lips and tongue are the sites most often affected.

Mental and Social Considerations

The social aspects of oral complications can make them the most difficult problems for cancer patients to cope with. Oral complications affect eating and speaking and may make the patient unable or unwilling to take part in mealtimes or to dine out. Patients may become frustrated, withdrawn, or depressed, and they may avoid other people. Some drugs that are used to treat depression may not be an option because they cause side effects that make oral complications worse.

Education, supportive care, and the treatment of symptoms are important for patients who have mouth problems that are related to cancer therapy. Patients will be closely monitored for pain, ability to cope, and response to treatment. Supportive care from health care providers and family can help the patient cope with cancer and its complications.

Special Considerations for Children

A change in dental growth and development is a special complication for cancer survivors who received high-dose chemotherapy or radiation therapy to the head and neck for childhood cancers. Changes may occur in the size and shape of the teeth; eruption of teeth may be delayed; and development of the head and face may not reach full maturity. The role and timing of orthodontic treatment for patients with altered dental growth and development is under study. Some treatments have been successful, but standard guidelines have not yet been established.

Chapter 29

Alopecia (Hair Loss)

A potential side effect of radiation therapy and chemotherapy is hair loss (alopecia). Hair loss may occur throughout the body, including the head, face, arms, legs, underarms, and pubic area. The hair may fall out entirely, gradually, or in sections. In some cases, the hair will simply thin—sometimes unnoticeably—and may become duller and dryer. Losing one's hair can be a psychologically and emotionally challenging experience and can affect a person's self-image and quality of life. However, the hair loss is usually temporary, and the hair grows back.

Causes

Radiation therapy and chemotherapy cause hair loss by damaging the hair follicles responsible for hair growth.

Chemotherapy: Not all chemotherapy causes hair loss. (A doctor can provide more information regarding which drugs are most likely to cause hair loss.) When hair loss does occur, it is usually not immediate, and the amount of hair loss varies from person to person, even among those taking the same medication. Hair loss most often starts after the first several weeks or rounds of chemotherapy treatment and tends to increase one to two months into treatment. The amount of hair loss depends on the type of drug, dose, and how the drug was given (orally, intravenously, or topically). Hair regrowth following chemotherapy usually occurs one to three months after maintenance treatment starts or intensive chemotherapy ends.

Radiation therapy: Radiation therapy only affects the portions of hair that are in the field of radiation. Hair loss depends on the dose and method of radiation treatment. When very high doses of radiation are used to treat cancer, the hair may become permanently lost or thinned in the treated area. If regrowth does occur, patients may find the regrown hair to be different in texture and thickness than the original hair.

Management

In some cases, hair loss due to cancer treatment is not preventable or treatable with stimulants, solutions, or special shampoos. Therefore, learning to deal with hair loss before it occurs can help a person better adjust to this change in physical appearance. Talking about feelings with a counselor, someone with a similar experience, family member, or friend may also provide comfort. Also, it may be helpful to talk about inevitable hair loss with family and friends, especially children, before it occurs. If children know to expect changes in the physical appearance of someone they are familiar with, it helps reduce feelings of anxiety.

Some people recommend cutting the hair shorter before treatment. This not only helps create volume and fullness for the shorter hairstyle, but also is less dramatic of a change when the hair falls out. Furthermore, when the hair begins to regrow, it takes less time to reach the shorter hairstyle. Having a hairstyle similar to the one before chemotherapy can help a person cope with the end of treatment and move forward.

Hair and scalp care: The following recommendations may help when caring for the hair and scalp during cancer treatment:

- Choose a mild shampoo, such as a baby shampoo, to clean the hair.
- Choose a soft hairbrush and gently style the remaining hair.
- Use sun protection on the scalp when outdoors, including sunscreen, hats, or a scarf.
- Cover the head during the cold months to prevent loss of body heat.

- Avoid blow-drying the hair with high heat.

- Avoid curling or straightening the hair with chemical products.

- Avoid permanent or semi-permanent hair coloring.

- Choose a soft, comfortable covering for the bed pillow.

Wig and hairpieces: The following information may be helpful if a patient chooses to wear a wig or hairpiece:

- Select the wig or hairpiece before the hair falls out if you prefer to match the current hair color and style. A hairdresser can style the wig/hairpiece to your liking.

- If shopping for a wig/hairpiece in a retail store is not appealing, there are wig and hairpiece shops specially designed for people with cancer. A home appointment can also be scheduled, or an order can be placed through a catalog or the internet.

- If finances are a concern, ask the patient's insurance provider if wigs/hairpieces are covered with cancer treatment or classified as a tax-deductible medical expense. To be covered by insurance, the doctor may have to prescribe the use of a wig/hairpiece with proper documentation. Free or loaner wigs/hairpieces may also be available. Ask an oncology social worker or nurse for resources within the hospital or local community.

- Be sure to have the wig/hairpiece fitted properly so that it does not irritate the scalp.

Caring for regrown hair: Complete hair regrowth often takes six to twelve months. When new hair regrows, at least temporarily, the texture may feel thinner than the hair that was lost. Pigment cells usually restore themselves, however, and hair usually returns to its original color. When caring for regrown hair:

- Limit washing the hair to twice a week.

- Massage the scalp to remove dry skin and flakes.

- Style hair with care and limit the amount of hard brushing, pinning, curling, or blow-drying with high heat, as new hair will initially be much finer and more prone to breaking than the original hair.

- Gently use a wide-tooth comb to style the regrown hair.

- Avoid curling or straightening the hair with chemical products (as in permanent wave solutions) until the hair is at least three inches long or until it is comfortable. Some individuals may need to wait for up to one year before they can chemically curl or straighten their hair.

- Avoid permanent or semi-permanent hair coloring for at least three months following treatment.

Chapter 30

Nervous System Disturbances

The nervous system is made up of the central nervous system (CNS) and the peripheral nervous system (PNS). The CNS is made up of the brain and spinal cord. The PNS is made up of the nerves outside of the CNS that carry information back and forth between the body and the brain. The PNS is involved in movement, sensing (touching, hearing, seeing, tasting, and smelling), and functioning of the internal organs, (for example, the stomach, lungs, and heart).

Nervous system disturbances are common side effects of cancer and cancer treatments and can affect any part of the nervous system. This chapter will outline nervous system disturbances, possible causes, and management.

Types of Nervous System Disturbances

Some of the different types of nervous system disturbances that may result from cancer or cancer treatment include the following:

- Hearing loss or tinnitus (ringing in the ears)
- Vision loss or vision disturbances (such as blurred or double vision)
- Speech difficulties, such as slurred speech
- Changes in taste and smell

- Problems with balance, dizziness, vertigo (feeling like the room is spinning), and nausea

- Problems with coordination (known as ataxia) and movement, including problems with posture, walking, or holding objects; clumsiness

- Generalized weakness (known as asthenia), characterized by an overall lack of bodily strength; drowsiness

- Paralysis of different parts of the body, ranging from paralysis of one side of the body (known as hemiplegia) to paralysis of a smaller area, such as the facial muscles

- Seizures

- Changes in the functioning of organs, resulting in symptoms, such as constipation, incontinence (inability to control bodily elimination), and erectile dysfunction (also called impotence or an inability to achieve or maintain an erection)

- Pain, resulting from damage to the nerves

- Peripheral neuropathy, a condition caused by damage or irritation to the peripheral nerves causing symptoms, such as numbness, tingling ("pins and needles"), or burning pain in the arms, hands, legs, or feet; decreased ability to sense hot and cold; difficulty lifting the feet or toes; difficulty picking up small objects; decreased muscle strength; vision or hearing changes; or constipation

Causes

Nervous system disturbances can be caused by many different factors, including cancer, cancer treatments, medications, or other disorders. Symptoms that are caused by disruption or damage to the nerves caused by cancer treatment (such as surgery, radiation treatment, or chemotherapy) can appear soon after treatment or many years later. Possible causes include the following:

- Cancers that affect the nervous system, such as brain cancer and sarcomas of the nerves (for example, neurofibrosarcoma, malignant peripheral nerve sheath tumor, peripheral primitive neuroectodermal tumor)

- Cancerous tumors growing in other parts of the body that press on nerves

- Cancers that metastasize (spread) to the brain

- Chemotherapy medications, such as vincristine (Oncovin), vinblastine (Velban), paclitaxel (Taxol), cisplatin (Platinol), carboplatin (Paraplatin), oxaliplatin (Eloxatin), fluorouracil (5-FU), cytarabine (Ara-C)

- Radiation treatment, especially to the head and neck or total body irradiation

- Surgery—nerves may be damaged or disrupted during surgery to remove cancerous tumors or perform biopsies

- Medications, including some antinausea drugs, antibiotics, heart medications, diuretics, and nonsteroidal anti-inflammatory drugs

- Infections causing swelling or inflammation of the brain, spinal cord, or inner ear

- Other conditions or symptoms related to cancer or cancer treatments, including anemia, dehydration, fatigue, stress, and depression

- Other conditions or disorders not related to cancer, such as diabetes, multiple sclerosis, and nerve injury

Management

Nervous system disturbances can be very distressing for patients and, in serious cases, can make it difficult for patients to complete normal, daily activities. Some symptoms caused by cancer treatment will resolve after treatment ends, but some may continue indefinitely. Although nerve damage and nervous system disturbances may not be preventable, most are effectively treated if diagnosed early. Early treatment can also prevent symptoms from becoming more problematic. It is important to tell your doctor immediately if you experience any symptoms that could indicate a nervous system disturbance. Once diagnosed, management of nervous system disturbances may include the following:

- Medications, such as antinausea/antivertigo drugs like meclizine (Antivert, Bonine), prochlorperazine (Compazine), or scopolamine patch (Transderm-Scop); antibiotics; and corticosteroids (to reduce inflammation and swelling)

- Pain medications, including opioid (strong) pain killers, as well as tricyclic antidepressants like nortriptyline (Pamelor, Aventyl)

273

amitriptyline (Elavil, Endep), or seizure medications like gabapentin (Neurontin) used to treat peripheral neuropathy and other types of nerve pain (known as neuropathic pain)

- Nerve blocks and transcutaneous electric nerve stimulation (TENS), which provide pain relief

- Occupational therapy, to enhance motor skills needed for daily activities, such as getting dressed, picking up small objects, writing, or doing household chores

- Physical therapy, to enhance physical strength, balance, coordination, and mobility

- Changes to the home environment to increase safety, such as installing hand rails in the bathroom, using nonskid rugs, adding extra lighting, and checking water temperature with the elbow rather than the hands

Chapter 31

Cancer-Related Fatigue

What is the difference between fatigue and tiredness?

Fatigue is often confused with tiredness. Tiredness happens to everyone. It is an expected feeling after certain activities or at the end of the day. Usually, you know why you are tired, and a good night's sleep solves the problem.

Fatigue is a daily lack of energy; an unusual or excessive whole-body tiredness not relieved by sleep. It can be acute (lasting a month or less) or chronic (lasting from one month to six months or longer). Fatigue can prevent a person from functioning normally and impacts a person's quality of life.

What is cancer-related fatigue?

Cancer-related fatigue (CRF) is one of the most common side effects of cancer and its treatment. It is not predictable by tumor type, treatment, or stage of illness. Usually, it comes on suddenly, does not result from activity or exertion, and is not relieved by rest or sleep. It is often described as "paralyzing." It might continue even after treatment is complete.

"Cancer-Related Fatigue," © 2003 The Cleveland Clinic Foundation, 9500 Euclid Avenue, Cleveland, OH 44195, www.clevelandclinic.org. Additional information is available from the Cleveland Clinic Health Information Center, 216-444-3771, toll-free 800-223-2273 extension 43771, or at http://www.clevelandclinic.org/health.

What causes CRF?

The exact reason for CRF is unknown. CRF might be related to the disease process or its treatments.

Cancer Treatments Commonly Associated with Fatigue

- *Chemotherapy:* Any chemotherapy drug might cause fatigue, but it might be a more common side effect of drugs such as vincristine, vinblastine, and cisplatin. Patients frequently experience fatigue after several weeks of chemotherapy, but this varies among patients. In some patients, fatigue lasts a few days, while others report fatigue persisting throughout the course of treatment and continuing after the treatment is complete.

- *Radiation therapy:* Radiation therapy can cause cumulative fatigue (fatigue that increases over time). This can occur regardless of the treatment site. Fatigue usually lasts from three to four weeks after treatment stops but can continue for up to two to three months.

- *Bone marrow transplant:* This aggressive form of treatment can cause fatigue that lasts up to one year.

- *Biological therapy:* Interferons and interleukins are cytokines, natural cell proteins that are normally released by white blood cells in response to infection. These cytokines carry messages that regulate other elements of the immune and endocrine systems. In high amounts, these cytokines can be toxic and lead to persistent fatigue.

- *Combination therapy:* More than one cancer treatment at the same time or one after the other increases the chances of developing fatigue.

Other Factors That May Contribute to Cancer-Related Fatigue

- In a tumor-induced "hypermetabolic" state, tumor cells compete for nutrients, often at the expense of the normal cells' growth. In addition to fatigue, weight loss and decreased appetite are common effects.

- Decreased nutrition from the side effects of treatments (such as nausea, vomiting, mouth sores, taste changes, heartburn, and diarrhea) can cause fatigue.

- Cancer treatments can cause reduced blood counts, which might lead to anemia, a blood disorder that occurs when there is not enough hemoglobin in the blood. Hemoglobin is a substance in the red blood cells that enables the blood to transport oxygen through the body. When the blood cannot transport enough oxygen to the body, fatigue can result.

- If the thyroid gland is under-active (hypothyroidism), metabolism might slow down so that the body does not burn food fast enough to provide adequate energy. This is a common condition in general, but it might happen after radiation therapy to the lymph nodes in the neck.

- Medicines used to treat side effects such as nausea, pain, depression, anxiety, and seizures can cause fatigue.

- Research shows that chronic, severe pain increases fatigue.

- Stress can worsen feelings of fatigue. Stress can result from dealing with the disease and the "unknowns," as well as from worrying about daily accomplishments or trying to meet the expectations of others.

- Fatigue might result when patients try to maintain their normal daily routines and activities during treatments. Modification might be necessary in order to conserve energy.

- Depression and fatigue often go hand-in-hand. It might not be clear which started first. One way to sort this out is to try to understand your depressed feelings and how they affect your life. If you are depressed all the time, were depressed before your cancer diagnosis, are preoccupied with feeling worthless and useless, you might need treatment for depression.

What can I do to combat fatigue?

The best way to combat fatigue is to treat the underlying medical cause. Unfortunately, the exact cause is often unknown or there might be multiple causes.

There are some medical treatments that might help improve fatigue caused by hypothyroidism or anemia. Other causes of fatigue must be managed on an individual basis.

The following are tips you can use to combat fatigue.

Assessment

1. Evaluate your level of energy

- Think of your personal energy stores as a "bank." Deposits and withdrawals have to be made over the course of the day or the week to balance energy conservation, restoration, and expenditure.

- Keep a diary for one week to identify the time of day when you are either most fatigued or have the most energy. Note what you think might be contributing factors.

2. Be alert to your personal warning signs of fatigue.

- Fatigue warning signs might include tired eyes, tired legs, whole-body tiredness, stiff shoulders, decreased energy or a lack of energy, inability to concentrate, weakness or malaise, boredom or lack of motivation, sleepiness, increased irritability, nervousness, anxiety, or impatience.

Energy Conservation

1. Plan ahead and organize your work.

- Change storage of items to reduce trips or reaching.
- Delegate tasks when needed.
- Combine activities and simplify details.

2. Schedule rest.

- Balance periods of rest and work.
- Rest before you become fatigued. Frequent, short rests are beneficial.

3. Pace yourself.

- A moderate pace is better than rushing through activities.
- Reduce sudden or prolonged strains.
- Alternate sitting and standing.

4. Practice proper body mechanics.

- When sitting, use a chair with good back support. Sit up with your back straight and your shoulders back.
- Adjust the level of your work. Work without bending over.
- When bending to lift something, bend your the knees and use your leg muscles, not your back, to lift. Do not bend forward at the waist with your knees straight.

- Carry several small loads instead of one large one, or use a cart.

5. Limit work that requires reaching over your head.
   - Use long-handled tools.
   - Store items lower.
   - Delegate activities whenever possible.

6. Limit work that increases muscle tension (isometric work).
   - Breathe evenly, do not hold your breath.
   - Wear comfortable clothes to allow for free and easy breathing.

7. Identify effects of your environment.
   - Avoid extremes of temperature.
   - Eliminate smoke or harmful fumes.
   - Avoid long, hot showers or baths.

8. Prioritize your activities.
   - Decide which activities are important to you, and what could be delegated.
   - Use your energy on important tasks.

Nutrition

Cancer-related fatigue is often made worse if you are not eating enough or if you are not eating the right foods. Maintaining good nutrition can help you feel better and have more energy. The following are strategies to help improve nutritional intake:

1. Meet your basic calorie needs. The estimated calorie needs for someone with cancer is 15 calories per pound of weight if your weight has been stable. Add 500 calories per day if you have lost weight. Example: A person who weighs 150 lbs. needs about 2250 calories per day to maintain his or her weight.

2. Include protein in your diet. Protein rebuilds and repairs damaged (and normally aging) body tissue. The estimated protein needs are 0.5–0.6 grams of protein per pound of body weight. Example: A 150 lb. person needs 75–90 grams of protein per day. The best sources of protein include foods from the dairy group

(8 oz. milk = 8 grams protein) and meats (meat, fish, or poultry = 7 grams of protein per ounce).

3. Drink plenty of fluids. A minimum of 8 cups of fluid per day will prevent dehydration. (That's 64 ounces, 2 quarts or 1 half-gallon). Fluids can include juice, milk, broth, milkshakes, gelatin, and other beverages. Of course, water is fine, too. Beverages containing caffeine do NOT count. Keep in mind that you'll need more fluids if you have treatment side effects such as vomiting or diarrhea.

4. Make sure you are getting enough vitamins. Take a vitamin supplement if you are not sure you are getting enough nutrients. A recommended supplement would be a multivitamin that provides at least 100 percent of the recommended daily allowances (RDA) for most nutrients. Note: vitamin supplements do not provide calories, which are essential for energy production. So vitamins cannot substitute for adequate food intake.

5. Make an appointment with a dietitian. A registered dietitian provides suggestions to work around any eating problems that might be interfering with proper nutrition (such as early feeling of fullness, swallowing difficulty, or taste changes). A dietitian can also suggest ways to maximize calories and include proteins in smaller amounts of food (such as powdered milk, instant breakfast drinks, and other commercial supplements or food additives).

Exercise

Decreased physical activity, which might be the result of illness or of treatment, can lead to tiredness and lack of energy. Scientists have found that even healthy athletes forced to spend extended periods in bed or sitting in chairs develop feelings of anxiety, depression, weakness, fatigue, and nausea.

Regular, moderate exercise can decrease these feelings, help you stay active, and increase your energy. Even during cancer therapy, it is often possible to continue exercising.

Here are some exercise guidelines:

*   Every patient should consult with his or her health care provider before beginning an exercise program.

*   A good exercise program starts slowly, allowing your body time to adjust.

- Keep a regular exercise schedule—exercise at least three times a week. Even more dangerous than not exercising at all is exercising only occasionally.

- The right kind of exercise never makes you feel sore, stiff, or exhausted. If you experience soreness, stiffness, exhaustion, or feel out of breath as a result of your exercise, you are overdoing it.

- Most exercises are safe, as long as you exercise with caution and you don't overdo it. The safest and most productive activities are swimming, brisk walking, indoor stationary cycling, and low-impact aerobics (taught by a certified instructor). These activities carry little risk of injury and benefit your entire body.

Stress Management

Managing stress can play an important role in combating fatigue. The following are some suggestions:

1. Adjust your expectations. For example, if you have a list of 10 things you want to accomplish today, pare it down to two and leave the rest for other days. A sense of accomplishment goes a long way to reducing stress.

2. Help others understand and support you. Family and friends can be helpful if they can "put themselves in your shoes" and understand what fatigue means to you. Cancer support groups can be a source of support as well. Other people with cancer understand what you are going through.

3. Relaxation techniques such as audio tapes that teach deep breathing or visualization can help reduce stress.

4. Activities that divert your attention away from fatigue can also be helpful. For example, activities such as knitting, reading, or listening to music require little physical energy but require attention.

If your stress seems out of control, talk to a health care professional. They are here to help.

Talk to Your Health Care Providers

Although cancer-related fatigue is a common, and often expected, side effect of cancer and its treatments, you should feel free to mention your concerns to your health care providers. There are times when fatigue might be a clue to an underlying medical problem. Other times, there might be medical interventions to assist in controlling some of the causes of fatigue. Finally, there might be suggestions that are more specific to your situation that would help in combating your fatigue. Be sure to let your doctor or nurse know if you have any of these symptoms:

- Increased shortness of breath with minimal exertion
- Uncontrolled pain
- Inability to control side effects from treatments (such as nausea, vomiting, diarrhea, or loss of appetite)
- Uncontrollable anxiety or nervousness
- Ongoing depression

Chapter 32

Cancer Pain

Cancer pain can be managed effectively in most patients with cancer or with a history of cancer. Although cancer pain cannot always be relieved completely, therapy can lessen pain in most patients. Pain management improves the patient's quality of life throughout all stages of the disease.

Flexibility is important in managing cancer pain. As patients vary in diagnosis, stage of disease, responses to pain and treatments, and personal likes and dislikes, management of cancer pain must be individualized. Patients, their families, and their health care providers must work together closely to manage a patient's pain effectively.

Assessment

To treat pain, it must be measured. The patient and the doctor should measure pain levels at regular intervals after starting cancer treatment, at each new report of pain, and after starting any type of treatment for pain. The cause of the pain must be identified and treated promptly.

PDQ® Cancer Information Summary. National Cancer Institute (NCI); Bethesda, MD. Pain (PDQ®): Supportive Care - Patient. Updated 02/2006. Available at http://cancer.gov. Accessed April 2006. Text under the heading "Exercises for Relieving Pain" is reprinted from *Pain: Clinical Manual For Nursing Practice*, by McCaffery M, Beebe A, pages 177, 201 and 206 © 1989 Mosby, reprinted with permission from Elsevier. Text under the heading "Relaxation Skills for Pain Relief" is excerpted from "Facing Forward Series: Life After Cancer Treatment," NCI, April 2002.

Patient Self-Report

To help the health care provider determine the type and extent of the pain, cancer patients can describe the location and intensity of their pain, any aggravating or relieving factors, and their goals for pain control. The family/caregiver may be asked to report for a patient who has a communication problem involving speech, language, or a thinking impairment. The health care provider should help the patient describe the following:

- **Pain:** The patient describes the pain, when it started, how long it lasts, and whether it is worse during certain times of the day or night.

- **Location:** The patient shows exactly where the pain is on his or her body or on a drawing of a body and where the pain goes if it travels.

- **Intensity or severity:** The patient keeps a diary of the degree or severity of pain.

- **Aggravating and relieving factors:** The patient identifies factors that increase or decrease the pain.

- **Personal response to pain:** Feelings of fear, confusion, or hopelessness about cancer, its prognosis, and the causes of pain can affect how a patient responds to and describes the pain. For example, a patient who thinks pain is caused by cancer spreading may report more severe pain or more disability from the pain.

- **Behavioral response to pain:** The health care provider and/or caregivers note behaviors that may suggest pain in patients who have communication problems.

- **Goals for pain control:** With the health care provider, the patient decides how much pain he or she can tolerate and how much improvement he or she may achieve. The patient uses a daily pain diary to increase awareness of pain, gain a sense of control of the pain, and receive guidance from health care providers on ways to manage the pain.

Assessment of the Outcomes of Pain Management

The results of pain management should be measured by monitoring for a decrease in the severity of pain and improvement in thinking ability, emotional well-being, and social functioning. The results of taking pain medication should also be monitored. Drug addiction is rare in cancer patients. Developing a higher tolerance for a drug and becoming physically dependent on the drug for pain relief does not mean that the patient is addicted. Patients should take pain medication as prescribed by the doctor. Patients who have a history of drug abuse may tolerate higher doses of medication to control pain.

Management with Drugs

Basic Principles of Cancer Pain Management

The World Health Organization developed a three-step approach for pain management based on the severity of the pain:

- For mild to moderate pain, the doctor may prescribe a Step 1 pain medication such as aspirin, acetaminophen, or a nonsteroidal anti-inflammatory drug (NSAID). Patients should be monitored for side effects, especially those caused by NSAIDs, such as kidney, heart and blood vessel, or stomach and intestinal problems.

0 No pain	1	2	3	4	5	6	7	8	9	10 Worst pain imaginable

Date	Time	Pain Rating (0-10) scale	Pain medication (name, dose, how often taken)	Other pain-relief methods tried	Side effects from pain medication
June 6 (example)	8 am	6	Morphine 30 mg every 4 hrs	massage	constipation

Figure 32.1. Pain diary and pain rating scale (Source: From "Facing Forward Series: Life After Cancer Treatment," NCI, April 2002.)

- When pain lasts or increases, the doctor may change the prescription to a Step 2 or Step 3 pain medication. Most patients with cancer-related pain will need a Step 2 or Step 3 medication. The doctor may skip Step 1 medications if the patient initially has moderate to severe pain.

- At each step, the doctor may prescribe additional drugs or treatments (for example, radiation therapy).

- The patient should take doses regularly, "by mouth, by the clock" (at scheduled times), to maintain a constant level of the drug in the body; this will help prevent recurrence of pain. If the patient is unable to swallow, the drugs are given by other routes (for example, by infusion or injection).

- The doctor may prescribe additional doses of drug that can be taken as needed for pain that occurs between scheduled doses of drug.

- The doctor will adjust the pain medication regimen for each patient's individual circumstances and physical condition.

Acetaminophen and NSAIDs

NSAIDs are effective for relief of mild pain. They may be given with opioids for the relief of moderate to severe pain. Acetaminophen also relieves pain, although it does not have the anti-inflammatory effect that aspirin and NSAIDs do. Patients, especially older patients, who are taking acetaminophen or NSAIDs should be closely monitored for side effects. Aspirin should not be given to children to treat pain.

Opioids

Opioids are very effective for the relief of moderate to severe pain. Many patients with cancer pain, however, become tolerant to opioids during long-term therapy. Therefore, increasing doses may be needed to continue to relieve pain. A patient's tolerance of an opioid or physical dependence on it is not the same as addiction (psychological dependence). Mistaken concerns about addiction can result in under treating pain.

Types of opioids: There are several types of opioids. Morphine is the most commonly used opioid in cancer pain management. Other commonly used opioids include hydromorphone, oxycodone, methadone, and fentanyl. The availability of several different opioids allows the doctor flexibility in prescribing a medication regimen that will meet individual patient needs.

Guidelines for giving opioids: Most patients with cancer pain will need to receive pain medication on a fixed schedule to manage the pain and prevent it from getting worse. The doctor will prescribe a dose of the opioid medication that can be taken as needed along with the regular fixed-schedule opioid to control pain that occurs between the scheduled doses. The amount of time between doses depends on which opioid the doctor prescribes. The correct dose is the amount of opioid that controls pain with the fewest side effects. The goal is to achieve a good balance between pain relief and side effects by gradually adjusting the dose. If opioid tolerance does occur, it can be overcome by increasing the dose or changing to another opioid, especially if higher doses are needed.

Occasionally, doses may need to be decreased or stopped. This may occur when patients become pain free because of cancer treatments such as nerve blocks or radiation therapy. The doctor may also decrease the dose when the patient experiences opioid-related sedation along with good pain control.

Medications for pain may be given in several ways. When the patient has a working stomach and intestines, the preferred method is by mouth, since medications given orally are convenient and usually inexpensive. When patients cannot take medications by mouth, other less invasive methods may be used, such as rectally or through medication patches placed on the skin. Intravenous methods are used only when simpler, less demanding, and less costly methods are inappropriate, ineffective, or unacceptable to the patient. Patient-controlled analgesia (PCA) pumps may be used to determine the opioid dose when starting opioid therapy. Once the pain is controlled, the doctor may prescribe regular opioid doses based on the amount the patient required when using the PCA pump. Intraspinal administration of opioids combined with a local anesthetic may be helpful for some patients who have uncontrollable pain.

Side effects of opioids: Patients should be watched closely for side effects of opioids. The most common side effects of opioids include nausea, sleepiness, and constipation. The doctor should discuss the side effects with patients before starting opioid treatment. Sleepiness and nausea are usually experienced when opioid treatment is started and tend to improve within a few days. Other side effects of opioid treatment include vomiting, difficulty in thinking clearly, problems with breathing, gradual overdose, and problems with sexual function.

Opioids slow down the muscle contractions and movement in the stomach and intestines resulting in hard stools. The key to effective prevention of constipation is to be sure the patient receives plenty of fluids to keep the stool soft. The doctor should prescribe a regular stool softener at the beginning of opioid treatment. If the patient does not respond to the stool softener, the doctor may prescribe additional laxatives.

Patients should talk to their doctor about side effects that become too bothersome or severe. Because there are differences between individual patients in the degree to which opioids may cause side effects, severe or continuing problems should be reported to the doctor. The doctor may decrease the dose of the opioid, switch to a different opioid, or switch the way the opioid is given (for example intravenous or injection rather than by mouth) to attempt to decrease the side effects.

Drugs Used with Pain Medications

Other drugs may be given at the same time as the pain medication. This is done to increase the effectiveness of the pain medication, treat symptoms, and relieve specific types of pain. These drugs include antidepressants, anticonvulsants, local anesthetics, corticosteroids, bisphosphonates, and stimulants. There are great differences in how patients respond to these drugs. Side effects are common and should be reported to the doctor. Certain bisphosphonates given for bone pain are linked to a risk of bone loss after dental work. Patients taking bisphosphonates should check with their doctor before having dental work done.

Physical and Psychosocial Interventions

Noninvasive physical and psychological methods can be used along with drugs and other treatments to manage pain during all phases of cancer treatment. The effectiveness of the pain interventions depends on the patient's participation in treatment and his or her ability to tell the health care provider which methods work best to relieve pain.

Physical Interventions

Weakness, muscle wasting, and muscle/bone pain may be treated with heat (a hot pack or heating pad); cold (flexible ice packs); massage, pressure, and vibration (to improve relaxation); exercise (to strengthen weak muscles, loosen stiff joints, help restore coordination and balance, and strengthen the heart); changing the position of the patient; restricting the movement of painful areas or broken bones; stimulation; controlled low-voltage electrical stimulation; or acupuncture.

Thinking and Behavioral Interventions

Thinking and behavior interventions are also important in treating pain. These interventions help give patients a sense of control and help them develop coping skills to deal with the disease and its symptoms. Beginning these interventions early in the course of the disease is useful so that patients can learn and practice the skills while they have enough strength and energy. Several methods should be tried, and one or more should be used regularly.

- **Relaxation and imagery:** Simple relaxation techniques may be used for episodes of brief pain (for example, during cancer treatment procedures). Brief, simple techniques are suitable for periods when the patient's ability to concentrate is limited by severe pain, high anxiety, or fatigue. (See Relaxation exercises below.)

- **Hypnosis:** Hypnotic techniques may be used to encourage relaxation and may be combined with other thinking/behavior methods. Hypnosis is effective in relieving pain in people who are able to concentrate and use imagery and who are willing to practice the technique.

- **Redirecting thinking:** Focusing attention on triggers other than pain or negative emotions that come with pain may involve distractions that are internal (for example, counting, praying, or saying things like "I can cope") or external (for example, music, television, talking, listening to someone read, or looking at something specific). Patients can also learn to monitor and evaluate negative thoughts and replace them with more positive thoughts and images.

- **Patient education:** Health care providers can give patients and their families information and instructions about pain and pain management and assure them that most pain can be controlled effectively. Health care providers should also discuss the major barriers that interfere with effective pain management.

- **Psychological support:** Short-term psychological therapy helps some patients. Patients who develop clinical depression or adjustment disorder may see a psychiatrist for diagnosis.

- **Support groups and religious counseling:** Support groups help many patients. Religious counseling may also help by providing spiritual care and social support.

Exercises for Relieving Pain

The following relaxation exercises may be helpful in relieving pain (Reprinted from *Pain: Clinical Manual For Nursing Practice*, by

McCaffery M, Beebe A, pages 177, 201 and 206 © 1989 Mosby, reprinted with permission from Elsevier.)

Exercise 1. Slow rhythmic breathing for relaxation:

1. Breathe in slowly and deeply, keeping your stomach and shoulders relaxed.

2. As you breathe out slowly, feel yourself beginning to relax; feel the tension leaving your body.

3. Breathe in and out slowly and regularly at a comfortable rate. Let the breath come all the way down to your stomach, as it completely relaxes.

4. To help you focus on your breathing and to breathe slowly and rhythmically: Breathe in as you say silently to yourself, "in, two, three." OR Each time you breathe out, say silently to yourself a word such as "peace" or "relax."

5. Do steps 1 through 4 only once or repeat steps 3 and 4 for up to 20 minutes.

6. End with a slow deep breath. As you breathe out say to yourself, "I feel alert and relaxed."

Exercise 2. Simple touch, massage, or warmth for relaxation:

Touch and massage are traditional methods of helping others relax. Some examples are:

*   Brief touch or massage, such as hand holding or briefly touching or rubbing a person's shoulders.

*   Soaking feet in a basin of warm water or wrapping the feet in a warm, wet towel.

*   Massage (3 to 10 minutes) of the whole body or just the back, feet, or hands. If the patient is modest or cannot move or turn easily in bed, consider massage of the hands and feet.

*   Use a warm lubricant. A small bowl of hand lotion may be warmed in the microwave oven or a bottle of lotion may be warmed in a sink of hot water for about 10 minutes.

*   Massage for relaxation is usually done with smooth, long, slow strokes. Try several degrees of pressure along with different types of massage, such as kneading and stroking, to determine which is preferred.

Especially for the elderly person, a back rub that effectively produces relaxation may consist of no more than 3 minutes of slow, rhythmic stroking (about 60 strokes per minute) on both sides of the spine, from the crown of the head to the lower back. Continuous hand contact is maintained by starting one hand down the back as the other hand stops at the lower back and is raised. Set aside a regular time for the massage. This gives the patient something pleasant to anticipate.

Exercise 3. Peaceful past experiences:

Something may have happened to you a while ago that brought you peace or comfort. You may be able to draw on that experience to bring you peace or comfort now. Think about these questions:

- Can you remember any situation, even when you were a child, when you felt calm, peaceful, secure, hopeful, or comfortable?

- Have you ever daydreamed about something peaceful? What were you thinking?

- Do you get a dreamy feeling when you listen to music? Do you have any favorite music?

- Do you have any favorite poetry that you find uplifting or reassuring?

- Have you ever been active religiously? Do you have favorite readings, hymns, or prayers? Even if you haven't heard or thought of them for many years, childhood religious experiences may still be very soothing.

Additional points: Some of the things that may comfort you, such as your favorite music or a prayer, can probably be recorded for you. Then you can listen to the tape whenever you wish. Or, if your memory is strong, you may simply close your eyes and recall the events or words.

Exercise 4. Active listening to recorded music:

- Obtain the following:
  - A cassette player or tape recorder. (Small, battery-operated ones are more convenient.)
  - Earphones or a headset. (Helps focus the attention better than a speaker a few feet away, and avoids disturbing others.)

- A cassette of music you like. (Most people prefer fast, lively music, but some select relaxing music. Other options are comedy routines, sporting events, old radio shows, or stories.)

- Mark time to the music; for example, tap out the rhythm with your finger or nod your head. This helps you concentrate on the music rather than on your discomfort.

- Keep your eyes open and focus on a fixed spot or object. If you wish to close your eyes, picture something about the music.

- Listen to the music at a comfortable volume. If the discomfort increases, try increasing the volume; decrease the volume when the discomfort decreases.

- If this is not effective enough, try adding or changing one or more of the following: massage your body in rhythm to the music; try other music; or mark time to the music in more than one manner, such as tapping your foot and finger at the same time.

Additional points: Many patients have found this technique to be helpful. It tends to be very popular, probably because the equipment is usually readily available and is a part of daily life. Other advantages are that it is easy to learn and not physically or mentally demanding. If you are very tired, you may simply listen to the music and omit marking time or focusing on a spot.

Relaxation Skills for Pain Relief

Before trying the full exercise below, first practice steps 1 through 5 so you can get used to deep breathing and muscle relaxation.

1. Find a quiet place where you can rest undisturbed for 20 minutes. Let others know you need this time for yourself.

2. Make sure the setting is relaxing. For example, dim the lights if you like, and find a comfortable chair or couch.

3. Get into a comfortable position where you can relax your muscles. Close your eyes and clear your mind of distractions.

4. Breathe deeply, at a slow and relaxing pace. People usually breathe shallowly, high in their chests. Concentrate on breathing deeply and slowly, raising your belly, rather than just your chest, with each breath.

5. Next, go through each of your major muscle groups, tensing (squeezing) them for 10 seconds and then relaxing. If tensing any particular muscle group is painful, skip the tensing step and concentrate just on relaxing. Focus completely on releasing all the tension from your muscles and notice the differences you feel when they are relaxed. Focus on the pleasant feeling of relaxation. In turn, tense, hold, and relax your:

- Right and left arms. Make a fist and bring it up to your shoulder, tightening your arm.

- Lips, eyes, and forehead. Scowl, raise your eyebrows, pucker your lips, and then grin.

- Jaws and neck. Clench your teeth and relax, then tilt your chin down toward your chest.

- Shoulders. Shrug your shoulders upward toward your ears.

- Chest. Push out your chest.

- Stomach. Suck in your stomach.

- Lower back. Stretch your lower back so that it forms a gentle arch, with your stomach pushed outward. Make sure to do this gently, as these muscles are often tight.

- Buttocks. Squeeze buttocks together.

- Thighs. Press thighs together.

- Calves. Point your toes up, toward your knees.

- Feet. Point your toes down, like a ballet dancer's.

You may find that your mind wanders. When you notice yourself thinking of something else, gently direct your attention back to your deepening relaxation. Be sure to maintain your deep breathing.

6. Review these parts of your body again, and release any tension that remains. Be sure to maintain your deep breathing.

7. Now that you are relaxed, imagine a calming scene. Choose a spot that is particularly pleasant to you. It may be a favorite comfortable room, a sandy beach, a chair in front of a fireplace, or any other relaxing place. Concentrate on the details:

- What can you see around you?

- What do you smell?

- What are the sounds that you hear? For example, if you are on the beach, how does the sand feel on your feet, how do the waves sound, and how does the air smell?

- Can you taste anything?

Continue to breathe deeply, as you imagine yourself relaxing in your safe, comfortable place.

8. Some people find it helpful at this point to focus on thoughts that enhance their relaxation. For example: "My arms and legs are very comfortable. I can just sink into this chair and focus only on the relaxation."

9. Spend a few more minutes enjoying the feeling of comfort and relaxation.

10. When you are ready, start gently moving your hands and feet and bringing yourself back to reality. Open your eyes, and spend a few minutes becoming more alert. Notice how you feel now that you have completed the relaxation exercise, and try to carry these feelings with you into the rest of your day.

Here's another exercise you can try to develop your relaxation skills:

1. Sit comfortably. Loosen any tight clothes. Close your eyes. Clear your mind and relax your muscles using steps 4 and 5 above.

2. Focus your mind on your right arm. Repeat to yourself, "My right arm feels heavy and warm." Stick with it until your arm does feel heavy and warm.

3. Repeat with the rest of your muscles until you are fully relaxed.

Keep in mind: These exercises don't work right away for everyone. It can take some time to feel these exercises are working, so practicing may help. If any of these steps makes you feel uncomfortable, feel free to leave it out. Ask your doctor or nurse about other ways to relax if these exercises don't work for you.

Anticancer Interventions for Pain Relief

Radiation therapy, radiofrequency ablation, and surgery may be used for pain relief rather than as treatment for primary cancer. Certain chemotherapy drugs may also be used to manage cancer-related pain.

Radiation therapy: Local or whole-body radiation therapy may increase the effectiveness of pain medication and other noninvasive therapies by directly affecting the cause of the pain (for example, by reducing tumor size). A single injection of a radioactive agent may relieve pain when cancer spreads extensively to the bones.

Radiofrequency ablation: Radiofrequency ablation uses a needle electrode to heat tumors and destroy them. This minimally invasive procedure may provide significant pain relief in patients who have cancer that has spread to the bones.

Surgery: Surgery may be used to remove part or all of a tumor to reduce pain directly, relieve symptoms of obstruction or compression, and improve outcome, even increasing long-term survival.

Invasive Interventions

Less invasive methods should be used for relieving pain before trying invasive treatment. Some patients, however, may need invasive therapy.

Nerve blocks: A nerve block is the injection of either a local anesthetic or a drug that inactivates nerves to control otherwise uncontrollable pain. Nerve blocks can be used to determine the source of pain, to treat painful conditions that respond to nerve blocks, to predict how the pain will respond to long-term treatments, and to prevent pain following procedures.

Neurologic interventions: Surgery can be performed to implant devices that deliver drugs or electrically stimulate the nerves. In rare cases, surgery may be done to destroy a nerve or nerves that are part of the pain pathway.

Management of procedural pain: Many diagnostic and treatment procedures are painful. Pain related to procedures may be treated before it occurs. Local anesthetics and short-acting opioids can be used to manage procedure-related pain, if enough time is allowed for the drug to work. Anti-anxiety drugs and sedatives may be used to reduce anxiety or to sedate the patient. Treatments such as imagery or relaxation are useful in managing procedure-related pain and anxiety.

Patients usually tolerate procedures better when they know what to expect. Having a relative or friend stay with the patient during the procedure may help reduce anxiety.

Patients and family members should receive written instructions for managing the pain at home. They should receive information regarding whom to contact for questions related to pain management.

Treating Older Patients

Older patients are at risk for under-treatment of pain because their sensitivity to pain may be underestimated, they may be expected to tolerate pain well, and misconceptions may exist about their ability to benefit from opioids. Issues in assessing and treating cancer pain in older patients include the following:

- Multiple chronic diseases and sources of pain: Age and complicated medication regimens put older patients at increased risk for interactions between drugs and between drugs and the chronic diseases.

- Visual, hearing, movement, and thinking impairments may require simpler tests and more frequent monitoring to determine the extent of pain in the older patient.

- Nonsteroidal anti-inflammatory drug (NSAID) side effects, such as stomach and kidney toxicity, thinking problems, constipation, and headaches, are more likely to occur in older patients.

- Opioid effectiveness: Older patients may be more sensitive to the pain-relieving and central nervous system effects of opioids resulting in longer periods of pain relief.

- Patient-controlled analgesia must be used cautiously in older patients, since drugs are slower to leave the body and older patients are more sensitive to the side effects.

- Other methods of administration, such as rectal administration, may not be useful in older patients since they may be physically unable to insert the medication.

- Pain control after surgery requires frequent direct contact with health care providers to monitor pain management.

- Reassessment of pain management and required changes should be made whenever the older patient moves (for example, from hospital to home or nursing home).

Chapter 33

Sexuality and Reproductive Concerns Related to Cancer Treatment

The Prevalence and Types of Sexual Dysfunction in People with Cancer

Sexuality is a complex characteristic that involves the physical, psychological, interpersonal, and behavioral aspects of a person. Recognizing that "normal" sexual functioning covers a wide range is important. Ultimately, sexuality is defined by each patient and his/her partner according to sex, age, personal attitudes, and religious and cultural values.

Many types of cancer and cancer therapies can cause sexual dysfunction. Research shows that approximately one-half of women who have been treated for breast and gynecologic cancers experience long-term sexual dysfunction. Men who have been treated for prostate cancer report problems with erectile dysfunction that varies depending on the type of treatment.

An individual's sexual response can be affected in many ways. The causes of sexual dysfunction are often both physical and psychological. The most common sexual problems for people who have cancer are loss of desire for sexual activity in both men and women, problems achieving and maintaining an erection in men, and pain with intercourse in women. Men may also experience inability to ejaculate, ejaculation

PDQ® Cancer Information Summary. National Cancer Institute; Bethesda, MD. Sexuality and Reproductive Issues (PDQ®): Supportive Care - Patient. Updated 07/2006. Available at http://cancer.gov. Accessed December 27, 2006.

going backward into the bladder, or the inability to reach orgasm. Women may experience a change in genital sensations due to pain, loss of sensation and numbness, or decreased ability to reach orgasm. Most often, both men and women are still able to reach orgasm; however, it may be delayed due to medications or anxiety.

Unlike many other physical side effects of cancer treatment, sexual problems may not resolve within the first year or two of disease-free survival and can interfere with the return to a normal life. Patients recovering from cancer should discuss their concerns about sexual problems with a health care professional.

Factors Affecting Sexual Function in People with Cancer

Both physical and psychological factors contribute to the development of sexual dysfunction. Physical factors include loss of function due to the effects of cancer therapies, fatigue, and pain. Surgery, chemotherapy, and radiation therapy may have a direct physical impact on sexual function. Other factors that may contribute to sexual dysfunction include pain medications, depression, feelings of guilt from misbeliefs about the origin of the cancer, changes in body image after surgery, and stresses due to personal relationships. Getting older is often associated with a decrease in sexual desire and performance, however, sex may be important to the older person's quality of life and the loss of sexual function can be distressing.

Surgery-Related Factors

Surgery can directly affect sexual function. Factors that help predict a patient's sexual function after surgery include age, sexual and bladder function before surgery, tumor location and size, and how much tissue was removed during surgery. Surgeries that affect sexual function include breast cancer, colorectal cancer, prostate cancer, and other pelvic tumors.

Breast cancer: Sexual function after breast cancer surgery has been the subject of much research. Surgery to save or reconstruct the breast appears to have little effect on sexual function compared with surgery to remove the whole breast. Women who have surgery to save the breast are more likely to continue to enjoy breast caressing, but there is no difference in areas such as how often women have sex, the ease of reaching orgasm, or overall sexual satisfaction. Having a mastectomy, however, has been linked to a loss of interest in sex. Chemotherapy has been linked to problems with sexual function.

Colorectal cancer: Sexual and bladder dysfunctions are common complications of surgery for rectal cancer. The main cause of problems with erection, ejaculation, and orgasm is injury to nerves in the pelvic cavity. Nerves can be damaged when their blood supply is disrupted or when the nerves are cut.

Prostate cancer: Newer nerve-sparing techniques for radical prostatectomy are being debated as a more successful approach for preserving erectile function than radiation therapy for prostate cancer. Long-term follow-up is needed to compare the effects of surgery with the effects of radiation therapy. Recovery of erectile function usually occurs within a year after having a radical prostatectomy. The effects of radiation therapy on erectile function are very slow and gradual occurring for two or three years after treatment. The cause of loss of erectile function differs between surgery and radiation therapy. Radical prostatectomy damages nerves that make blood vessels open wider to allow more blood into the penis. Eventually the tissue does not get enough oxygen, cells die, and scar tissue forms that interferes with erectile function. Radiation therapy appears to damage the arteries that bring blood to the penis.

Brachytherapy (internal radiation therapy using radioactive implants) is being used more often to treat prostate cancer. With brachytherapy alone, ejaculation and erectile function are better preserved than when external radiation or hormone therapy are added. Radiation damage to nerves and blood vessels may occur with brachytherapy, and higher doses of radiation may cause more damage.

Other pelvic tumors: Men who have surgery to remove the bladder, colon, or rectum may improve recovery of erectile function if nerve-sparing surgical techniques are used. The sexual side effects of radiation therapy for pelvic tumors are similar to those after prostate cancer treatment.

Women who have surgery to remove the uterus, ovaries, bladder, or other organs in the abdomen or pelvis may experience pain and loss of sexual function depending on the amount of tissue or organ removed. With counseling and other medical treatments, these patients may regain normal sensation in the vagina and genital areas and be able to have pain-free intercourse and reach orgasm.

Chemotherapy-Related Factors

Chemotherapy is associated with a loss of desire and decreased frequency of intercourse for both men and women. The common side effects of chemotherapy such as nausea, vomiting, diarrhea, constipation, mucositis, weight loss or gain, and loss of hair can affect an individual's sexual self-image and make him or her feel unattractive.

For women, chemotherapy may cause vaginal dryness, pain with intercourse, and decreased ability to reach orgasm. In older women, chemotherapy may increase the risk of ovarian cancer. Chemotherapy may also cause a sudden loss of estrogen production from the ovaries. The loss of estrogen can cause shrinking, thinning, and loss of elasticity of the vagina, vaginal dryness, hot flashes, urinary tract infections, mood swings, fatigue, and irritability. Young women who have breast cancer and have had surgeries, such as removal of one or both ovaries, may experience symptoms related to loss of estrogen. These women experience high rates of sexual problems since there is a concern that estrogen replacement therapy, which may decrease these symptoms, could cause the breast cancer to return. For women with other types of cancer, however, estrogen replacement therapy can usually resolve many sexual problems. Also, women who have graft-versus-host disease (a reaction of donated bone marrow or peripheral stem cells against a person's tissue) following bone marrow transplantation may develop scar tissue and narrowing of the vagina that can interfere with intercourse.

For men, sexual problems such as loss of desire and erectile dysfunction are more common after a bone marrow transplant because of graft-versus-host disease or nerve damage. Occasionally chemotherapy may interfere with testosterone production in the testicles. Testosterone replacement may be necessary to regain sexual function.

Radiation Therapy-Related Factors

Like chemotherapy, radiation therapy can cause side effects such as fatigue, nausea and vomiting, diarrhea, and other symptoms that can decrease feelings of sexuality. In women, radiation therapy to the pelvis can cause changes in the lining of the vagina. These changes eventually cause a narrowing of the vagina and formation of scar tissue that results in pain with intercourse, infertility and other long term sexual problems. Women should discuss concerns about these side effects with their doctor and ask about the use of a vaginal dilator.

For men, radiation therapy can cause problems with getting and keeping an erection. The exact cause of sexual problems after radiation therapy is unknown. Possible causes are nerve injury, a blockage of blood supply to the penis, or decreased levels of testosterone. Sexual changes occur very slowly over a period of six months to one year after radiation therapy. Men who had problems with erectile dysfunction before getting cancer have a greater risk of developing sexual problems after cancer diagnosis and treatment. Other risk factors that can contribute to a greater risk of sexual problems in men are cigarette smoking, history of heart disease, high blood pressure, and diabetes.

Hormone Therapy-Related Factors

Hormone therapy for prostate cancer can decrease normal hormone levels and cause a decrease in sexual desire, erectile dysfunction, and problems reaching orgasm. Younger men do not always experience the same degree of sexual dysfunction. Some treatment centers are experimenting with delayed or intermittent hormone therapy to prevent sexual problems. It is not yet known if these modified treatments affect the long-term survival of younger men.

The effects of tamoxifen on the sexuality and mood of women who have breast cancer are not clearly understood.

Psychological Factors

Patients recovering from cancer often have anxiety or guilt that previous sexual activities may have caused their cancer. Some patients believe that sexual activity may cause the cancer to return or pass the cancer to their partner. Discussing their feelings and concerns with a health care professional is important for patients. Misbeliefs can be corrected and patients can be reassured that cancer is not passed on through sexual contact.

Loss of sexual desire and a decrease in sexual pleasure are common symptoms of depression. Depression is more common in patients with cancer than in the general healthy population. It is important that patients discuss their feelings with their doctor. Getting treatment for depression may be helpful in relieving sexual problems.

Cancer treatments may cause physical changes that affect how an individual sees his or her physical appearance. This view can make a man or woman feel sexually unattractive. It is important that patients discuss these feelings and concerns with a health care professional. Patients can learn how to deal effectively with these problems.

The stress of being diagnosed with cancer and undergoing treatment for cancer can make existing problems in relationships even worse. The sexual relationship can also be affected. Patients who do not have a committed relationship may stop dating because they fear being rejected by a potential new partner who learns about their history of cancer. One of the most important factors in adjusting after cancer treatment is the patient's feeling about his or her sexuality before being diagnosed with cancer. If patients had positive feelings about sexuality, they may be more likely to resume sexual activity after treatment for cancer.

Assessment of Sexual Function in People with Cancer

Sexual function is an important factor that adds to quality of life. Patients should discuss their problems and concerns about sexual function with their doctor. Some doctors may not have the appropriate training to discuss sexual problems. Patients should ask for other information resources or for a referral to a health care professional who is comfortable with discussing sexuality issues.

General Factors Affecting Sexual Functioning

When a possible sexual problem is identified, the health care professional will do a detailed interview either with the patient alone or with the patient and his or her partner. The patient may be asked any of the following questions about his or her current and past sexual functioning:

- How often do you feel a spontaneous desire to have sex?

- Do you enjoy sex?

- Do you become sexually aroused (for men, are you able to get and keep an erection, or for women, does your vagina expand and become lubricated)?

- Are you able to reach orgasm during sex? What types of stimulation can trigger an orgasm (for example, self-touch, use of a vibrator, shower massage, partner caressing, oral stimulation, or intercourse)?

- Do you have any pain during sex? Where do you feel the pain? What does the pain feel like? What kinds of sexual activity trigger the pain? Does this cause pain every time? How long does the pain last?

- When did your sexual problems begin? Was it around the same time that you were diagnosed with cancer or received treatment for cancer?

- Are you taking any medications? Did you start taking any new medications or did the doctor change the dose of any medications around the time that these sexual problems began?

- What was your sexual functioning like before you were diagnosed with cancer? Did you have any sexual problems before you were diagnosed with cancer?

Psychosocial Aspects of Sexuality

Patients may also be asked about the significance of sexuality and relationships whether or not they have a partner. Patients who have a partner may be asked about the length and stability of the relationship before being diagnosed with cancer. They may also be asked about their partner's response to the diagnosis of cancer and if they have any concerns about how their partner may be affected by their treatment. It is important that patients and their partners discuss their sexual problems, concerns, and fears about their relationship with a health care professional with whom they feel comfortable.

Medical Aspects of Sexuality

Patients may be asked about current and past medical history since many medical illnesses can affect sexual function. Lifestyle risk factors such as smoking and high alcohol intake can also affect sexual function as well as prescribed and over-the-counter medications. Patients may be asked to fill out questionnaires to help identify sexual problems and may undergo a variety of physical examinations, blood tests, ultrasound studies, measurement of nighttime erections, and hormone tests.

Effects of Medicines on Sexual Function

The side effects of medicines can add to the sexual side effects of surgery, radiation therapy, and chemotherapy. Cancer patients may receive drug therapy that can affect nerves, blood vessels, and hormones that control normal sexual function. Mental alertness and moods may also be affected. These side effects may occur in cancer patients who take opioids for pain and drugs to treat depression, for example.

Treatment of Sexual Problems in People with Cancer

Many patients are fearful or anxious about their first sexual experience after cancer treatment. Fear and anxiety can cause patients to avoid intimacy, touch, and sexual activity. The partner may also feel fearful or anxious about initiating any activity that might be thought of as pressuring to be intimate or that might cause physical discomfort. Patients and their partners should discuss concerns with their doctor or other qualified health professional. Honest communication of feelings, concerns, and preferences is important.

In general, a wide variety of treatment modalities are available for patients with sexual dysfunction after cancer. Patients can learn to adapt to changes in sexual function through reading books, pamphlets, and internet resources or listening to and watching videos and CD-ROMs. Health professionals who specialize in sexual dysfunction can provide patients with these resources as well as information on national organizations that may provide support. Some patients may need medical intervention such as hormone replacement, medications, medical devices, or surgery. Patients who have more serious problems may need sexual counseling on an individual basis, with his or her partner, or in a group. Further testing and research is needed to compare the effectiveness of various treatment programs that combine medical and psychological approaches for people who have had cancer.

Fertility Issues

Radiation therapy and chemotherapy treatments may cause temporary or permanent infertility. These side effects are related to a number of factors including the patient's sex, age at time of treatment, the specific type and dose of radiation therapy or chemotherapy, the use of single therapy or many therapies, and length of time since treatment.

When cancer or its treatment may cause infertility or sexual dysfunction, every effort should be made to inform and educate the patient about this possibility. When the patient is a child, this can be difficult. The child may be too young to understand issues involving infertility or sexuality, or parents may choose to shield the child from these issues.

Chemotherapy: For patients receiving chemotherapy, age is an important factor and recovery improves the longer the patient is off chemotherapy. Chemotherapy drugs that have been shown to affect fertility include: busulfan, melphalan, cyclophosphamide, cisplatin, chlorambucil, mustine, carmustine, lomustine, vinblastine, cytarabine, and procarbazine.

Radiation: For men and women receiving radiation therapy to the abdomen or pelvis, the amount of radiation directly to the testes or ovaries is an important factor. In women older than 40 years, infertility may occur at lower doses of radiation. Fertility may be preserved by the use of modern radiation therapy techniques and the use of lead shields to protect the testes. Women may undergo surgery to protect the ovaries by moving them out of the field of radiation.

Procreative alternatives: Patients who are concerned about the effects of cancer treatment on their ability to have children should discuss this with their doctor before treatment. The doctor can recommend a counselor or fertility specialist who can discuss available options and help patients and their partners through the decision-making process. Options may include freezing sperm, eggs, or ovarian tissue before cancer treatment.

Chapter 34

Fever, Sweats,
and Hot Flashes

Fever

Normal human body temperature changes during each 24-hour period according to a definite pattern. It is lowest in the morning before dawn and highest in the afternoon. Normal body temperature is maintained by temperature control activities in the body that keep a balance between heat loss and heat production.

An abnormal increase in body temperature is caused by either hyperthermia (an unusual increase in body temperature above normal) or fever. Hyperthermia is caused by a breakdown in the body's temperature control activities. In fever, the temperature controls in the body are working correctly, but body temperature increases as the body responds to chemicals produced by microorganisms that cause infection or works to kill harmful microorganisms such as bacteria or viruses. There are three phases to fever. In the first phase, the body raises its temperature to a new level by causing the blood vessels in the skin to constrict and move blood from the skin surface to the interior of the body which helps to retain heat. The skin becomes cool, the muscles contract causing shivering or chills, and the body produces more heat. The body's efforts to retain and produce heat continue until a new higher temperature is reached. In the second phase, heat production

PDQ® Cancer Information Summary. National Cancer Institute; Bethesda, MD. Fever, Sweats, and Hot Flashes (PDQ®): Supportive Care - Patient. Updated 11/2005. Available at http://cancer.gov. Accessed November 10, 2006.

and heat loss are equal, shivering stops, and the body maintains the new higher temperature. In the third phase, body temperature is lowered to normal as the body gets rid of the excess heat by causing the blood vessels in the skin to open and move blood from the interior of the body to the skin surface. Sweating occurs and helps to cool the body.

Fever is most likely to cause harmful effects in older persons or the very young. In older persons, the hypothalamus's temperature regulating centers do not work as well and the body temperature may rise above normal causing irregular heartbeat, lack of blood flow, changes in the ability to think clearly, or heart failure. Children between six months and six years old may have seizures due to a fever.

Description and Causes

The main causes of fever in cancer patients are infections, tumors, reactions to drugs or blood transfusions, and graft-versus-host-disease. Graft-versus-host-disease occurs when transplanted bone marrow or peripheral stem cells attack the patient's tissue. Infection is a common cause of fever in cancer patients and can cause death. Tumor cells can produce various substances that can cause fever. A wide variety of medications can cause fever including chemotherapy drugs, biological response modifiers, and antibiotics, such as vancomycin and amphotericin.

Other causes of fever in cancer patients include drug withdrawal; neuroleptic malignant syndrome; blockages of the bladder, bowel, or kidney; and blockage of an artery by tumor fragments. Other medical conditions occurring at the same time as the cancer such as blood clots, connective tissue disorders, and central nervous system hemorrhage or stroke, may also cause fever.

Assessment

The doctor will ask questions about past medical problems, review all medications the patient is taking, and perform a thorough physical examination to determine the cause of fever. Patients who are suspected of having an infection, especially those who have neutropenia (a very low white blood cell count) and fever, will undergo very careful inspection of the skin, body openings (mouth, ears, nose, throat, urethra, vagina, rectum), needle stick sites, biopsy sites, and skin folds (for example, the breasts, armpits, or groin). The teeth, gums, tongue, nose, throat, and sinuses will be carefully examined. Any tubes that are inserted into veins or arteries or other tubes placed in the body, such as stomach tubes, are common sources of infection. Urine, sputum, and blood specimens will be examined for signs of infection. Patients with neutropenia may not show the usual symptoms of infection, so they should be examined frequently.

Treatment

The symptoms of fever in very weakened cancer patients may include fatigue, muscle pain, sweating, and chills. Possible treatments to manage fever include those that treat the underlying cause, giving intravenous fluids, nutritional support, and other measures to make the patient more comfortable. The specific treatments are determined by the stage of cancer and the patient's goals for care. For example, some patients who are nearing the end of life may decide not to be treated for the underlying cause such as pneumonia or other infections, but may still request general comfort measures and fluids to maintain their quality of life. Other patients may choose antibiotics to relieve symptoms such as cough, fever, or shortness of breath that occur because of the infection.

Antibiotics may be used to treat fever caused by infection. Antibiotic therapy regimens and drugs to treat fungal infections are prescribed by the doctor. Fever caused by a tumor is usually treated by prescribing standard therapies for the specific type of cancer. If the therapy is not successful, the therapy takes awhile to work, or there is no therapy available, the doctor may prescribe nonsteroidal anti-inflammatory drugs (NSAIDs).

Sometimes fever may be caused by a reaction to drugs given to treat the cancer or prevent infection. Drugs that are known to cause fever include biological response modifiers, amphotericin B, and bleomycin. Suspected drug-related fever may be treated by stopping the drug that is causing the fever. When a biological response modifier, certain chemotherapy drugs, or antibiotics cause the fever, the doctor may control the fever by adjusting the type of drug, how the drug is given, the amount of drug given, or how often the drug is given. Acetaminophen, NSAIDs, and steroids may also be given before the patient receives the drug that causes the fever. Meperidine may be given to stop chills associated with a drug-related fever.

Neuroleptic malignant syndrome (NMS) is a rare but sometimes fatal reaction to drugs that a patient is given for psychotic conditions, delirium, or nausea and vomiting. The symptoms of NMS are fever, muscle stiffness, confusion, loss of control of body functions, and an increase in white blood cell count. A delirious patient who does not improve when treated with medication should be examined for NMS. Treatment for NMS includes stopping the drug, treating the symptoms, and sometimes using other drugs.

Cancer patients may develop a fever as a reaction to blood products (for example, receiving a blood transfusion). Removing white blood cells from the blood or treating the blood product with radiation before transfusing it into the patient can lessen the reaction. The possibility of fever due to receiving blood products can also be lessened by giving patients acetaminophen or antihistamines before the transfusion.

General Treatments to Relieve Fever

Along with treatment of the underlying cause of fever, comfort measures may also be helpful in relieving the discomfort that goes along with fever, chills, and sweats. During periods of fever, giving the patient plenty of liquids, removing excess clothing and linens, and bathing or sponging the patient with lukewarm water may give relief. During periods of chills, replace wet blankets with warm, dry blankets, keep the patient away from drafts, and adjust the room temperature to improve patient comfort.

Nonsteroidal anti-inflammatory drugs (NSAIDs) or acetaminophen may also be prescribed to relieve symptoms. Aspirin may be effective in decreasing fever, but should be used with caution in patients with Hodgkin lymphoma and cancer patients who are at risk for developing a decrease in the number of platelets in the blood. Aspirin is not recommended in children with fever because of the risk of developing Reye syndrome.

Sweats

Sweat is made by sweat glands in the skin. Sweating helps to keep the body cool and can occur with disease or fever, when in a warm environment, exercising, or as part of hot flashes experienced with menopause. Most breast cancer and prostate cancer patients report having moderate to severe hot flashes. Distressing hot flashes seem to be less frequent and gradually decrease with time in most post-menopausal women who do not have breast cancer. In breast cancer survivors, however, hot flash intensity does not decrease with time. Most men with prostate cancer who have had surgery to remove the testicles experience hot flashes.

Causes

Sweats in the cancer patient may be associated with the tumor, cancer treatment, or other medical conditions that are not related to the cancer. Sweats are a typical symptom of certain types of tumors such as Hodgkin lymphoma, pheochromocytoma, or tumors involving the nervous system and endocrine system. Sweats may also be caused by the following conditions:

- Fever

- Female menopause (natural menopause, surgical removal of the ovaries, or damage to ovaries from chemotherapy, radiation, or hormone therapy)

- Male menopause (surgical removal of the testicles or hormone therapy)

- Drugs such as tamoxifen, opioids, antidepressants, and steroids

- Problems in the hypothalamus in the brain

- Sweating disorders

Treatments

Sweats: Treatment of sweats caused by fever is directed at the underlying cause of the fever. (Refer to the fever Treatment section for more information.) Sweats caused by a tumor are usually controlled by treatment of the tumor.

Hot flashes: Hot flashes associated with natural or treatment-related menopause can be effectively controlled with estrogen replacement. Many women are not able to take estrogen replacement (for example, women with breast cancer). Hormone replacement therapy that combines estrogen with progestin may increase the risk of breast cancer or breast cancer recurrence. A variety of other medications to treat hot flashes have varying degrees of effectiveness or have unacceptable side effects. The most effective drugs include megestrol (a drug similar to progesterone) and certain antidepressants such as venlafaxine. Many other drugs as well as vitamin E and soy are less effective in relieving hot flashes. Relaxation training may be effective in decreasing hot flash intensity in postmenopausal women who are in general good health.

Treatment of hot flashes in men may include estrogens, progesterone, and antidepressants. Certain hormones (such as estrogen) can make some cancers grow. The effect of hormone use on the growth of prostate cancer is being studied.

General Treatments to Relieve Symptoms

A variety of other medications are being used for general treatment of cancer-related sweats. The use of loose-fitting cotton clothing, fans, and behavioral techniques such as relaxation training is also recommended.

Chapter 35

Pruritus (Itching)

Pruritus is an itching sensation that triggers the desire to scratch. It is a distressing symptom that can cause discomfort. Scratching may cause breaks in the skin that may result in infection. Pruritus can be related to anything from dry skin to undiagnosed cancer. It can occur in people who have cancer or in those who have received cancer treatment.

Risk Factors

Pruritus may occur in some people with cancer but not in others. However, the following persons with cancer may be at a higher risk for developing pruritus:

- Persons with various malignant diseases that are known to produce symptoms of pruritus, including, but not limited to AIDS-related Kaposi sarcoma, Hodgkin lymphoma and other lymphomas, leukemias, adenocarcinomas, and cancer of the stomach, pancreas, lung, colon, brain, breast, and prostate. Pruritus tends to disappear when cancer is cured or in remission. It may reappear when the disease recurs.

- Persons who have had chemotherapy. Usually the itching subsides within 30–90 minutes and does not require treatment. The

PDQ® Cancer Information Summary. National Cancer Institute; Bethesda, MD. Pruritus (PDQ®): Supportive Care - Patient. Updated 10/2005. Available at http://cancer.gov. Accessed November 10, 2006.

313

development of pruritus may be a sign that the patient is especially sensitive to the chemotherapy drug.

- Persons who have had radiation therapy. Radiation can kill skin cells and cause burning and itching. As the skin peels off, scratching can damage it further, which creates the potential for infection. Treatment may need to be interrupted to allow the skin time to heal.

- Persons who have had radiation therapy plus chemotherapy. The combined effects of these drugs can cause an increased skin reaction.

- Persons who have had biological response modifier therapy (a treatment to try to improve the body's natural immune response to disease).

- Persons who have had bone marrow transplantation. Patients may experience changes in skin condition that include dryness, itching, and rashes.

Drugs given at any time during cancer treatment may cause pruritus. Itching may be caused by sensitivity to the drug, or the drug may interfere with normal nerve function.

Pruritus can be a symptom of infection. The infection may or may not be related to cancer treatment. Infections involving itching may be caused by a tumor, fungus, discharge from a wound, or drainage after surgery.

Pruritus is a symptom, not a diagnosis or disease. If you feel itching, let your doctor know. The doctor will ask for your medical history and give you a thorough physical examination. This assessment will enable the doctor to discover the problem that is causing the itching and find the best treatment for it.

Treatment

Maintaining healthy skin may relieve pruritus. Good skin care includes adequate nutrition and daily fluid intake, protection from the environment, and cleansing practices that don't dry the skin.

Some specific factors that may relieve itching are the following:

- **Moisturizing creams and lotions:** These water-containing products form films over the skin surface and encourage the production of moisture beneath the film. This prevents dryness, which can cause itching. These products should be carefully chosen for each person's needs. Some ingredients, such as petrolatum, lanolin, and mineral oil can cause allergic reactions in some people.

- **Powders, bubble baths, and cornstarch:** These products should be used with caution because they can irritate the skin and cause itching. Cornstarch is an effective treatment for itching that is associated with dry skin due to radiation therapy but should not be applied to moist surfaces, to areas with hair, sweat glands, skin folds, or to areas close to mucosal surfaces, such as the vagina or rectum. When cornstarch becomes moist, it can promote fungal growth. Some powders such as those that contain talcum and aluminum can cause skin irritation during radiation therapy and should be avoided when you are receiving radiation treatment. Alcohol or menthol, which are found in some creams and over-the-counter lotions, may also produce skin reactions. Topical steroid creams may reduce itching but may cause thinning of the skin and can make it more prone to injury.

- **Tepid baths:** Baths that are moderately warm and last no longer than one half hour every day or every two days can help relieve itching. Frequent bathing can aggravate dry skin, and hot baths can promote itching.

- **Mild soaps:** Mild soaps contain less soap or detergent that can irritate skin. Oil can be added to the water at the end of a bath or applied to the skin before drying.

- **A cool humid environment:** Heat can cause itching. Your skin loses moisture when the humidity is low. A cool, humid environment may prevent your skin from itching.

- **Removal of detergent residue:** Residue left on clothing by detergent and fabric softeners may aggravate pruritus. The irritation can be reduced by adding vinegar (one teaspoon per quart of water) to the laundry rinse cycle or by using a mild laundry soap that is sold for washing baby clothes.

- **Cotton clothing and bed sheets:** Body heat, wool, and some synthetic fabrics can aggravate itching. It may be helpful to wear loose-fitting, lightweight cotton clothing and to use cotton bed sheets.

In addition to the skin-care factors, medications applied to the skin or taken by mouth may be necessary to treat pruritus. Antibiotics may relieve itching caused by infection. Antihistamines may be useful in some cases of pruritus. Sedatives, tranquilizers, and antidepressants may be useful treatments. Aspirin seems to have reduced itching in some patients but increases it for others. Aspirin combined with cimetidine may be effective for patients with Hodgkin lymphoma or polycythemia vera.

Interrupting the itch-scratch-itch cycle, an increase in itching that can result from the process of scratching, may also help to alleviate pruritus. The cycle may be broken by applying a cool washcloth or ice over the affected area. Rubbing the skin and applying pressure or vibration to the skin may also help. Other methods that may be useful in relieving symptoms include distraction, music therapy, relaxation, and imagery techniques.

Chapter 36

Lymphedema

Lymphedema is the buildup of lymph (a fluid that helps fight infection and disease) in the fatty tissues just under the skin. The buildup of lymph causes swelling in specific areas of the body, usually an arm or leg, with an abnormally large amount of tissue proteins, chronic inflammation, and thickening and scarring of tissue under the skin. Lymphedema is a common complication of cancer and cancer treatment and can result in long-term physical, psychological, and social issues for patients.

The Lymphatic System

The lymphatic system consists of a network of specialized lymphatic vessels and various tissues and organs throughout the body that contain lymphocytes (white blood cells) and other cells that help the body fight infection and disease. The lymphatic vessels are similar to veins but have thinner walls. Some of these vessels are very close to the skin surface and can be found near veins; others are just under the skin and in the deeper fatty tissues near the muscles and can be found near arteries. Muscles and valves within the walls of the lymphatic vessels near the skin surface help pick up fluid and proteins from tissues throughout the body and move the lymph in one direction, toward the heart. Lymph is slowly moved through larger

PDQ® Cancer Information Summary. National Cancer Institute; Bethesda, MD. Lymphedema (PDQ®): Supportive Care - Patient. Updated 07/2006. Available at http://cancer.gov. Accessed November 10, 2006.

and larger lymphatic vessels and passes through small bean-shaped structures called lymph nodes. Lymph nodes filter substances that can be harmful to the body and contain lymphocytes and other cells that activate the immune system to fight disease. Eventually, lymph flows into one of two large ducts in the neck region. The right lymphatic duct collects lymph from the right arm and the right side of the head and chest, emptying it into the large vein under the right collarbone. The left lymphatic duct or thoracic duct collects lymph from both legs, the left arm, and the left side of the head and chest, emptying it into the large vein under the left collarbone.

The lymphatic system collects excess fluid and proteins from the body tissues and carries them back to the bloodstream. Proteins and substances too big to move through the walls of veins can be picked up by the lymphatic vessels because they have thinner walls. Edema may occur when there is an increase in the amount of fluid, proteins, and other substances in the body tissues because of problems in the blood capillaries and veins or a blockage in the lymphatic system.

Understanding Lymphedema

Lymphedema may be either primary or secondary. Primary lymphedema is a rare inherited condition in which lymph nodes and lymph vessels are absent or abnormal. Secondary lymphedema can be caused by a blockage or cut in the lymphatic system, usually the lymph nodes in the groin area and the armpit. Blockages may be caused by infection, cancer, or scar tissue from radiation therapy or surgical removal of lymph nodes. This chapter discusses secondary lymphedema.

Acute Versus Gradual-Onset Lymphedema

There are four types of acute lymphedema. The first type of acute lymphedema is mild and lasts only a short time, occurring a few days after surgery to remove the lymph nodes or after injury to the lymphatic vessels or veins just under the collarbone. The affected limb may be warm and slightly red, but is usually not painful and gets better within a week by keeping the affected arm or leg supported in a raised position and by contracting the muscles in the affected limb (for example, making a fist and releasing it).

The second type of acute lymphedema occurs six to eight weeks after surgery or during a course of radiation therapy. This type may be caused by inflammation of either lymphatic vessels or veins. The affected limb is tender, warm or hot, and red and is treated by keeping the limb supported in a raised position and taking anti-inflammatory drugs.

The third type of acute lymphedema occurs after an insect bite, minor injury, or burn that causes an infection of the skin and the lymphatic vessels near the skin surface. It may occur on an arm or leg that is chronically swollen. The affected area is red, very tender, and hot and is treated by supporting the affected arm or leg in a raised position and taking antibiotics. A compression pump should not be used and the affected area should not be wrapped with elastic bandages during the early stages of infection. Mild redness may continue after the infection.

The fourth and most common type of acute lymphedema develops very slowly and may become noticeable 18 to 24 months after surgery or not until many years after cancer treatment. The patient may experience discomfort of the skin; aching in the neck, shoulders, spine, or hips caused by stretching of the soft tissues or overuse of muscles; or posture changes caused by increased weight of the arm or leg.

Temporary Versus Chronic Lymphedema

Temporary lymphedema is a condition that lasts less than six months. The skin indents when pressed and stays indented, but there is no hardening of the skin. A patient may be more likely to develop lymphedema if he or she has one of the following:

- Surgical drains that leak protein into the surgical site
- Inflammation
- Inability to move the limb(s)
- Temporary loss of lymphatic function
- Blockage of a vein by a blood clot or inflammation

Chronic (long-term) lymphedema is the most difficult of all types of edema to treat. The damaged lymphatic system of the affected area is not able to keep up with the increased need for fluid drainage from the body tissues. This may be caused by one of the following:

- Recurrence or spread of a tumor to the lymph nodes
- Infection of and/or injury to the lymphatic vessels
- Periods of not being able to move the limbs
- Radiation therapy or surgery

- Inability to control early signs of lymphedema
- Blockage of a vein by a blood clot

A patient who is in the early stages of developing lymphedema will have swelling that indents with pressure and stays indented but remains soft. The swelling may easily improve by supporting the arm or leg in a raised position, gently exercising, and wearing elastic support garments. Continued problems with the lymphatic system cause the lymphatic vessels to expand, allowing lymph to flow back into the body tissues and make the condition worse. Pain, heat, redness, and swelling result as the body tries to get rid of the extra fluid. The skin becomes hard and stiff and no longer improves with raised support of the arm or leg, gentle exercise, or elastic support garments.

Patients with chronic lymphedema are at increased risk of infection. No effective treatment is yet available for patients who have advanced chronic lymphedema. Once the body tissues have been repeatedly stretched, lymphedema may recur more easily.

Risk Factors

Factors that can lead to the development of lymphedema include radiation therapy to an area where the lymph nodes were surgically removed, problems after surgery that cause inflammation of the arm or leg, a larger number of lymph nodes removed in surgery, and being older.

Risk factors for lymphedema include the following:

- Breast cancer, if the patient received radiation therapy or had lymph nodes removed. Radiation therapy to the underarm area after surgical removal of the lymph nodes and having a larger number of lymph nodes removed increases the risk of lymphedema.

- Surgical removal of lymph nodes in the underarm, groin, or pelvic regions

- Radiation therapy to the underarm, groin, pelvic, or neck regions

- Scar tissue in the lymphatic ducts or veins and under the collarbones, caused by surgery or radiation therapy

- Cancer that has spread to the lymph nodes in the neck, chest, underarm, pelvis, or abdomen

- Tumors growing in the pelvis or abdomen that involve or put pressure on the lymphatic vessels and/or the large lymphatic duct in the chest and block lymph drainage

- Having an inadequate diet or being overweight. These conditions may delay recovery and increase the risk for lymphedema.

Diagnosis

Specific criteria for diagnosing lymphedema do not yet exist. About half of patients with mild edema describe their affected arm or leg as feeling heavier or fuller than usual. To evaluate a patient for lymphedema, a medical history and physical examination of the patient should be completed. The medical history should include any past surgeries, problems after surgery, and the time between surgery and the onset of symptoms of edema. Any changes in the edema should be determined, as should any history of injury or infection. Knowing which medications a patient is taking is also important for diagnosis.

Management of Lymphedema

Patients at risk for lymphedema should be identified early, monitored, and taught self-care. A patient may be more likely to develop lymphedema if he or she eats an inadequate diet, is overweight, is inactive, or has other medical problems. To detect the condition early, the following should be examined:

- Comparison of actual weight to ideal weight

- Measurements of the arms and legs

- Protein levels in the blood

- Ability to perform activities of daily living

- History of edema, previous radiation therapy, or surgery

- Other medical illnesses such as diabetes, high blood pressure, kidney disease, heart disease, or phlebitis (inflammation of the veins)

It is important that the patient know about his or her disease and the risk of developing lymphedema. Poor drainage of the lymphatic system due to surgical removal of the lymph nodes or to radiation therapy may make the affected arm or leg more susceptible to serious infection. Even a small infection may lead to serious lymphedema. Patients should be taught about arm, leg, and skin care after surgery and/or radiation therapy. It is important that patients take precautions to prevent injury and infection in the affected arm or leg because lymphedema can occur 30 or more years after surgery. Breast cancer patients who follow instructions about skin care and proper exercise after mastectomy are less likely to experience lymphedema.

Lymphatic drainage is improved during exercise; therefore, exercise is important in preventing lymphedema. Breast cancer patients should do hand and arm exercises as instructed after mastectomy. Patients who have surgery that affects pelvic lymph node drainage should do leg and foot exercises as instructed. The doctor decides how soon after surgery the patient should start exercising. Physiatrists (doctors who specialize in physical medicine and rehabilitation) or physical therapists should develop an individualized exercise program for the patient.

Better recovery occurs when lymphedema is discovered early, so patients should be taught to recognize the early signs of edema and to tell the doctor about any of the following symptoms:

- Feelings of tightness in the arm or leg

- Rings or shoes that become tight

- Weakness in the arm or leg

- Pain, aching, or heaviness in the arm or leg

- Redness, swelling, or signs of infection

Prevention and Control of Lymphedema

- Keep the arm or leg raised above the level of the heart, when possible. Avoid making rapid circles with the arm or leg to keep blood from collecting in the lower part of the limb.

- Clean the skin of the arm or leg daily and moisten with lotion.

- Avoid injury and infection of the arm or leg.

  - Arms: Use an electric razor for shaving; wear gardening and cooking gloves; use thimbles for sewing; take care of fingernails; do not cut cuticles.

  - Legs: Keep the feet covered when outdoors; keep the feet clean and dry, wear cotton socks; cut toenails straight across; see a podiatrist as needed to prevent ingrown nails and infections.

  - Either arms or legs: Suntan gradually, use sunscreen; clean cuts with soap and water, then use antibacterial ointment;

use gauze wrapping instead of tape, do not wrap so tight that circulation is cut off; talk to the doctor about any rashes; avoid needle sticks of any type in the affected arm or leg; avoid extreme hot or cold such as ice packs or heating pads; do not overwork the affected arm or leg.

- Do not put too much pressure on the arm or leg.
    - Do not cross legs while sitting.
    - Wear loose jewelry; wear clothes without tight bands.
    - Carry a handbag on the unaffected arm.
    - Do not use blood pressure cuffs on the affected arm.
    - Do not use elastic bandages or stockings with tight bands.
    - Do not sit in one position for more than 30 minutes.
- Watch for signs of infection, such as redness, pain, heat, swelling, and fever. Call the doctor immediately if any of these signs appear.
- Do prescribed exercises regularly as instructed by the doctor or therapist.
- Keep regular follow-up appointments with the doctor.
- Check all areas of the arms and legs every day for signs of problems.
    - Measure around the arm or leg at regular intervals as suggested by the doctor or therapist.
    - Measure the arm or leg at the same two places each time.
    - Tell the doctor if the limb suddenly gets larger.
- The ability to feel sensations such as touch, temperature, or pain in the affected arm or leg may be lessened. Use the unaffected limb to test temperatures for bath water or cooking.

Treatment for Lymphedema

Lymphedema is treated by physical methods and with medication. Physical methods include supporting the arm or leg in a raised position, manual lymphatic drainage (a specialized form of very light massage that helps to move fluid from the end of the limb toward the trunk of the body), wearing custom-fitted clothes that apply controlled pressure around the affected limb, and cleaning the skin carefully to prevent infection. Lymphedema may be treated by combining several therapies. This is known as complex physical therapy (or complex decongestive therapy), which consists of manual lymphedema treatment, compression wrapping, individualized exercises, and skin care followed by a maintenance program. Complex physical therapy must be performed by a professional trained in the techniques.

Surgery for treating lymphedema usually results in complications and is seldom recommended for cancer patients.

Compression Garments

When pressure garments are used, they should cover the entire area of edema. For example, a stocking that reaches only to the knee tends to become tight and block the lymphatic vessels and veins if there is edema in the thigh. Pumps connected to cuffs that wrap around the arm or leg and apply pressure on and off may be helpful; however, some physicians and therapists feel these pumps are not effective and may make the edema worse. The cuff is inflated and deflated according to a controlled time cycle. This pumping action is believed to increase the movement of fluid in the veins and lymphatic vessels and keeps fluid from collecting in the arm or leg. Compression pumps should be used only under the supervision of a trained health care professional because high external pressure can damage the lymphatic vessels near the skin surface.

Drug Therapy

Antibiotics may be used to treat and prevent infections. Other types of drugs such as diuretics or anticoagulants (blood thinners) are generally not helpful, and may make the problem worse.

Finding the exact cause of the swelling and treating it correctly is important. Edema often leads to infection, which then increases fluid and protein deposits in the tissues. If an infection is diagnosed, appropriate antibiotics should be given. Blood clots should be ruled out because massage and other therapy techniques to encourage drainage may cause the clots to move through the bloodstream and cause more serious heart or lung problems. If blood clots are found, they should be treated with anticoagulants.

Coumarin is a dietary supplement that has been studied as a treatment for lymphedema. In the United States, dietary supplements are regulated as foods, not drugs. Supplements are not required to be approved by the Food and Drug Administration (FDA) before being put on the market. Because there are no standards for manufacturing consistency, dose, or purity, one lot of dietary supplements may differ considerably from the next.

Coumarin was once used in some foods and medications in the United States. It was found to cause liver damage, and its use in foods and medications in the United States has been banned since the 1950s. Coumarin is available in several countries, but has not been approved for use in the United States or Canada.

Dietary Management

The nutritional status of the patient should be evaluated and appropriate dietary recommendations should be made. Blood protein levels and weight should be monitored regularly, and patients should be encouraged to eat protein-rich foods.

Pain Management

Patients with lymphedema may experience pain caused by the swelling and pressure on nerves; loss of muscle tissue and function; or scar tissue causing shortening of muscles and less movement at joints. Pain may be treated with medications, relaxation techniques, and/or transcutaneous electric nerve stimulation (TENS); however, the most successful treatment is to decrease the lymphedema.

Complications

Edema can make tissues less able to take in nutrients and more likely to be damaged if the affected limb is not moved for long periods. Therefore, patients with lymphedema should be monitored for areas of skin breakdown, especially over areas with very little tissue between the skin and bone (hips, knees, and elbows).

Bladder emptying problems can develop from lymphedema in the pelvic or groin areas. Patients with lymphedema who are also taking opioids may develop bowel problems. Bowel and bladder status should be monitored regularly for any signs of urine retention or constipation.

Psychosocial Considerations

Because lymphedema is disfiguring and sometimes painful and disabling, it can create mental, physical, and sexual problems. Several studies have noted that women who develop lymphedema after treatment for breast cancer have more mental, physical, and sexual difficulties than women who do not develop lymphedema. The added stresses associated with lymphedema may interfere with treatment that is often painful, difficult, and time-consuming.

Coping with lymphedema in the arm after breast cancer treatment is especially difficult for patients who have little social support. Some patients may react to the problem by withdrawing. Coping is also difficult for patients with painful lymphedema. Patients with lymphedema may be helped by group and individual counseling that provides information about ways to prevent lymphedema, the role of diet and exercise, advice for picking comfortable and flattering clothes, and emotional support.

Lymphangiosarcoma

In addition to the complications associated with chronic lymphedema noted in previous sections, a rare but fatal complication of lymphedema is lymphangiosarcoma, a tumor of the lymphatic vessels. The average time between mastectomy and the appearance of lymphangiosarcoma is about 10 years. After a patient develops lymphangiosarcoma, the average survival time is a little more than one year.

The cause of lymphangiosarcoma is not known. It appears as one or more bluish-red bumps on the affected arm or leg. First, one purplered, slightly raised area in the skin of the arm or leg appears. The patient usually describes it as a bruise. Later, more tumors appear, and the bumps grow. Death usually results from metastases to the lungs.

Chapter 37

Blood Cell Deficiencies: Cytopenias

Cancer patients frequently develop cytopenia, a disorder in which the production of one or more blood cell type ceases or is greatly reduced. Cancer and chemotherapy used to treat cancer, and sometimes radiation therapy, can cause cytopenia.

Types

A deficiency of red blood cells is called anemia; a deficiency of white blood cells, or leukocytes, leukopenia or neutropenia (neutrophils make up over half of all white blood cells); and deficiency of platelets, thrombocytopenia.

Pancytopenia is the deficiency of all three blood cell types and is characteristic of aplastic anemia, a potentially life-threatening disorder that requires a stem cell transplant.

Blood Cells

The blood consists of three types of cells: red blood cells (erythrocytes), white blood cells (leukocytes), and platelets. Erythrocytes contain hemoglobin, the protein that carries oxygen from the lungs to all cells in the body. Proper cell function depends on an adequate oxygen supply. When cells are oxygen deprived, organ function can be seriously impaired.

Leukocytes (white blood cells) protect the body against viral, bacterial, and parasitic infection and detect and remove damaged, dying, or dead tissues. Someone with a deficiency of white blood cells is extremely vulnerable to infection.

The term "leukocyte" refers to all six types of white blood cells; each plays a unique role in the immune system:

- Basophils circulate in the blood and initiate the inflammatory response.

- Eosinophils kill infecting parasites and produce allergic reactions.

- Lymphocytes produce antibodies and regulate immune responses.

- Mast cells are fixed in tissues and initiate the inflammatory response.

- Monocytes capture infecting organisms for identification, ingest infecting organisms, and remove damaged or dying cells and cell debris. When monocytes become fixed in tissue, they are called macrophages.

- Neutrophils identify and kill infecting organisms, and remove dead tissue.

Platelets are essential factors for blood clotting. Sudden blood loss triggers platelet activity at the site of the wound. Exposure to oxygen in the air causes platelets to break apart and combine with a substance called fibrinogen to form fibrin. Fibrin has a thread-like structure and forms a scab, or external clot, as it dries. Platelet deficiency causes one to bruise and bleed easily. Blood does not clot at an open wound, and there is greater risk for internal bleeding.

All blood cells have a lifespan: erythrocytes have a lifespan of about 120 days; leukocytes, 1 to 3 days; and platelets, approximately 10 days. The body continually replenishes the blood supply through a process called hematopoiesis.

Blood cell formation: Hematopoiesis, the formation and development of blood cells, occurs in bone marrow. Bone marrow is a nutrient-rich spongy tissue located mainly in the central portions of long flat bones (e.g., sternum, pelvic bones) in adults and all bones in infants.

All blood cells derive from blood-forming stem cells that reside in bone marrow. Stem cells replicate indefinitely and develop into mature, specialized cells. A hormone produced in the kidneys, erythropoietin, stimulates blood stem cells to produce all three types of blood cells.

Causes and Risk Factors

Chemotherapy and radiation therapy both reduce the number of blood-forming stem cells in cancer patients, but chemotherapeutic agents have a greater adverse effect because they suppress bone marrow function in several ways. The degree of damage is related to the particular drug(s) and the dose.

Chemotherapeutic agents can produce deficiencies in all blood cell types by:

- damaging blood-forming stem cells,

- suppressing the kidneys' production of erythropoietin (hormone that stimulates blood cell production), and

- triggering red cell destruction (hemolysis) by inducing an immune response that causes the body to mistakenly identify erythrocytes as foreign bodies and destroy them.

Malignant tumors can cause anemia and other cytopenias when they directly invade bone marrow and suppress marrow function. Malignant cells also can migrate from tumors in other parts of the body to bone marrow. Tumors also can replace normal blood-forming stem cells with abnormal clones.

Medications used to treat bacterial infection and other illnesses also can contribute to immune system suppression. Some of these are listed here:

- Antacids: cimetidine (Tagamet®)

- Antibiotics: chloramphenicol (Chloromycetin®), sulfonamide (Thiosulfil®, Gantanol®); cephalosporin (Cephalexin®), vancomycin (Vancocin®)

- Anticonvulsants: phenytoin/hydantoin (Dilantin®), felbamate (Felbatol®), carbamazepine (Tegretol®)

- Antimalarials: chloroquine (Aralen®)

- Antivirals: ganciclovir (Vitrasert®), zidovudine (AZT®)

- Cardiac drugs: diltiazem (Cardizem®), nifedipine (Procardia®), verapamil (Calan®)

- Diabetes drugs: glipizide (Glucotrol®), glyburide (Micronase®)
- Hyperthyroid drug: propylthiouracil
- NSAIDs (nonsteroidal anti-inflammatory drugs): phenylbutazone (Butazolidin®), indomethacin (Indocin®, Indochron E-R®) (Due to potentially severe gastrointestinal and cardiovascular side effects, NSAIDs should only be used as instructed.)
- Rheumatoid arthritis drugs: auranofin (Ridaura®), aurothioglucose (Solganal®), gold sodium thiomalate (Myochrysine®)

Signs and Symptoms

Anemia

A deficiency in erythrocytes reduces the amount of oxygen reaching all cells in the body, thus impairing all tissue and organ function. Severe fatigue is the most common symptom of anemia and is experienced by approximately 75% of chemotherapy patients. Patients find it more disabling than other treatment side effects, including nausea and depression.

Anemia also produces these symptoms:

- Confusion
- Dizziness
- Headache
- Lightheadedness
- Loss of concentration
- Pallor (pale skin, nail beds, gums, linings of eyelids)
- Rapid heart rate (tachycardia)
- Shortness of breath (dyspnea)

Neutropenia

Patients with a white blood cell deficiency experience frequent or severe bacterial, viral, and fungal infections; fever; and mouth and throat ulcers.

Complications: Bacteremia, the form of sepsis characterized by the presence of bacteria in the blood, can develop in immunocompromised patients who have neutropenia. Fever, rapid heart rate, and quick shallow breathing are signs of early sepsis, usually a reversible condition.

Untreated bacteremia can lead to severe sepsis, in which one or more organs become dysfunctional. Septic shock is severe sepsis with low blood pressure. The risk for death increases with the development of septic shock. Even aggressive treatment can fail to reverse the condition.

Thrombocytopenia

Platelet deficiency causes patients to bruise and bleed easily. Bleeding occurs most often in the mucous membranes lining the mouth, nose, colon, and vagina. Tiny reddish-purple skin lesions (petechiae), evidence of pinpoint hemorrhages, may appear on the skin or in the mouth.

Pancytopenia

Patients who are deficient in all blood cell types experience signs and symptoms associated with each, but bleeding from the nose and gums, and easy bruising usually appear first. Symptoms of anemia (e.g., fatigue, shortness of breath) are also common. Patients may look and feel well, otherwise, despite the seriousness of their condition.

Diagnosis

Diagnosis of cytopenia in the cancer patient requires a complete blood count (CBC) and the identification of any blood and bone marrow abnormalities.

Complete Blood Count

A complete blood count (CBC) is performed to identify anemia, neutropenia, or thrombocytopenia. A sample of the patient's blood is drawn and examined under a microscope to obtain the CBC.

Red blood cell count (RBC) is the number of red blood cells capable of carrying hemoglobin in a cubic millimeter of blood. The normal RBC for men is 4.5 to 6 million cubic millimeter; for women, 4 to 5.5 million per cubic millimeter. Reticulocytes (young red blood cell) are also counted.

White blood cell count (WBC) is the total number of all five types of white blood cells. The normal WBC for men and women is 5,000 to 10,000 per milliliter of blood.

Five types of cells are counted and then reported as a percentage of the WBC. This is called the differential. (Mast cells are not included because they are not present in the blood.) Typical reports show the normal range:

- Basophils < 1%
- Eosinophils 1–4%
- Lymphocytes 20–40%
- Monocytes or macrophages 2–8%
- Neutrophils 55–70%

Cell counts above or below the normal range are highlighted for the physician. The normal platelet count ranges from 150,000 to 450,000 platelets per milliliter of blood.

Monitoring the Blood Count

Because chemotherapeutic agents adversely affect bone marrow cells, a complete blood count (CBC) is necessary prior to each treatment. The effects on bone marrow are temporary and normal functioning usually returns within 4–10 days.

Because mature red blood cells have a relatively long life (120 days), cell production usually resumes before symptoms of deficiency develop. White blood cells, however, have a life span of 1 to 3 days only. Those in circulation remain unaffected, but the production of new leukocytes may be slow, creating a period of increased risk for infection.

White blood cell production usually recovers before the next treatment. If it does not, treatment is delayed until the cell count increases sufficiently.

Thrombocytopenia (below normal platelet count of 15,000 to 300,000 per milliliter) and the risk of increased bleeding usually peaks 10 to 14 days following a course of chemotherapy. Damage to these cells is not permanent and their full recovery is expected within 2-weeks after treatment.

Bone Marrow Aspiration and Needle Biopsy

Both of these tests involve taking samples of bone marrow for examination under a microscope. Samples are usually obtained from the pelvic bone but may be taken from the breastbone.

The puncture site for marrow extraction from the pelvic bone is located in the lower back. Both procedures present a risk for bleeding at the puncture site and infection, although infection is rare.

Aspiration: Bone marrow aspiration is performed with a thin aspirating needle (needle with a syringe) to obtain a sample of bone marrow fluid.

The puncture site is cleansed with antiseptic and then a local anesthetic is given to the patient. Once the anesthetic has taken effect, the aspirating needle is inserted into the bone. The plunger is then pulled to suction out a sample of bone marrow fluid into the syringe. The sample is put between glass slides for examination under a microscope.

Pressure is applied to the puncture site to stop any bleeding, and then the wound is covered with a bandage.

Needle biopsy: A bone marrow biopsy needle is used to remove a sample of bone marrow tissue. Sometimes marrow aspirate is taken before the biopsy is performed.

First, the puncture site is cleansed with antiseptic, and then a local anesthetic is given to the patient. Once the anesthetic has taken effect, a small incision is made in the lower back. The biopsy needle is inserted through the incision and into the bone. The solid core of the needle is removed from the shaft, and the needle turned back and forth to collect a tissue sample.

Pressure is applied to the puncture site to stop any bleeding. The wound is then covered with a bandage.

Treatment

Anemia

People with anemia (reduced red cell production) are advised to:

- rest and
- eat foods high in iron (meat, fish, poultry, lentils, legumes, iron-enriched grains and flours).

If immediate remedy is necessary, treatment includes:

- medication that helps restore the red blood supply and
- a transfusion of packed red blood cells.

Epoetin alpha (Epogen®, Procrit®)is a synthetic erythropoietin (normally produced by the kidneys) that stimulates stem cells to produce red blood cells. Restoration of the red blood cell supply with medication is gradual.

Darbepoetin alfa (Aranesp®) also stimulates red blood cell production but requires fewer doses and less disruption of daily living.

Thrombocytopenia

People with an abnormally low platelet count should avoid bruising or breaking the skin, and should carefully brush their teeth. A persistently decreased platelet count may be treated with a transfusion of platelets.

Neutropenia

The patient with a low white blood cell count is advised to:

* avoid contact with people who are ill,

* monitor closely for signs of infection (e.g., fever), and

* take antibiotics when appropriate.

Medication, a colony-stimulating factor (CSF), may be prescribed to speed the development of white blood cells and shorten the period of susceptibility to infection.

Growth Factors

Growth factors are synthetic versions of substances involved in stimulating red and white blood cell production. Physicians exercise caution when prescribing these medications for people with tumors that involve the bone marrow, because growth factors might stimulate malignant cell growth.

These medications include:

* Epoetin alpha (Procrit®, Epogen®) stimulates red blood cell production,

* G-CSF (granulocyte colony-stimulating factor; filgrastim, Neupogen®) stimulates neutrophil production, and

* GM-CSF (granulocyte-macrophage colony-stimulating factor) stimulates production of several white blood cells, including macrophages.

Leukocytes and other cells that contain granules are also called granulocytes.

Side effects: Fever, fatigue, dizziness, diarrhea, nausea, vomiting, weakness, and paresthesia (prickling sensation) are side effects associated with epoetin alpha.

Bone pain, malaise, headache, flu-like symptoms, muscle ache, redness at the injection site, and skin rash may occur with GM-CSF.

G-CSF commonly produces bone pain.

Bone Marrow and Stem Cell Transplantation

The treatment of choice for the pancytopenic patient with a matched bone marrow donor is stem cell transplantation. The goal of transplantation is to restore blood-forming stem cells to the marrow.

Immunosuppressive Therapy

When a compatible bone marrow donor cannot be found, immuno-suppression is the treatment of choice for patients with pancytope-nia.

Antilymphocyte globulin (ALG) or antithymocyte globulin (ATG) combined with cyclosporine is given. Improvement in blood counts is slow, taking a couple of months, and relapse is common. Follow-up includes an annual bone marrow examination.

Side effects: Flu-like symptoms and joint pain are common early side effects of ALG and ATG. Long-term treatment with cyclosporine can cause hypertension, seizures, opportunistic infections, and nephro-toxicity (poisoning of the kidney).

Prognosis

Anemia, thrombocytopenia, and neutropenia caused by cancer treatment usually resolve once the course of treatment is over.

Pancytopenia patients who receive a marrow transplant from a matched donor also have a good prognosis for recovering satisfactory cell counts. Recipients of marrow from imperfectly matched donors are at high risk for complications caused by the transplant. Survival rates of patients who receive immunosuppressive therapy are similar to those who receive transplants.

Chapter 38

Hypercalcemia

Understanding Hypercalcemia

Hypercalcemia occurs in 10%–20% of people with cancer, although it occurs much less often in children. The cancers most often associated with hypercalcemia are cancer of the breast and lung, as well as certain cancers of the blood, particularly multiple myeloma. Early diagnosis and treatment with fluids and drugs that lower calcium levels in the blood can improve symptoms in a few days, but diagnosis may be difficult. Symptoms of hypercalcemia can appear gradually and may resemble symptoms of many cancers and other diseases. Early diagnosis and treatment are not only lifesaving in the short term, but may also increase the patient's ability to complete cancer therapy and improve the patient's quality of life.

Patients who have advanced terminal cancer and are no longer receiving treatment for the cancer may choose not to be treated for hypercalcemia. This option should be considered by a patient and his or her family in advance, before symptoms of hypercalcemia occur.

Normal Calcium Regulation

Healthy people consume about the same amount of calcium in their diet as their bodies lose in urine, feces, and sweat. Hypercalcemia

PDQ® Cancer Information Summary. National Cancer Institute; Bethesda, MD. Hypercalcemia (PDQ®): Supportive Care - Patient. Updated 09/2005. Available at http://cancer.gov. Accessed November 10, 2006.

associated with cancer disrupts the body's ability to maintain a normal level of calcium.

Kidney Function

Normal, healthy kidneys are able to filter large amounts of calcium from the blood, excrete the excess not needed by the body, and retain the amount of calcium the body does need. However, hypercalcemia may cause such high levels of calcium in the body that the kidneys are overworked and become unable to excrete the excess. Some tumors produce a substance that can cause the kidneys to excrete too little calcium. This results in a large amount of urine being produced, which then causes dehydration. Dehydration may lead to appetite loss, nausea, and vomiting which make the dehydration worse. Inactivity caused by weakness and tiredness may increase the amount of calcium in the blood by increasing the amount of calcium that is absorbed from the bones. Calcium deposits may collect in the kidneys, causing permanent damage.

Causes of Hypercalcemia

The main causes of hypercalcemia due to cancer are an increase in the amount of calcium absorbed from the bones, and an inability of the kidneys to excrete excess calcium. Some cancer cells secrete substances that cause calcium to be absorbed into the bloodstream from bones. Immobility, dehydration, anorexia, nausea, and vomiting may also increase calcium levels.

Incidence

Hypercalcemia occurs most frequently in patients with lung and breast cancer. It may also occur in patients with multiple myeloma, head and neck cancer, cancer of unknown primary origin, lymphoma, leukemia, kidney cancer, and gastrointestinal cancer.

Symptoms

There is little relationship between symptoms of hypercalcemia and the actual level of calcium in the blood. Symptoms of hypercalcemia resemble symptoms of other illnesses, making an early and rapid diagnosis difficult. The severity of the symptoms may depend on other factors, such as previous cancer treatment, reactions to drugs, or other illnesses a patient may have.

Most patients do not experience all of the symptoms of hypercalcemia, and some patients may not have any symptoms at all. However, most patients with high calcium levels in the blood do have symptoms. Some patients develop signs of hypercalcemia when calcium levels are only slightly high, while patients who have had higher calcium levels for a long time may show few symptoms.

The most common symptoms of hypercalcemia are feeling tired, difficulty thinking clearly, lack of appetite, pain, frequent urination, increased thirst, constipation, nausea, and vomiting.

Symptoms may be classified by the affected body part:

Nervous system: Calcium plays a major role in the normal functioning of the central nervous system (the brain and spinal cord). Symptoms of hypercalcemia may include weakness, loss of reflexes in the muscles, and decreased stamina. Patients with central nervous system symptoms may have changes in personality, difficulty thinking or speaking clearly, disorientation, or hallucinations. Eventually, coma may result. Headaches can also occur, which can be made worse by vomiting and dehydration.

Heart: Hypercalcemia affects normal heart rhythms and increases sensitivity to some heart medications (such as digoxin). As calcium levels increase, irregular heartbeats may develop, and may lead to a heart attack.

Gastrointestinal: Increased stomach acid often is produced with hypercalcemia and may intensify loss of appetite, nausea, and vomiting. Constipation may result from the dehydration associated with hypercalcemia.

Kidney: Hypercalcemia causes the kidneys to not function correctly, leading to the production of large volumes of urine. The large amount of urine combined with less liquid intake leads to symptoms of dehydration, including thirst, dry mouth, little or no sweating, and concentrated urine. Patients with myeloma often have kidney problems due to hypercalcemia. Kidney stones may result from long-term hypercalcemia.

Bone: Hypercalcemia of cancer can result from bone metastases or bone loss, and may contribute to broken bones, bone disfigurement, and pain.

Assessment

Laboratory assessment: A blood test is done to check the level of calcium. Other blood tests may be done to check kidney function.

Clinical assessment: Patients with high calcium levels should be examined for the following:

- Symptoms:
  - Nerves and muscles (muscle strength, muscle tone, reflexes, tiredness, indifference, depression, confusion, restlessness)
  - Heart (high blood pressure, heart changes, irregular heartbeat, digitalis poisoning)
  - Kidneys (production of too much urine, night-time urinating, sugar in the urine, excess thirst)
  - Gastrointestinal (loss of appetite, nausea, abdominal pain, constipation, abdominal bloating)
  - Other (muscle and bone pain, itching)
- History:
  - How fast did the symptoms appear?
  - Is there x-ray evidence of primary or metastatic bone disease?
  - Has the patient been taking tamoxifen, estrogen, or androgens?
  - Is the patient taking digoxin?
  - Is the patient receiving calcium in intravenous fluids?
  - Is the patient receiving thiazide diuretics, vitamins A or D, or lithium?
  - Is there another disease present that could cause dehydration or lack of movement?
  - Are there effective treatments for the patient's cancer?

Decision to Treat

The decision to treat hypercalcemia depends on the treatment goals determined by the patient, caregivers, and the physician. The natural course of untreated hypercalcemia progresses to loss of consciousness and coma. This may be preferred by some patients at the end of life who have unrelieved suffering or untreatable symptoms.

Treatment

Prevention

Patients at risk of developing hypercalcemia may be the first to recognize its symptoms, such as fatigue. Measures to prevent hypercalcemia include drinking enough fluids, controlling nausea and vomiting, walking and being active, and cautious use or elimination of drugs that can contribute to the development of hypercalcemia or affect its treatment. Calcium in the diet should not be reduced or eliminated, however, because the body's absorption of calcium is reduced in patients with hypercalcemia.

Managing Hypercalcemia

Fluids are given to treat dehydration. Medication is given to stop the breakdown of bone. The cancer causing the hypercalcemia should be treated effectively.

The severity of the hypercalcemia determines the amount of treatment necessary. Severe hypercalcemia should be treated immediately and aggressively. Less severe hypercalcemia should be treated according to the symptoms. Response to treatment is shown by the disappearance of the symptoms of hypercalcemia and a decrease in the level of calcium in the blood.

Mild hypercalcemia does not usually need to be treated aggressively. Patients with mild hypercalcemia and central nervous system symptoms are harder to treat. Younger patients are especially difficult to treat because they tolerate hypercalcemia better. Other causes of the central nervous system symptoms should be ruled out before deciding that they are caused by hypercalcemia alone.

Treatment for hypercalcemia can improve symptoms. Increased urination and thirst, central nervous system symptoms, nausea, vomiting, and constipation improve with treatment more easily than other symptoms, such as loss of appetite, and tiredness. Pain may be more easily controlled once calcium levels are normal. Effective therapy that lowers calcium usually improves symptoms, enhances the quality of life, and may allow the patient to leave the hospital.

After calcium levels return to normal, urine and blood should continue to be checked often to make sure the treatment is still working.

Mild Hypercalcemia

Giving fluids by vein and observing the patient is an accepted treatment for patients with mild hypercalcemia (but no symptoms) and who also have cancer that responds well to anticancer treatment (such as lymphoma, breast cancer, ovarian cancer, head and neck cancers, or multiple myeloma). If the patient has symptoms, or has a cancer that is expected to respond slowly to treatment, then drugs to treat the hypercalcemia should be started. Other treatments should focus on controlling nausea, vomiting, and fever, encouraging continued activity, and limiting use of drugs that cause sleepiness.

Moderate to Severe Hypercalcemia

Replacing fluids is the first and most important step in treating moderate or severe hypercalcemia. Replacing fluids will not restore normal calcium levels in all patients, but it is still important to do first. The patient's mental state should improve, and nausea and vomiting should decrease within the first 24 hours, but this improvement is only temporary. If cancer therapy (surgery, radiation, or chemotherapy) is not able to be started immediately, then drugs to lower the calcium levels must be used to control the hypercalcemia.

Drugs that may help stop the breakdown of bone include calcitonin, plicamycin (mithramycin), bisphosphonates (etidronate, pamidronate, and clodronate), and gallium nitrate. Steroids and phosphate may also be used to treat hypercalcemia. Dialysis is used as a treatment for hypercalcemia in patients with kidney failure. Other drugs are currently being studied as possible treatments for hypercalcemia. Combinations of drugs may also be used.

Patient and Family Education

Because hypercalcemia affects quality of life and can be life-threatening if not treated, patients and their caregivers should be aware of the symptoms. They should also learn how to prevent hypercalcemia, what can make it worse, and when to see the doctor.

Supportive Care

Even with improved treatment for hypercalcemia, many patients do not survive this complication of cancer. Only effective anticancer therapy improves the patient's chances for long-term survival.

Supportive care includes measures to provide the patient with protection from injury, prevention of fractures, and treatment of symptoms.

Treatment of symptoms is important, especially the prevention of accidental or self-inflicted injury if a patient is confused. Nausea, vomiting, and constipation may also need to be controlled until calcium levels go down. Broken bones may occur due to weakening, so patients need to be moved gently, and falling must be prevented. Activity and weight-bearing exercises should be encouraged. Any new bone pain should be reported so that it can be evaluated for possible fractures.

Supportive care to comfort terminally ill patients and their family members becomes necessary in the last stages of the disease. Changes in the patient's thinking and behavior may especially upset the family.

Psychosocial Management

Usually, treatment of the hypercalcemia will eliminate delirium, agitation, or mental changes, but some patients may need other medications to treat these symptoms. Mental changes may take some time to get better, even after calcium levels return to normal.

Lethargy (mental and physical sluggishness) is often a symptom of hypercalcemia. Family members (and sometimes medical staff) may think that the patient is depressed until the actual cause is determined. Most patients will not have symptoms of depression (such as hopelessness, helplessness, guilt, worthlessness, or thoughts of suicide) and instead will appear to be indifferent.

Patients and family members should report symptoms of hypercalcemia such as lethargy, fatigue, confusion, loss of appetite, nausea/vomiting, constipation, and excessive thirst to the health care provider.

Prognosis

Hypercalcemia usually develops as a late complication of cancer, and its appearance is very serious. However, it is not clear if death occurs due to a hypercalcemia crisis (uncontrolled or one that comes back and gets worse) or due to the advanced cancer.

Chapter 39

Late Effects of Treatment for Childhood Cancer

Late effects are treatment-related health problems that appear months or years after treatment has ended. The treatment of cancer may damage healthy cells at the same time it destroys cancer cells. Some cancer treatments, such as chemotherapy, radiation therapy, and bone marrow or stem cell transplant, stop the growth of rapidly dividing cells, such as cancer cells. Since bones, tissues, and organs that are growing with the child have cells that are also dividing rapidly, cancer treatment can prevent them from developing normally. Other cancer treatments include surgery to remove all or part of certain organs that have cancer in them. The damage from these cancer treatments can be mild or serious, and the effects may be seen during treatment or months to years later.

Side effects that continue or appear after cancer treatment has ended are called late effects. It is important for the parents and the patient to know that children treated for cancer (childhood cancer survivors) may develop late effects from their treatment.

Late effects of cancer treatment may affect the following in childhood cancer survivors:

- Organs, bones, or body tissues
- Mood, feelings, and actions
- Thinking, learning, and memory

PDQ® Cancer Information Summary. National Cancer Institute; Bethesda, MD. Late Effects of Treatment for Childhood Cancer (PDQ®): Treatment - Patient. Updated 03/2005. Available at http://cancer.gov. Accessed November 10, 2006.

The risk that a cancer treatment will cause late effects depends on many things, including the following:

- The type of cancer and where it is in the body
- The child's age (when treated)
- The type and amount of treatment
- The area treated
- Genetic factors or health problems the child had before the cancer

Regular follow-up by health professionals who are expert in finding and treating late effects is important for the long-term health of childhood cancer survivors. Records about the cancer diagnosis and treatment, including all test results, should be kept by childhood cancer survivors (or their caregivers). This information may be used to help find and treat late effects.

Doctors are studying the late effects that cancer treatments cause in childhood cancer survivors. They are trying to find out if changing treatment can help prevent or lessen late effects in childhood cancer survivors.

Central Nervous System

Cancer treatments to the central nervous system (CNS) may affect the child's brain. Childhood cancer survivors who received radiation therapy to the head, brain surgery, or intrathecal chemotherapy are at risk of having problems in the following areas:

- Thinking
- Learning
- Problem solving
- Speech
- Reading
- Writing
- Memory
- Coordinating movement between the eyes, hands, and other muscles

Survivors may have learning disabilities or a lower IQ.

The following factors may increase the risk of CNS late effects:

- Being young at the time of treatment (the younger the child, the greater the risk)
- Having a tumor in the CNS
- Receiving certain combinations of treatment, such as high-dose chemotherapy and radiation therapy to the brain

Treatment for these and other childhood cancers may cause CNS late effects:

- Acute lymphoblastic leukemia (ALL)
- Central nervous system (CNS) tumors
- Head and neck cancers

Survivors of childhood cancer may have anxiety and depression related to physical changes, appearance, or the fear of cancer coming back. These problems may prevent survivors from returning to their normal routines and activities. They may also cause problems with personal relationships, education, employment, and health.

Being diagnosed with a life-threatening disease and receiving treatment for it is often traumatic. This trauma may cause a group of symptoms called post-traumatic stress disorder (PTSD). PTSD is defined as having certain symptoms following a stressful event that involved death or the threat of death, serious injury, or a threat to oneself or others. People who have survived very stressful situations, such as military combat or natural disasters, may also have PTSD.

PTSD can affect cancer survivors in the following ways:

- Reliving the time they were diagnosed and treated for cancer, in nightmares or flashbacks, and thinking about it all the time
- Avoiding places, events, and people that remind them of the cancer experience
- Being constantly overexcited, fearful, irritable, or unable to sleep, or having trouble concentrating

Family problems, little or no social support from family or friends, and stress not related to the cancer may increase the chances of having PTSD. Because avoiding places and persons connected to the cancer is part of PTSD, survivors with PTSD may not try to get the medical treatment they need.

Senses

Ears

Childhood cancer survivors may have late effects that affect hearing. The risk of hearing loss may be increased in childhood cancer survivors who received either of the following:

- Certain anticancer drugs, such as cisplatin or carboplatin
- Radiation therapy to the brain

Risk may also be increased in childhood cancer survivors who were young at the time of treatment (the younger the child, the greater the risk).

Treatment for these and other childhood cancers may cause hearing late effects:

- Central nervous system (CNS) tumors
- Neuroblastoma
- Head and neck cancers

Eyes

Childhood cancer survivors may have late effects that affect the eyes. Eye late effects may include the following:

- Bone growth problems around the eye socket that affect the shape of the child's face as it grows
- Dry eye
- Cataracts
- Damage to the optic nerve and retina
- Poor vision
- Drooping eyelids
- Eyelid tumors

The following may increase the risk of damage to the eye or eye socket:

- Being younger than one year at the time of treatment
- Tumor of the retina

The risk may also be increased in childhood cancer survivors who had either of the following:

- An eye removed by surgery
- Radiation therapy to the eye or eye socket

Radiation therapy for these and other childhood cancers may cause eye late effects:

- Retinoblastoma, rhabdomyosarcoma, and other tumors of the eye
- Central nervous system (CNS) tumors
- Head and neck cancers

Digestive System

Teeth and Jaw

Childhood cancer survivors may have late effects that affect the teeth and jaw. Teeth and jaw late effects may include the following:

- Teeth are small or do not have a normal shape
- The roots of the teeth are short
- Missing teeth
- New teeth come in at a later than normal age
- The head and face do not reach full growth
- Tooth enamel is not normal
- Salivary glands do not make enough saliva
- Tooth decay (including cavities) and gum disease

The risk of teeth and jaw late effects may be increased in childhood cancer survivors who received any of the following:

- Radiation therapy to the head and neck
- Chemotherapy to treat leukemia
- High-dose chemotherapy with stem cell transplant and total-body irradiation (TBI) to treat neuroblastoma

Risk may also be increased in survivors who were younger than three years at the time of treatment.

It is important that childhood cancer survivors have regular dental checkups to help prevent or detect infection or decay.

Treatment for these and other childhood cancers may cause teeth and jaw late effects:

- Central nervous system (CNS) leukemia
- Neuroblastoma
- Hodgkin lymphoma
- Head and neck cancers
- Nasopharyngeal cancer

Liver

Childhood cancer survivors may have late effects that affect the liver. Liver late effects may include the following:

- Hepatic fibrosis (an overgrowth of connective tissue in the liver)
- Liver failure
- Portal hypertension
- Hepatitis C infection
- Permanent liver damage caused by veno-occlusive disease

Hepatic fibrosis, hepatitis C infection, and veno-occlusive disease can cause long-term problems.

The risk of liver late effects may be increased in childhood cancer survivors who received any of the following:

- A blood transfusion before 1992
- Radiation therapy together with chemotherapy
- Chemotherapy with thioguanine to treat acute lymphoblastic leukemia (ALL)

Risk may also be increased in survivors who had liver disease before treatment or developed veno-occlusive disease during treatment.

Treatment for these and other childhood cancers may cause liver late effects:

- Acute lymphoblastic leukemia (ALL)
- Neuroblastoma
- Wilms tumor

Digestive Tract

Childhood cancer survivors may have late effects that affect the digestive tract. Digestive tract late effects may include the following:

- Ulcers
- Bowel perforation (a hole in the intestine)
- Pain in the abdomen
- Inability of the intestine to absorb nutrients from food
- A narrowing of the intestine
- Blocked bowel (chronic)
- Infection
- Diarrhea (chronic)

These effects may be caused by damage to the blood vessels, which may lead to long-term problems. Radiation therapy to the abdomen may damage blood vessels and increase the risk of digestive tract late effects.

Treatment for these and other childhood cancers may cause digestive tract late effects:

- Paratesticular rhabdomyosarcoma
- Wilms tumor

Spleen

Childhood cancer survivors may have late effects that affect the spleen. Spleen late effects may increase the risk of life-threatening bacterial infections.

The risk of spleen late effects may be increased in childhood cancer survivors who received either of the following:

- Splenectomy (surgery to remove the spleen)
- High-dose radiation therapy to the spleen

It is very important that childhood cancer survivors who received either of these treatments keep immunizations up-to-date and receive antibiotics before having any dental work.

Spleen late effects may be caused by treatment for childhood Hodgkin lymphoma and other childhood cancers.

Heart

Childhood cancer survivors may have late effects that affect the heart. Heart late effects may include the following:

- Abnormal heartbeat
- Disease of the heart muscle
- Congestive heart failure
- Increased risk of stroke, blood clots, and chest pains
- Tiring quickly during exercise
- Coronary artery disease (hardening of the heart arteries)

The following may increase the risk of heart late effects:

- Being female
- Being young at the time of treatment (the younger the child, the greater the risk)
- Having other risk factors for heart disease, such as a family history of heart disease, being overweight, smoking, or having high blood pressure, high cholesterol, or diabetes
- Having received a stem cell transplant
- This risk may also increase as the amounts of anthracycline drugs and radiation used increase and as the time since treatment gets longer.

Treatment for these and other childhood cancers may cause heart late effects:

- Acute lymphoblastic leukemia (ALL)
- Central nervous system (CNS) tumors
- Hodgkin lymphoma
- Wilms tumor

Lung

Childhood cancer survivors may have late effects that affect the lungs. Lung late effects may include the following:

- Shortness of breath

- Cough (chronic)
- Pulmonary fibrosis (the build-up of scar tissue in the lung)
- Pneumonia (chronic)
- Inflamed lungs or pleura

The risk of lung late effects may be increased in childhood cancer survivors who had either of the following:

- Infections or graft-versus-host disease after a bone marrow transplant
- Lung disease, such as asthma, before cancer treatment

Risk may also be increased in survivors who received any of the following:

- Certain anticancer drugs, such as bleomycin or doxorubicin
- Radiation therapy to the chest
- Stem cell transplant

Treatment for these and other childhood cancers may cause lung late effects:

- Acute lymphoblastic leukemia (ALL)
- Hodgkin lymphoma
- Non-Hodgkin lymphoma
- Wilms tumor

Kidney

Childhood cancer survivors may have late effects that affect the kidneys. Kidney late effects may include the following:

- Renal tubular acidosis
- Fanconi syndrome
- Kidney failure
- Hypertension (high blood pressure)

The following may increase the risk of kidney late effects:

- Having cancer in both kidneys

- Being young at the time of treatment (the younger the child, the greater the risk)
- Having a genetic syndrome that increases the risk of kidney problems, such as Denys-Drash syndrome

Risk may also be increased in childhood cancer survivors who received any of the following:

- Certain anticancer drugs, such as cisplatin, carboplatin, or ifosfamide
- Certain antibiotics or antifungal drugs
- Radiation therapy to the kidney or areas near the kidney

Kidney late effects may be caused by treatment for Wilms tumor and other childhood cancers.

Thyroid

Childhood cancer survivors may have late effects that affect the thyroid. Thyroid late effects may include the following:

- Hypothyroidism (not enough thyroid hormone)
- Hyperthyroidism (too much thyroid hormone)
- Goiter
- Lumps in the thyroid

The risk of thyroid late effects may be increased in childhood cancer survivors who received either of the following:

- Radiation therapy to the head and neck
- Total-body irradiation (TBI) as part of a stem cell transplant

The risk may also be greater in females and may increase as the amount of time since diagnosis gets longer.

Treatment for these and other childhood cancers may cause thyroid late effects:

- Acute lymphoblastic leukemia (ALL)
- Brain tumors
- Hodgkin lymphoma

- Head and neck cancers

Neuroendocrine System

Childhood cancer survivors may have late effects that affect the neuroendocrine system. Neuroendocrine late effects may include the following:

- Low levels of pituitary hormones, including growth hormone
- Early puberty (especially in females)
- Late puberty
- Disorders of the hypothalamus
- Pituitary gland problems

Childhood cancer survivors who received a stem cell transplant with total-body irradiation (TBI) have an increased risk of growth disorders.

Their risk is affected as follows:

- Low levels of growth hormone are more likely if the survivor:
  - is female; or
  - received radiation therapy to the head before the transplant; or
  - received TBI in a single dose instead of divided doses; or
  - had graft-versus-host disease; or
  - received busulfan and cyclophosphamide.
- Adult height that is shorter than normal is more likely if the survivor:
  - is male; or
  - received the transplant at a young age; or
  - received TBI in a single dose instead of divided doses.

Treatment for these and other childhood cancers may cause neuroendocrine late effects:

- Acute lymphoblastic leukemia (ALL)
- Central nervous system (CNS) tumors
- Lymphoma

Musculoskeletal System

Bone

Childhood cancer survivors may have late effects that affect the bones. Bone late effects may include the following:

- Bone pain
- Joint stiffness
- Weak or thin bones that can break easily
- Decreased amounts of calcium in bones
- Decreased bone and tissue growth in treated areas

The following may increase the risk of bone late effects:

- Being female
- Being older at the time of treatment
- Having low levels of estrogen or growth hormone

Risk may also be increased in childhood cancer survivors who received either of the following:

- Radiation therapy, especially to the head and spine
- Steroids, such as dexamethasone, with cancer treatment
- Bone late effects may be caused by treatment for certain childhood cancers

Treatment for these and other childhood cancers may cause bone late effects:

- Acute lymphoblastic leukemia (ALL)
- Central nervous system (CNS) tumors
- Bone cancer
- Wilms tumor

Body Weight

Childhood cancer survivors may have late effects that affect body weight and cause obesity. The following may increase the risk of obesity:

- Being female and having received treatment at age 4 years or younger, with high-dose radiation therapy to the head

- Being young at the time of treatment (the younger the child, the greater the risk)
- Being slender at the time of diagnosis
- Having an increase in body fat at an earlier than normal age

Treatment for these and other childhood cancers may cause obesity:

- Acute lymphoblastic leukemia (ALL)
- Brain tumors
- Hodgkin lymphoma
- Non-Hodgkin lymphoma

Reproductive System

Testicles

Childhood cancer survivors may have late effects that affect the testicles. Testicular late effects may cause infertility or a low sperm count. Low sperm counts may be temporary or permanent depending on the radiation dose and schedule, the area of the body treated, and the age when treated.

The risk of testicular late effects may be increased in childhood cancer survivors who received either of the following:

- Chemotherapy with alkylating agents, such as cyclophosphamide, procarbazine, and ifosfamide
- Radiation therapy to the abdomen

Treatment for these and other childhood cancers may cause testicular late effects:

- Acute lymphoblastic leukemia (ALL)
- Osteosarcoma
- Hodgkin lymphoma
- Sarcoma

Ovaries

Childhood cancer survivors may have late effects that affect the ovaries. Ovarian late effects may include the following:

- Infertility

- Irregular menstrual periods
- Ovarian failure
- Early menopause

The risk of ovarian late effects may be increased in childhood cancer survivors who received any of the following:

- Chemotherapy with alkylating agents, such as cyclophosphamide, mechlorethamine, procarbazine, and ifosfamide
- Radiation therapy together with alkylating agents
- Treatment at an older age

Uterus

Childhood cancer survivors may have late effects that affect the uterus. The uterus may become less elastic and grow to a size that is smaller than normal. This can cause an increased risk of miscarriage and premature birth. Growth of the fetus within the uterus may also be affected.

The risk of uterine late effects may be increased in women who received radiation therapy to the abdomen. Ovarian and uterine late effects may be caused by treatment for childhood osteosarcoma and other childhood cancers.

Reproduction

Childhood cancer survivors may have late effects that affect pregnancies. Late effects on pregnancies include increased risk of the following:

- Miscarriage
- Ending the pregnancy for medical reasons
- Low birth-weight babies
- Early labor
- Premature delivery
- Abnormal position of the fetus
- Birth defects

For male survivors of childhood cancer, there is an increased risk that their children may be stillborn.

Certain stem cell and bone marrow transplants increase the risk of infertility. Stem cell and bone marrow transplants that include total-body irradiation (TBI), cyclophosphamide, or busulfan may damage the ovaries. Problems with the ovaries, fertility, and the ability to carry a baby to term may occur.

The following methods may be used so that childhood cancer survivors can have children:

- Freezing the eggs or sperm before cancer treatment in patients who have reached puberty
- In vitro fertilization (IVF)

There is a risk that there may be cancer cells in the saved eggs, sperm, or embryo. This risk is highest in patients who had cancer of the blood, testicles, or ovaries.

Survivors of childhood cancer may wonder if their children will have birth defects, inherited diseases, or cancer. There is a small increase in the risk of birth defects in the children of females who received radiation therapy to the lower back, but most children of childhood cancer survivors are born healthy.

There may be an increased risk of birth defects in children whose embryos were created in the laboratory and an increased risk of cancer in the children of cancer survivors who had second cancers.

Second Cancers

Certain factors related to treatment increase the risk of second cancers. These include the following:

- Radiation therapy may cause solid tumors and leukemia.
- Risk of second cancers after radiation therapy is increased if alkylating agents were also used and if the patient is female, was younger at the time of diagnosis, or had Hodgkin lymphoma or soft tissue cancer.
- Certain anticancer drugs, such as alkylating agents or platinum drugs may cause leukemia.
- Survivors of childhood Hodgkin lymphoma have the highest risk of developing second cancers, especially breast or thyroid cancer. Young age at diagnosis and treatment for relapsed disease increase the risk.
- Bone marrow transplants increase the risk of tumors later in life.

Some childhood cancer survivors have an increased risk of developing a second cancer because they have certain genetic syndromes that also placed them at risk of developing the primary cancer. These include the following:

- Neurofibromatosis
- Li-Fraumeni syndrome
- Familial polyposis
- The genetic form of retinoblastoma

Frequent and careful follow-up exams are very important for these childhood cancer survivors.

Mortality

Improvements in cancer treatment have decreased the number of deaths from primary cancer. The number of late effects in childhood cancer survivors may increase with age, however, and survivors may not live as long as people who did not have cancer. The most common causes of death in childhood cancer survivors include the following:

- Relapse of the primary cancer
- Second cancer
- Heart damage

Studies of the causes of late effects have led to changes in treatment. This has improved the quality of life for cancer survivors and helped to prevent deaths from late effects.

Long-Term Follow-Up

Regular follow-up care is very important for survivors of childhood cancer. Follow-up care will be different for each person who has been treated for cancer, depending on the type of cancer, the type of treatment, and the person's general health. It is important that childhood cancer survivors receive regular exams by a health care provider who is familiar with their treatments and risks and who can recognize the early signs of late effects.

Childhood cancer survivors are more likely to need special education services, especially survivors of central nervous system tumors, leukemia, and Hodgkin disease.

The childhood cancer survivor's follow-up care will go on into adulthood. It ideally includes the survivor's primary doctor and specialists; educational, vocational, and social service systems; and the family.

Long-term follow-up improves the health and quality of life for cancer survivors and also helps doctors study the late effects of cancer treatments so that safer therapies for newly diagnosed children may be developed.

The quality of life enjoyed by cancer survivors may be improved by behaviors that promote their future health and well-being, such as a healthy diet, exercise, and regular medical and dental checkups. These self-care behaviors are especially important for cancer survivors because of their risk of treatment-related health problems. Healthy behaviors may make late effects less severe and lower the risk of other diseases.

Avoiding behaviors that are damaging to health is also important. Smoking, excess alcohol use, and the use of illegal drugs increase the risk of organ damage and, possibly, of second cancers.

Part Five

Emotional, Cognitive, and Mental Health Issues in Cancer Care

Chapter 40

Dealing with a Changing Self-Image

When you have cancer and when you are having treatment for cancer, changes occur.

- You don't have as much energy as you did before the cancer.
- Your body is not the same as it was.
- If you're single, your dating life may be awkward. You may face new challenges in your sex life.
- If you have a partner, you may face changes in your relationship.

These changes can be hard to accept. But most people with cancer find that, with time, they are able to develop a new self-image by following these suggestions:

- stay actively involved in life
- get help when needed
- talk openly about sex and intimacy with loved ones

Cancer and its treatment can change how you look and feel.

- Surgery can leave scars or change the way you look.

Excerpted from "Taking Time: Support for People with Cancer," National Cancer Institute, September 2003. The complete text of this document is available online at www.cancer.gov. The booklet can also be ordered by calling 800-4-CANCER.

- Chemotherapy can cause your hair to fall out.

- Radiation can make you feel very tired.

- Some drugs may cause you to gain weight or feel bloated.

- Treatments can make it hard to eat. They may upset your stomach and make you throw up. Or they can make you feel so sick that you do not want to eat.

- Some treatments can make it hard to get pregnant or father a child.

Cancer treatment can last for weeks or months. The good news is that most of these side effects go away when the treatment is over.

Many people want to know as much as they can about side effects, even before treatment begins. This way, they can talk with their doctor about ways to treat them. For example, a doctor can change a person's drugs or suggest new foods to eat.

If you think you might want to have children in the future, ask your doctor to refer you to a fertility doctor before you begin treatment for your cancer.

Fatigue

Many people feel fatigue (they are very tired or have little energy) when they are being treated for cancer. They may have good days with lots of energy and bad days when they are very tired. This fatigue is likely to last for a while after treatment is over. For some people, it can last for many months.

Let people know that you have both good and bad days. Try to do something special on days when you feel better. Let yourself rest on the days you are very tired. And don't be afraid to tell others if you feel fatigue, even if you need to change your plans.

Your Self-Image

Each of us has a mental picture of how we look, our "self-image." Although we may not always like how we look, we are used to and accept our self-image.

Cancer and its treatment can change your self-image. You may have changes such as hair loss or scars from surgery. Some of these changes (hair loss) will go away when treatment is over. Other changes (scars) will always be a part of how you look. Every person changes in different ways. Some changes people will notice and other changes only you will notice. Some changes you may like and with some others, you may need time to adjust.

Coping with these changes can be hard. But, over time, most people learn to accept them. Your family and friends can help by showing they love you the way you are.

Staying Active

Many people find that staying active can help. Whether you swim, play a sport, or take an exercise class, you may find that being active helps you accept your new self-image. Talk with your doctor about ways you can stay active.

Hobbies and volunteer work can also help improve your self-image. You may like to read, listen to music, or sew. You may also want to teach a child how to read or volunteer at a homeless shelter. You may find that you feel better about yourself when you get involved in helping others and doing things you enjoy.

Your Appearance

Reconstructive surgery: If cancer surgery changes the way you look, you may want to have reconstructive surgery (plastic surgery). Many patients feel that this type of surgery helps them cope better with their new self-image. For instance, you may choose to have surgery to improve the look of a surgical scar. Most insurance companies pay for reconstructive surgery.

Prosthetic devices: If a part of your body needs to be amputated (cut off) because of cancer, a prosthetic device (a fake or man-made body part) can replace what was cut off. For example, if your leg is amputated, you may want to have a prosthetic leg to replace the one you lost. Most insurance companies pay for prosthetic devices.

Wigs and scarves: Cancer treatment may cause you to lose your hair. You may want to cover your head to keep you warm and protected from the sun. You may also feel that wearing a wig or scarf improves how you look.

It is a good idea to buy your wig before treatment starts. This way, the wig will match the color and style of your own hair. You may want to start wearing your wig before losing your hair. Try to find a wig or scarf that fits well and is not scratchy, since your scalp may be tender and sore. You may be able to deduct the cost of your wig from your income taxes. Most of the time, your hair will grow back when treatment is over, even though it may be a different color and not feel like it did before.

Facing Cancer with Your Spouse or Partner

Some couples grow stronger when they face cancer together. They look at their lives in a new way. Problems that once seemed big don't feel that way now. Other couples facing cancer have more trouble.

Your Sex Life May Change

Sometimes people with cancer and their partners or spouses have trouble showing their love for each other. For instance, one man said that his wife wouldn't kiss him any more because she was afraid that she would catch cancer. In truth, people cannot give each other cancer. If your loved one is worried about catching cancer from you, suggest he or she talk with your doctor.

People can also have problems with sex because of cancer and its treatment. For instance, you may not like how you look and not want to have sex. If this happens, talk with your spouse or partner. Your partner probably loves you for more than your body.

Your spouse or partner may be afraid to have sex with you. He or she may be afraid of hurting you or having sex when you are not feeling well. Let your partner know if you want to have sex or would rather just hug, kiss, and cuddle.

Sometimes, cancer and its treatment causes other problems with sex.

- Fatigue can make you so tired that you don't want to have sex.
- Surgery can make certain positions painful.
- Prostate cancer treatments can make it hard for a man to have an erection.
- Some treatments cause women to have vaginal dryness.
- Orgasm is sometimes hard to achieve.

Even though you may feel awkward, talk about your sex life with people who can help. Let your doctor or nurse know if you are having problems. There may be drugs you can take or other ways you and your loved one can give each other pleasure. Some people also find it helpful to talk with other couples about how to stay close while dealing with cancer.

Remember that you are special for who you are, not how you look. Your sense of humor, intellect, sweetness, common sense, special talents, and loyalty, these and many other qualities make you special. Sex is not the only basis for a relationship. It is one of many ways to express love and respect.

Dating

If you are single, you may worry about dating. You may be afraid that you are not as good looking as you used to be. And you may not know how, or when, to talk with someone new about your cancer.

One woman with breast cancer said that dating was easier than she thought it would be. She felt like she knew when the time was right to talk about her disease. In fact, she said that her cancer never caused problems with people she dated.

Summing Up: Dealing with a New Self-Image

When you have cancer and when you are having treatment for cancer, you go through changes.

- You don't have as much energy as you did before the cancer.
- Your body is not the same as it was.
- If you're single, your dating life may be awkward.
- You may face new problems in your sex life.

These changes can be hard to accept. But most people with cancer find that, with time, they learn to accept their new self-image.

Chapter 41

Spirituality in Cancer Care

Many cancer patients rely on spiritual and/or religious beliefs and practices to help them cope with their disease. This is called spiritual coping. Some patients may want their doctors and caregivers to address spiritual concerns, not only for end-of-life issues but also during treatment. Medical staff may therefore ask patients to identify spiritual issues that are important to them during cancer care.

Definition of Spirituality and Religion

For many people, spirituality and religion have different meanings. The terms spirituality and religion are often used in place of each other, but for many people they have different meanings. Religion may be defined as a specific set of beliefs and practices, usually associated with an organized group. Spirituality may be defined as an individual's sense of peace, purpose, and connection to others, and beliefs about the meaning of life. Spirituality may be found and expressed through an organized religion or in other ways. Many patients consider themselves both spiritual and religious. Some patients may consider themselves spiritual, but not religious. Other patients may consider themselves religious, but not spiritual.

Spiritual distress is unresolved religious or spiritual conflict and doubt. A serious illness like cancer may challenge a patient's beliefs

PDQ® Cancer Information Summary. National Cancer Institute; Bethesda, MD. Spirituality in Cancer Care (PDQ®): Supportive Care - Patient. Updated 06/2006. Available at http://cancer.gov. Accessed November 20, 2006.

or religious values, resulting in high levels of spiritual distress. Some cancer patients may feel that cancer is a punishment by God or may suffer a loss of faith after being diagnosed.

Other patients may experience mild spiritual distress when coping with cancer. For example, when prayer is used as a coping method, some patients may worry about how to pray or may doubt their prayers are being answered.

Relation of Spirituality to Quality of Life

Spiritual and religious well-being may be associated with improved quality of life. It is not known for sure how spirituality is related to health. Some research shows that spiritual or religious beliefs and practices promote a positive mental attitude that may help a patient feel better. Spiritual and religious well-being may be associated with improved quality of life in the following ways:

- Reduced anxiety, depression, and discomfort
- Reduced sense of isolation (feeling alone)
- Better adjustment to the effects of cancer and its treatment
- Increased ability to enjoy life during cancer treatment
- A feeling of personal growth as a result of living with cancer
- Improved health outcomes

Spiritual distress may contribute to poorer health outcomes. High levels of spiritual distress may interfere with the patient's ability to cope with cancer and cancer treatment. This distress may contribute to poorer health outcomes and less satisfaction with life. Health care providers may encourage patients to seek advice from appropriate spiritual or religious leaders to help resolve their conflicts, which may improve their health, quality of life, and ability to cope.

Screening and Assessment

A spiritual assessment may help the doctor understand if a patient will use religious or spiritual beliefs to cope with the cancer diagnosis and treatment. Knowing the role that religion and spirituality play in the patient's life may help the doctor understand how religious and spiritual beliefs affect the patient's response to the cancer diagnosis and decisions about cancer treatment. Some doctors or caregivers may wait for the patient to bring up spiritual concerns. Others will ask for some initial information in an interview or on a form called a spiritual assessment.

A spiritual assessment will include asking about religious preference, beliefs, and spiritual practices. Medical staff may not ask about every issue the patient feels is important. The patient should feel comfortable bringing up other spiritual or religious issues that he or she thinks may affect cancer care. A spiritual assessment may include questions relating to the following issues:

- Religious denomination, if any
- Beliefs or philosophy of life
- Important spiritual practices or rituals
- Use of spirituality or religion as a source of strength
- Participation in a religious community
- Use of prayer or meditation
- Loss of faith
- Conflicts between spiritual or religious beliefs and cancer treatments
- Ways the caregivers may address the patient's spiritual needs
- Concerns about death and the afterlife
- End-of-life planning

Meeting the Patient's Spiritual and Religious Needs

In addressing a patient's spiritual needs during cancer care, medical staff will take their lead from the wishes of the patient. Spirituality and religion are very personal decisions. Patients can expect doctors and caregivers to respect their religious and spiritual beliefs and concerns. A cancer patient who relies on spirituality to cope with the disease may count on medical staff to respect that practice with support and referrals to appropriate spiritual or religious resources. Patients who do not choose to have spiritual issues addressed during cancer care may also count on medical staff to respect and support their views.

Doctors and caregivers will try to respond to their patients' concerns, but may avoid taking part in patients' religious rituals or debating religious beliefs. Doctors may address a patient's spiritual needs in setting goals and planning treatment. Doctors may address a patient's spiritual needs in the following ways:

- Identifying goals for care and making medical decisions that are consistent with the patient's spiritual and/or religious views and which also enable the doctor to maintain the integrity of his or her own spiritual and/or religious views.

- Respectfully supporting the patient's use of spiritual coping during the illness.

- Encouraging patients to speak with their clergy or spiritual leader.

- Referring the patient to a hospital chaplain, appropriate religious leader, or support group that addresses spiritual issues during illness.

Chapter 42

Cognitive Changes Related to Cancer

Cognitive disorders and delirium are conditions in which the patient experiences a confused mental state and changes in behavior. People who have cognitive disorders or delirium may fall in and out of consciousness and may have problems with the following:

- Attention
- Thinking
- Awareness
- Emotion
- Memory
- Muscle control
- Sleeping and waking

Delirium occurs frequently in cancer patients, especially in patients with advanced cancer. Delirium usually occurs suddenly and the patient's symptoms may come and go during the day. This condition can be treated and is often temporary, even in people with advanced illness. In the last 24 to 48 hours of life, however, delirium may be permanent due to problems such as organ failure.

PDQ® National Information Summary. National Cancer Institute; Bethesda, MD. Cognitive Disorders and Delirium (PDQ®) - Patient. Updated 05/19/2006. Available at: http://www.cancer.gov. Accessed 8/24/06.

Causes of Cognitive Disorders and Delirium

Cognitive disorders and delirium may be complications of cancer and cancer treatment, especially in people with advanced cancer.

In cancer patients, cognitive disorders and delirium may be due to the direct effects that cancer has on the brain, such as the pressure of a growing tumor. Cognitive disorders and delirium may also be caused by indirect effects of cancer or its treatment, including the following:

- Organ failure

- Electrolyte imbalances: Electrolytes are important minerals (including salt, potassium, calcium, and phosphorous) that are needed to keep the heart, kidneys, nerves, and muscles working correctly.

- Infection

- Medication side effects: Patients with cancer usually take many medications. Some drugs have side effects that include delirium and confusion. The effects of these drugs usually go away after the drug is stopped.

- Withdrawal from drugs that depress (slow down) the central nervous system (brain and spinal cord)

Other conditions besides having cancer may place a patient at risk for developing delirium. Risk factors include the following:

- Advanced cancer or other serious illness

- Having more than one disease

- Older age

- Previous mental disorder, such as dementia

- Low levels of albumin (protein) in the blood

- Infection

- Taking medications that affect the mind or behavior

- Taking high doses of pain medication

Early identification of risk factors may help prevent the onset of delirium or may reduce the length of time it takes to correct it.

Effects of Cognitive Disorders and Delirium on the Patient, Family, and Healthcare Providers

Cognitive disorders and delirium can be upsetting to the family and caregivers, and may be dangerous to the patient if judgment is affected. These conditions can cause the patient to act unpredictably and sometimes violently. Even a quiet or calm patient can suddenly experience a change in mood or become agitated, requiring increased care. The safety of the patient, family, and caregivers is most important.

Patients with cognitive disorders or delirium are more likely to fall, be incontinent (unable to control bladder and/or bowels), and become dehydrated (drink too little water to maintain health). They often require a longer hospital stay than patients without cognitive disorders or delirium.

The confused mental state of these patients may hinder their communication with family members and the healthcare providers. Assessment of the patient's symptoms becomes difficult and the patient may be unable to make decisions regarding care. Agitation in these patients may be mistaken as an expression of pain. Conflict can arise among the patient, family, and staff concerning the level of pain medication needed.

Diagnosis of Cognitive Disorders and Delirium

A patient who suddenly becomes agitated or uncooperative, experiences personality or behavior changes, has impaired thinking, decreased attention span, or intense, unusual anxiety or depression, may be experiencing cognitive disorders or delirium. Patients who develop these symptoms need to be assessed completely.

Early symptoms of delirium are similar to symptoms of anxiety, anger, depression, and dementia. Delirium that causes the patient to be very inactive may appear to be depression. Delirium and dementia are difficult to tell apart, since both may cause disorientation and impair memory, thinking, and judgment. Dementia may be caused by a number of medical conditions, including Alzheimer disease. Some differences in the symptoms of delirium and dementia include the following:

- Patients with delirium often go in and out of consciousness. Patients who have dementia usually remain alert.

- Delirium may occur suddenly. Dementia appears gradually and gets worse over time.

377

- Sleeping and waking problems are more common with delirium than with dementia.

In elderly patients who have cancer, dementia is often present along with delirium, making diagnosis difficult. The diagnosis is more likely dementia if symptoms continue after treatment for delirium is given.

In patients aged 65 or older who have survived cancer for more than five years, the risk for cognitive disorders and dementia is increased, apart from the risk for delirium.

Regular screening of the patient and monitoring of the patient's symptoms can help in the diagnosis of delirium.

Treatment of Delirium

Patient and family concerns are addressed when deciding the treatment of delirium. Deciding if, when, and how to treat a person with delirium depends on the setting, how advanced the cancer is, the wishes of the patient and family, and how the delirium symptoms are affecting the patient.

Monitoring alone may be all that is necessary for patients who are not dangerous to themselves. In other cases, symptoms may be treated or causes of the delirium may be identified and treated.

Treatment of the Symptoms of Delirium by Changing the Patient's Surroundings

Controlling the patient's surroundings may help reduce mild symptoms of delirium. The following changes may be effective:

- Putting the patient in a quiet, well-lit room with familiar objects
- Placing a clock or calendar where the patient can see it
- Reducing noise
- Having family present
- Limiting changes in caregivers

To prevent a patient from harming himself or herself or others, physical restraints also may be necessary.

Treatment of the Causes of Delirium

The standard approach to managing delirium is to find and treat the causes. Symptoms may be treated at the same time. Identifying the causes of delirium will include a physical examination to check general signs of health, including checking for signs of disease. A medical history of the patient's past illnesses and treatments will also be taken. In a terminally ill delirious patient being cared for at home, the doctor may do a limited assessment to determine the cause or may treat just the symptoms.

Treatment may include the following:

- Stopping or reducing medications that cause delirium

- Giving fluids into the bloodstream to correct dehydration

- Giving drugs to correct hypercalcemia (too much calcium in the blood)

- Giving antibiotics for infections

Treatment of the Symptoms of Delirium with Medication

Drugs called antipsychotics may be used to treat the symptoms of delirium. Drugs that sedate (calm) the patient may also be used, especially if the patient is near death. All of these drugs have side effects and the patient will be monitored closely by a doctor. The decision to use drugs that sedate the patient will be made in cooperation with family members after efforts have been made to reverse the delirium.

Delirium and Sedation

The decision to use drugs to sedate the patient who is near death and has symptoms of delirium, pain, and difficult breathing presents ethical and legal issues for both the doctor and the family. When the symptoms of delirium are not relieved with standard treatment approaches and the patient is experiencing severe distress and suffering, the doctor may discuss the option to give drugs that will sedate the patient. This decision is guided by the following principles:

- Healthcare professionals who have experience in palliative care make repeated assessments of the patient's response to treatments. The family is always included.

- The need to use drugs that sedate the patient is evaluated by a multidisciplinary team of healthcare professionals.

- Temporary sedation should be considered.

- A multidisciplinary team of healthcare professionals will work with the family to ensure that the family's views are assessed and understood.

Chapter 43

Normal Adjustment and Adjustment Disorders in Cancer Patients

Normal Adjustment

Adjusting to cancer is an ongoing process in which the patient learns to cope with emotional distress, solve cancer-related problems, and gain control over cancer-related life events. Patients are faced with many challenges that change as the disease and its treatment change. Common periods of crisis and significant challenge include hearing the diagnosis, receiving treatment (for example, surgery, radiation therapy, and chemotherapy), completing treatment, hearing that the cancer is in remission, hearing that the cancer has come back, and becoming a cancer survivor. Each of these events involves specific coping tasks, questions about life and death, and common emotional problems.

Patients are better able to adjust to a cancer diagnosis if they are able to continue fulfilling normal responsibilities, cope with emotional distress, and stay actively involved in activities that are meaningful and important to them.

Coping is the use of thoughts and behaviors to adjust to life situations. A person's coping style is usually related to his or her personality (for example, always expecting the best, always expecting the worst, being shy or reserved, or being outgoing).

PDQ® Cancer Information Summary. National Cancer Institute; Bethesda, MD. Normal Adjustment and the Adjustment Disorders (PDQ®): Supportive Care - Patient. Updated 07/18/2006. Available at http://cancer.gov. Accessed August 30, 2006.

Coping strategies are thoughts and behaviors that are used in rare situations, for example, when one must change his or her daily routine or work schedule to adjust to the side effects of cancer treatment. Developing coping strategies can help a patient learn how to change problem situations, manage emotional distress, and understand why cancer has happened and what impact cancer may have on his or her life. Patients who adjust well are usually committed and actively involved in coping with cancer. They are still able to find meaning and importance in their lives. Patients who do not adjust well become less involved with coping, withdraw, and feel hopeless. Studies are looking at how different types of coping strategies affect the quality of life for cancer survivors.

Distress can occur when a person feels that he or she does not have the resources to manage or control the cancer. Distress experienced by patients who have the same diagnosis and are undergoing the same treatment may be very different. A doctor or health care professional can help the patient adjust to the treatment schedule and help the patient cope with treatment by, for example, providing medication for nausea.

General Factors Influencing Adjustment

Many individual differences affect how a patient adjusts to cancer. It is difficult to predict how a person will cope with cancer. The following factors influence how a patient adjusts to cancer:

- The type of cancer, cancer stage, and chance of recovery
- The phase of cancer such as newly diagnosed, being treated, in remission, or recurrent cancer
- Individual coping abilities
- Friends and family available to support the patient
- The patient's age
- The availability of treatment
- Beliefs about the cause of cancer

Specific Influences on Adjustment

Hearing the diagnosis: The process of adjusting to cancer can begin even before hearing the diagnosis. Patients may experience normal levels of fear, worry, and concern when they have unexplained symptoms or are undergoing testing to determine if they have cancer. When a patient hears the diagnosis of cancer, many patients wonder, "Could I die from this?"

Receiving a diagnosis of cancer can cause expected and normal emotional distress. Some patients may feel disbelief and ask, "Are you sure you have the right test results?" Most patients feel they are unable to think clearly. They may feel numb or in shock, or as if "This can't be happening to me." Many patients may not understand or remember important information that the doctor gave them about the diagnosis and treatment options. Patients should have a way to review this information by having someone with them at appointments, requesting that the session be taped, or by requesting a second appointment to ask the doctor questions and go over the treatment plan. As the patient gradually accepts the reality of the diagnosis, he or she may begin to experience depression, anxiety, lack of appetite, inability to sleep, poor concentration, and varying degrees of inability to function in daily activities. When the patient receives and understands information about treatment options, he or she may gradually feel more hopeful and optimistic. Eventually, patients develop ways to cope and be able to adjust to the cancer diagnosis.

Cancer treatments: When cancer treatment begins, patients may experience fears about painful procedures, unwanted side effects (for example hair loss, nausea and vomiting, fatigue, pain), and interruptions to normal activities and responsibilities (for example, being unable to work). Patients who can weigh the discomforts of short-term loss against the benefits of long-term gain (for example, living longer) and decide, "It's worth it," usually adjust well. Questions that patients may ask during treatment include, "Will I survive this?" "Will they get it all?" or "What side effects will I experience?" As these questions arise, patients will learn to adjust with them. Developing ways to cope with specific problems (for example fatigue, transportation to treatment, and work schedule changes) is helpful.

Post-treatment: Completing cancer treatment can cause mixed feelings. It may be a time of celebration and relief or a time of increased anxiety with awareness that the cancer could return once the treatment is stopped. Patients who can balance their positive expectations with the realities of ongoing fears adjust well. Many patients experience increased anxiety and fear of the cancer returning as they have less frequent contact with their physician. Other adjustment concerns include living with uncertainty, resuming previous responsibilities, and being overly concerned about health. During remission, patients often experience normal anxiety and worry as the dates of regular follow-up appointments with their oncologist approach with the possibility that the cancer has returned.

Normal adjustment to post-treatment and remission may involve using the following coping strategies to help control normal emotional distress:

- Being honest with one's emotions

- Being aware of one's feelings and able to express them to others

- Having a nonjudgmental acceptance of one's feelings and a willingness to work through these emotions

- Having support from others who are willing to listen and accept

Patients who can express a wide range of both positive and negative emotions usually adjust well.

The return of cancer: Changing from a treatment plan that focuses on curing the cancer to one that provides comfort and relief of symptoms can cause extreme anxiety. Patients may experience shock, disbelief, and denial followed by a period of significant distress (for example, depressed moods, difficulty concentrating, and frequent thoughts of death). Normal adjustment may include periods of sadness and crying, feelings of anger at God or a higher power, periods of withdrawal and isolation, and thoughts of giving up. Patients gradually adjust to the return of cancer over a period of weeks by changing expectations from curing to healing. Healing is a process of "becoming whole again" by transforming one's life in many ways in the face of death. It is very important that the patient maintain hope throughout this process. Patients who believe that pain and suffering can be controlled will have hope for future quality of life. Those who believe they are loved and cared for will have hope in future relationships. Religion and spirituality are very important in helping patients maintain hope.

Survivorship: The adjustment from completing cancer treatment to a long-term survivorship is a gradual process that extends over many years. Some common problems reported by cancer survivors as they face the future include fear of the cancer coming back, lasting physical effects such as tiredness, problems sleeping, and concerns about sexual function. Most patients adjust well and some even report benefits of having cancer such as a greater appreciation of life, changes in life values, and stronger spiritual or religious beliefs. Patients who do not adjust well usually have more medical problems, fewer friends and family who provide support, fewer financial resources, and problems with psychological adjustment unrelated to the cancer.

Psychological and Social Distress

Most patients experience some level of distress, however, only a small percentage receives help. Distress is an unpleasant emotional, psychological, social, or spiritual experience that interferes with the patient's ability to cope with cancer treatment. Patients may experience a range of feelings from normal sadness and fear to deep depression, anxiety, panic, or isolation. These feelings can interfere with a person's ability to relate to family, friends, coworkers, and others during the normal routines of daily living. This is called social distress.

Screening

Health care professionals may have patients complete questionnaires periodically to identify the need for referral to a mental health professional. Key times that distress may become disabling include the time of diagnosis, during cancer treatment, at the end of a long course of treatment, during remission, when the cancer returns, or when beginning palliative care. Patients who are experiencing mild distress may benefit from a referral to a self-help group. Patients who are experiencing moderate to severe distress may require a referral to a mental health professional such as a psychiatrist, psychologist, social worker, or pastoral counselor.

Psychological and Social Assessment

It is important that patients understand the benefits of talking with a mental health professional about their concerns and worries. A patient can expect the health professional to help in the following ways:

- Listen closely to his or her concerns
- Show an interest in his or her experiences with cancer
- Ask about his or her family, friends, and other persons who provide support
- Ask how he or she has been adjusting to the cancer

- Encourage him or her to continue using coping strategies that are successful

- Suggest other coping strategies to address his or her concerns

Patients will be encouraged to continue counseling or psychotherapy as needed.

Psychological and Social Therapies for Distress

Recent studies of psychological and social therapies have shown benefits for cancer patients. These therapies are defined as non-drug treatments offering psychological and educational support:

- Relaxation training

- Coping strategies

- Cancer education/information sessions

- Group social support

These therapies may be combined in different ways for various lengths of time, in both individual and group formats. To date, these therapies have most commonly been studied in white, middle-to-higher income American women with breast cancer, though they are currently being studied in more patient groups. Cancer patients who receive such therapies show positive benefits compared to those who do not, including lower levels of depression, anxiety, and disease-related symptoms, as well as improved immune system functioning and health habits like exercise. The size of these benefits and how they affect patients' recovery will need more study.

The Adjustment Disorders

Adjustment disorders include behaviors or moods more extreme than expected in reaction to a cancer diagnosis, treatment, recurrence or side effects. These behaviors or moods may result in significant problems in functioning with family, friends, and at work. An adjustment disorder usually begins within three months of the first signs of distress, for example a cancer diagnosis. Some patients may develop a chronic adjustment disorder because they experience multiple causes of distress, one right after another (for example, the cancer diagnosis, the start of treatment, side effects of treatment, completion of treatment, and returning to work). Chronic adjustment disorders may become a more serious mental disorder (for example, major depression). This is more common in children and adolescents than in adults.

Treatment

Individual and group counseling and psychotherapy: Treatment that focuses on the patient's thoughts, feelings, and behaviors may be used to relieve emotional distress in individual patients or groups. The following are examples of these techniques:

- Relaxation training
- Biofeedback
- Problem-solving
- Distraction
- Thought stopping
- Coping self-statements
- Mental imagery exercises

Medications: Counseling or psychotherapy should be tried before medication. If the patient does not improve with short-term psychotherapy or develops a more severe mental disorder, such as depression, the doctor will then prescribe the appropriate medication.

Chapter 44

Depression in Cancer Patients

Depression is a disabling illness that affects about 15% to 25% of cancer patients. It affects men and women with cancer equally. People who face a diagnosis of cancer will experience different levels of stress and emotional upset.

Everyone who is diagnosed with cancer will react to these issues in different ways and may not experience serious depression or anxiety.

Just as patients need to be evaluated for depression throughout their treatment, so do family caregivers. Caregivers have been found to experience a good deal more anxiety and depression than people who are not caring for cancer patients.

There are many misconceptions about cancer and how people cope with it, such as the following:

- All people with cancer are depressed.

- Depression in a person with cancer is normal.

- Treatment does not help the depression.

- Everyone with cancer faces suffering and a painful death.

Sadness and grief are normal reactions to the crises faced during cancer, and will be experienced at times by all people. Because sadness

Excerpted from PDQ® Cancer Information Summary. National Cancer Institute; Bethesda, MD. Depression (PDQ®): Supportive Care - Patient. Updated 01/2006. Available at http://cancer.gov. Accessed April 30, 2006.

is common, it is important to distinguish between normal levels of sadness and depression. An important part of cancer care is the recognition of depression that needs to be treated. Some people may have more trouble adjusting to the diagnosis of cancer than others may. Major depression is not simply sadness or a blue mood. Major depression affects about 25% of patients and has common symptoms that can be diagnosed and treated. Symptoms of depression that are noticed when a patient is diagnosed with cancer may be a sign that the patient had a depression problem before the diagnosis of cancer.

All people will experience reactions of sadness and grief periodically throughout diagnosis, treatment, and survival of cancer. When people find out they have cancer, they often have feelings of disbelief, denial, or despair. They may also experience difficulty sleeping, loss of appetite, anxiety, and a preoccupation with worries about the future. These symptoms and fears usually lessen as a person adjusts to the diagnosis. Signs that a person has adjusted to the diagnosis include an ability to maintain active involvement in daily life activities, and an ability to continue functioning as spouse, parent, employee, or other roles by incorporating treatment into his or her schedule. If the family of a patient diagnosed with cancer is able to express feelings openly and solve problems effectively, both the patient and family members have less depression. Good communication within the family reduces anxiety. A person who cannot adjust to the diagnosis after a long period of time, and who loses interest in usual activities, may be depressed. Mild symptoms of depression can be distressing and may be helped with counseling. Even patients without obvious symptoms of depression may benefit from counseling; however, when symptoms are intense and long-lasting, or when they keep coming back, more intensive treatment is important.

Diagnosis

The symptoms of major depression include the following:

- Having a depressed mood for most of the day and on most days
- Loss of pleasure and interest in most activities
- Changes in eating and sleeping habits
- Nervousness or sluggishness
- Tiredness
- Feelings of worthlessness or inappropriate guilt

- Poor concentration
- Constant thoughts of death or suicide

To make a diagnosis of depression, these symptoms should be present for at least two weeks. The diagnosis of depression can be difficult to make in people with cancer due to the difficulty of separating the symptoms of depression from the side effects of medications or the symptoms of cancer. This is especially true in patients undergoing active cancer treatment or those with advanced disease. Symptoms of guilt, worthlessness, hopelessness, thoughts of suicide, and loss of pleasure are the most useful in diagnosing depression in people who have cancer.

Some people with cancer may have a higher risk for developing depression. The cause of depression is not known, but the risk factors for developing depression are known. Risk factors may be cancer-related and noncancer-related.

Cancer-Related Risk Factors

- Depression at the time of cancer diagnosis
- Poorly controlled pain
- An advanced stage of cancer
- Other life events that produce stress
- Increased physical impairment or pain
- Pancreatic cancer
- Being unmarried and having head and neck cancer
- Treatment with some anticancer drugs

Noncancer-Related Risk Factors

- History of depression
- Lack of family support
- Family history of depression or suicide
- Previous suicide attempts
- History of alcoholism or drug abuse
- Having many illnesses at the same time that produce symptoms of depression (such as stroke or heart attack)

The evaluation of depression in people with cancer should include a careful evaluation of the person's thoughts about the illness; medical history; personal or family history of depression or suicide; current mental status; physical status; side effects of treatment and the disease; other stresses in the person's life; and support available to the patient.

The most common type of depression in people with cancer is called reactive depression. This shows up as feeling moody and being unable to perform usual activities. The symptoms last longer and are more pronounced than a normal and expected reaction but do not meet the criteria for major depression. When these symptoms greatly interfere with a person's daily activities, such as work, school, shopping, or caring for a household, they should be treated in the same way that major depression is treated (such as crisis intervention, counseling, and medication, especially with drugs that can quickly relieve distressing symptoms). Basing the diagnosis on just these symptoms can be a problem in a person with advanced cancer since the illness may be causing decreased functioning. It is important to identify the difference between fatigue and depression since they can be assessed and treated separately. In more advanced illness, focusing on despair, guilty thoughts, and a total lack of enjoyment of life is helpful in diagnosing depression.

Medical factors may also cause depression in cancer patients. Medication usually helps this type of depression more effectively than counseling, especially if the medical factors cannot be changed (for example, dosages of the medications that are causing the depression cannot be changed or stopped). Some medical causes of depression in cancer patients include uncontrolled pain; abnormal levels of calcium, sodium, or potassium in the blood; anemia; vitamin B_{12} or folate deficiency; fever; and abnormal levels of thyroid hormone or steroids in the blood.

Treatment

Treatment with Drugs

Major depression may be treated with a combination of counseling and medications (drugs), such as antidepressants. A primary care doctor may prescribe medications for depression and refer the patient to a psychiatrist or psychologist for the following reasons:

- A physician or oncologist is not comfortable treating the depression (for example, the patient has suicidal thoughts)

- The symptoms of depression do not improve after two to four weeks of treatment

- The symptoms are getting worse

- The side effects of the medication keep the patient from taking the dosage needed to control the depression

- The symptoms are interfering with the patient's ability to continue medical treatment

Antidepressants are usually effective in the treatment of depression and its symptoms. Unfortunately, antidepressants are not prescribed often for cancer patients. About 25% of all cancer patients are depressed, but only about 16% receive medication for the depression. The choice of antidepressant depends on the patient's symptoms, potential side effects of the antidepressant, and the person's individual medical problems and previous response to antidepressant drugs.

Most antidepressants take three to six weeks to begin working. The side effects must be considered when deciding which antidepressant to use. For example, a medication that causes sleepiness may be helpful in an anxious patient who is having problems sleeping, since the drug is both calming and sedating. Patients who cannot swallow pills may be able to take the medication as a liquid or as an injection. If the antidepressant helps the symptoms, treatment should continue for at least six months. Electroconvulsive therapy (ECT) is a useful and safe therapy when other treatments have been unsuccessful in relieving major depression.

Treatment with Psychotherapy

Several psychiatric therapies have been found to be helpful in the treatment of depression related to cancer. Most therapy programs for depression are given in four to 30 hours and are offered in both individual and group settings. They may include sessions about cancer education or relaxation skills. These therapies are often used in combination and include crisis intervention, psychotherapy, and thought/behavior techniques. Patients explore methods of lowering distress, improving coping and problem-solving skills; enlisting support; reshaping negative and self-defeating thoughts; and developing a close personal bond with an understanding health care provider. Talking with a clergy member may also be helpful for some people.

Specific goals of these therapies include the following:

- Assist people diagnosed with cancer and their families by answering questions about the illness and its treatment, explaining information, correcting misunderstandings, giving reassurance about the situation, and exploring with the patient how the diagnosis relates to previous experiences with cancer.

- Assist with problem solving, improve the patient's coping skills, and help the patient and family to develop additional coping skills. Explore other areas of stress, such as family role and lifestyle changes, and encourage family members to support and share concern with each other.

- Ensure that the patient and family understand that support will continue when the focus of treatment changes from trying to cure the cancer to relieving symptoms. The health care team will treat symptoms to help the patient control pain and remain comfortable, and will help the patient and his or her family members maintain dignity.

Cancer support groups may also be helpful in treating depression in cancer patients, especially adolescents. Support groups have been shown to improve mood, encourage the development of coping skills, improve quality of life, and improve immune response. Support groups can be found through the wellness community, the American Cancer Society, and many community resources, including the social work departments in medical centers and hospitals.

Evaluation and Treatment of Suicidal Cancer Patients

The incidence of suicide in cancer patients may be as much as 10 times higher than the rate of suicide in the general population. One study has shown that the risk of suicide in cancer patients is highest in the first months after diagnosis, and that this risk decreases significantly over decades. Passive suicidal thoughts are fairly common in cancer patients. The relationships between suicidal tendency and the desire for hastened death, requests for physician-assisted suicide, or euthanasia are complicated and poorly understood. Men with cancer are at an increased risk of suicide compared with the general population, with more than twice the risk. Overdosing with painkillers and sedatives is the most common method of suicide by cancer patients, with most cancer suicides occurring at home. The occurrence of suicide is higher in patients with oral, pharyngeal, and lung cancers and in HIV-positive patients with Kaposi sarcoma. The actual incidence of suicide in cancer patients is probably underestimated, since there may be reluctance to report these deaths as suicides.

General risk factors for suicide in a person with cancer include the following:

- A history of mental problems, especially those associated with impulsive behavior (such as borderline personality disorders)
- A family history of suicide
- A history of suicide attempts
- Depression
- Substance abuse
- Recent death of a friend or spouse
- Having little social support

Cancer-specific risk factors for suicide include the following:

- A diagnosis of oral, throat, or lung cancer (often associated with heavy alcohol and tobacco use)
- Advanced stage of disease and poor prognosis
- Confusion/delirium
- Poorly controlled pain
- Physical impairments such as the following
  - Loss of mobility
  - Loss of bowel and bladder control
  - Amputation
  - Loss of eyesight or hearing
  - Paralysis
  - Inability to eat or swallow
- Tiredness
- Exhaustion

Patients who are suicidal require careful evaluation. The risk of suicide increases if the patient reports thoughts of suicide and has a plan to carry it out. Risk continues to increase if the plan is "lethal," that is, the plan is likely to cause death. A lethal suicide plan is more likely to be carried out if the way chosen to cause death is available to the person, the attempt cannot be stopped once it is started, and help is unavailable. When a person with cancer reports thoughts of death, it is important to determine whether the underlying cause is depression or a desire to control unbearable symptoms. Prompt identification and treatment of major depression is important in decreasing the risk for suicide. Risk factors, especially hopelessness (which is a better predictor for suicide than depression) should be carefully determined. The assessment of hopelessness is not easy in the person who has advanced cancer with no hope of a cure. It is important to determine the basic reasons for hopelessness, which may be related to cancer symptoms, fears of painful death, or feelings of abandonment.

Talking about suicide will not cause the patient to attempt suicide; it actually shows that this is a concern and permits the patient to describe his or her feelings and fears, providing a sense of control. A crisis intervention-oriented treatment approach should be used which involves the patient's support system. Contributing symptoms, such as pain, should be aggressively controlled and depression, psychosis, anxiety, and underlying causes of delirium should be treated. These problems are usually treated in a medical hospital or at home. Although not usually necessary, a suicidal cancer patient may need to be hospitalized in a psychiatric unit.

The goal of treatment of suicidal patients is to attempt to prevent suicide that is caused by desperation due to poorly controlled symptoms. Patients close to the end of life may not be able to stay awake without a great amount of emotional or physical pain. This often leads to thoughts of suicide or requests for aid in dying. Such patients may need sedation to ease their distress.

Other treatment considerations include using medications that work quickly to alleviate distress (such as, antianxiety medication or stimulants) while waiting for the antidepressant medication to work; limiting the quantities of medications that are lethal in overdose; having frequent contact with a health care professional who can closely observe the patient; avoiding long periods of time when the patient is alone; making sure the patient has available support; and determining the patient's mental and emotional response at each crisis point during the cancer experience.

Pain and symptom treatment should not be sacrificed simply to avoid the possibility that a patient will attempt suicide. Patients often have a method to commit suicide available to them. Incomplete pain and symptom treatment might actually worsen a patient's suicide risk.

Frequent contact with the health professional can help limit the amount of lethal drugs available to the patient and family. Infusion devices that limit patient access to medications can also be used at home or in the hospital. These are programmable, portable pumps with coded access and a locked cartridge containing the medication. These pumps are very useful in controlling pain and other symptoms. Some pumps can give multiple drug infusions, and some can be programmed over the phone. The devices are available through home care agencies, but are very expensive. Some of the expense may be covered by insurance.

Considerations for Depression in Children

Most children cope with the emotions related to cancer and not only adjust well, but show positive emotional growth and development. A small number of children, however, develop psychologic problems including depression, anxiety, sleeping problems, relationship problems, and are uncooperative about treatment. A mental health specialist should treat these children.

Children with severe late effects of cancer have more symptoms of depression. Anxiety usually occurs in younger patients, while depression is more common in older children. Most cancer survivors are generally able to adapt and adjust successfully to cancer and its treatment; however, a small number of cancer survivors have difficulty adjusting.

Diagnosis of Childhood Depression

The term depression refers to a symptom or a set of symptoms or conditions that occur together and suggest the presence of depression, or an illness. A diagnosis of depression as an illness depends on how severe the symptoms are and how long they last. For example, a child may be sad in response to trauma, and the sadness usually lasts a short time. Depression, however, is marked by a response that lasts a long time, and is associated with sleeplessness, irritability, changes in eating habits, and problems at school and with friends. Depression should be considered whenever any behavior problem continues. Depression does not refer to temporary moments of sadness, but rather to a disorder that affects development and interferes with the child's progress. Childhood depression and adult depression are different illnesses due to the developmental issues involved in childhood.

Some signs of depression in the school-aged child include the following:

- Not eating
- Inactivity

- Looking sad
- Aggressive behavior
- Crying
- Hyperactivity
- Physical complaints
- Fear of death
- Frustration
- Feelings of sadness or hopelessness
- Self-criticism
- Frequent daydreaming
- Low self-esteem
- Refusing to go to school
- Learning problems
- Slow movements
- Showing anger towards parents and teachers
- Loss of interest in activities that were previously enjoyed

Some of these signs can occur in response to normal developmental stages; therefore, it is important to determine whether they are related to depression or a developmental stage.

Determining a diagnosis of depression includes evaluating the child's family situation, as well as his or her level of emotional maturity and ability to cope with illness and treatment; the child's age and state of development; and the child's self esteem and prior experience with illness.

A comprehensive assessment for childhood depression is necessary for effective diagnosis and treatment. Evaluation of the child and family situation focuses on the child's health history; observations of the behavior of the child by parents, teachers, or health care workers; interviews with the child; and use of psychological tests.

Treatment of Childhood Depression

Individual and group counseling are usually used as the first treatment for a child with depression, and are directed at helping the child to master his or her difficulties and develop in the best way possible. Play therapy may be used as a way to explore the younger child's view of himself or herself, the disease, and treatment. From the beginning of treatment, a child needs help to understand, at his or her developmental level, the diagnosis of cancer and the treatment involved. A doctor may prescribe medications, such as antidepressants, for children. Some of the same antidepressants prescribed for adults may also be prescribed for children.

Suicide and Children

Suicide is as rare among adolescents who have no other mental disorders as it is among adults. The adolescent often believes that his or her disease is outside the realm of control and is in the hands of God or some other force. Refusing treatment is not a way of attempting suicide, but comes from his or her belief that fate, luck, or God determines life and death.

Some adolescent cancer survivors may be overwhelmed by feelings of hopelessness. This may lead to thoughts of suicide. Suicide is treated by the careful evaluation of the child with cancer and his or her family. The multiple factors that can make a child's life unbearable need to be examined. Suicide prevention must include individual evaluation; referral to the correct health professionals; treatment with medications; and both individual counseling and family therapy.

Chapter 45

Anxiety Disorders in Cancer Patients

Anxiety is a normal reaction to cancer. One may experience anxiety while undergoing a cancer screening test, waiting for test results, receiving a diagnosis of cancer, undergoing cancer treatment, or anticipating a recurrence of cancer. Anxiety associated with cancer may increase feelings of pain, interfere with one's ability to sleep, cause nausea and vomiting, and interfere with the patient's (and his or her family's) quality of life. If left untreated, severe anxiety may even shorten a patient's life.

Persons with cancer will find that their feelings of anxiety increase or decrease at different times. A patient may become more anxious as cancer spreads or treatment becomes more intense. The level of anxiety experienced by one person with cancer may differ from the anxiety experienced by another person. Most patients are able to reduce their anxiety by learning more about their cancer and the treatment they can expect to receive. For some patients, particularly those who have experienced episodes of intense anxiety before their cancer diagnosis, feelings of anxiety may become overwhelming and interfere with cancer treatment. Most patients who have not had an anxiety condition before their cancer diagnosis will not develop an anxiety disorder associated with cancer.

PDQ® Cancer Information Summary. National Cancer Institute; Bethesda, MD. Anxiety Disorder (PDQ®): Supportive Care - Patient. Updated 10/2005. Available at: http://cancer.gov. Accessed August 30, 2006.

Intense anxiety associated with cancer treatment is more likely to occur in patients with a history of anxiety disorders and patients who are experiencing anxiety at the time of diagnosis. Anxiety may also be experienced by patients who are in severe pain, are disabled, have few friends or family members to care for them, have cancer that is not responding to treatment, or have a history of severe physical or emotional trauma. Central nervous system metastases and tumors in the lungs may create physical problems that cause anxiety. Many cancer medications and treatments can aggravate feelings of anxiety.

Contrary to what one might expect, patients with advanced cancer experience anxiety due not to fear of death, but more often from fear of uncontrolled pain, being left alone, or dependency on others. Many of these factors can be alleviated with treatment.

Description and Cause

Some persons may have already experienced intense anxiety in their life because of situations unrelated to their cancer. These anxiety conditions may recur or become aggravated by the stress of a cancer diagnosis. Patients may experience extreme fear, be unable to absorb information given to them by caregivers, or be unable to follow through with treatment. In order to plan treatment for a patient's anxiety, a doctor may ask the following questions about the patient's symptoms:

- Have you had any of the following symptoms since your cancer diagnosis or treatment? When do these symptoms occur (how many days prior to treatment, at night, or at no specific time) and how long do they last?

- Do you feel shaky, jittery, or nervous?

- Have you felt tense, fearful, or apprehensive?

- Have you had to avoid certain places or activities because of fear?

- Have you felt your heart pounding or racing?

- Have you had trouble catching your breath when nervous?

- Have you had any unjustified sweating or trembling?

- Have you felt a knot in your stomach?

- Have you felt like you have a lump in your throat?

- Do you find yourself pacing?

- Are you afraid to close your eyes at night for fear that you may die in your sleep?

- Do you worry about the next diagnostic test, or the results of it, weeks in advance?

- Have you suddenly had a fear of losing control or going crazy?

- Have you suddenly had a fear of dying?

- Do you often worry about when your pain will return and how bad it will get?

- Do you worry about whether you will be able to get your next dose of pain medication on time?

- Do you spend more time in bed than you should because you are afraid that the pain will intensify if you stand up or move about?

- Have you been confused or disoriented lately?

Anxiety disorder includes adjustment disorder, panic disorder, phobias, obsessive-compulsive disorder, post-traumatic stress disorder, generalized anxiety disorder, and anxiety disorder caused by other general medical conditions.

Adjustment Disorder

Adjustment disorder includes behaviors or moods more extreme than expected in a reaction to a cancer diagnosis. Symptoms include severe nervousness, worry, jitteriness, and the inability to go to work, attend school, or be with other people. Adjustment disorder is more likely to occur in cancer patients during critical times of the disease. These include being tested for the disease, learning the diagnosis, and experiencing a relapse of the disease. Many cancer patients can achieve relief from adjustment disorder in several ways, including receiving reassurance from caregivers, exercising relaxation techniques, taking medication, and participating in support and education programs.

Panic Disorder

Patients with panic disorder experience intense anxiety. Patients may suffer shortness of breath, dizziness, rapid heart beat, trembling, profuse sweating, nausea, tingling sensations, or fears of "going crazy." Attacks may last for several minutes or several hours and are treated with medication. Symptoms of panic disorder may be very similar to other medical conditions.

Phobias

Phobias are ongoing fears about or avoidance of a situation or object. People with phobias usually experience intense anxiety and avoid situations that may frighten them. Cancer patients may fear needles. They may also fear small spaces and avoid having tests in confined spaces, such as magnetic resonance imaging (MRI) scans.

Obsessive-Compulsive Disorder

A person with obsessive-compulsive disorder has persistent thoughts, ideas, or images (obsessions) that are accompanied by repetitive behaviors (compulsions). Patients with obsessive-compulsive disorder may be unable to follow through with cancer treatment because they are disabled by thoughts and behaviors that interfere with their ability to function normally. Obsessive-compulsive disorder is treated with medication and psychotherapy. Obsessive-compulsive disorder is rare in patients with cancer who did not have the disorder before being diagnosed with cancer.

Post-Traumatic Stress Disorder

The diagnosis of cancer may cause a person who has previously experienced a life-threatening event to relive the trauma associated with that event. Patients with cancer who have post-traumatic stress disorder may experience extreme anxiety before surgery, chemotherapy, painful medical procedures, or bandage changes. Post-traumatic stress disorder is treated with psychotherapy.

Generalized Anxiety Disorder

Patients with generalized anxiety disorder may experience extreme and constant anxiety or unrealistic worry. For example, patients with supportive family and friends may fear that no one will care for them. Patients may worry that they cannot pay for their treatment, although they have adequate financial resources and insurance. Generalized anxiety disorder may happen after a patient has been very depressed. A person who has generalized anxiety may feel irritable or restless, have tense muscles, shortness of breath, heart palpitations, sweating, dizziness, and be easily fatigued.

Anxiety Disorder Caused by Other General Medical Conditions

Patients with cancer may experience anxiety that is caused by other medical conditions. Patients who are experiencing severe pain feel anxious, and anxiety can increase pain. The sudden appearance of extreme anxiety may be a symptom of infection, pneumonia, or an imbalance in the body's chemistry. It may also occur before a heart attack or blood clot in the lung and be accompanied by chest pain or trouble breathing. A decrease in the amount of oxygen that the blood is able to carry may also make the patient feel as though he or she is suffocating; this can cause anxiety.

Anxiety is a direct or indirect side effect of some medications. Some medications can cause anxiety, while others may cause restlessness, agitation, depression, thoughts of suicide, irritability, or trembling.

Certain tumors may cause anxiety or produce symptoms that resemble anxiety and panic by creating chemical imbalances or shortness of breath.

Treatment

It may be difficult to distinguish between normal fears associated with cancer and abnormally severe fears that can be classified as an anxiety disorder. Treatment depends on how the anxiety is affecting daily life for the patient. Anxiety that is caused by pain or another medical condition, a specific type of tumor, or as a side effect of medication, is usually controlled by treating the underlying cause.

Treatment for anxiety begins by giving the patient adequate information and support. Developing coping strategies such as the patient viewing his or her cancer from the perspective of a problem to be solved, obtaining enough information in order to fully understand his or her disease and treatment options, and utilizing available resources and support systems, can help to relieve anxiety. Patients may benefit from other treatment options for anxiety, including: psychotherapy, group therapy, family therapy, participating in self-help groups, hypnosis, and relaxation techniques such as guided imagery (a form of focused concentration on mental images to assist in stress management), or biofeedback (a method of early detection of the symptoms of anxiety in order to take preventative action). Medications may be used alone or in combination with these techniques. Patients should not avoid anxiety-relieving medications for fear of becoming addicted. Their doctors will give them sufficient medication to alleviate the symptoms and decrease the amount of the drug as the symptoms diminish.

Post-Treatment Considerations

After cancer therapy has been completed, a cancer survivor may be faced with new anxieties. Survivors may experience anxiety when they return to work and are asked about their cancer experience, or when confronted with insurance-related problems. A survivor may fear subsequent follow-up examinations and diagnostic tests, or they may fear a recurrence of cancer. Survivors may experience anxiety due to changes in body image, sexual dysfunction, reproductive issues, or post-traumatic stress. Survivorship programs, support groups, counseling, and other resources are available to help people readjust to life after cancer.

Chapter 46

Post-Traumatic Stress
Disorder in Cancer Patients

Some survivors of cancer experience trauma-related symptoms similar to symptoms experienced by people who have survived highly stressful situations, such as military combat, natural disasters, violent personal attack (such as rape), or other life-threatening events. This group of symptoms is called posttraumatic stress disorder (PTSD) and includes avoiding situations related to the trauma, continuously thinking of the trauma, and being overexcited.

People with histories of cancer are considered to be at risk for PTSD. The physical and mental shock of having a life-threatening disease, of receiving treatment for cancer, and living with repeated threats to one's body and life are traumatic experiences for many cancer patients.

Diagnosis and Symptoms

Posttraumatic stress disorder (PTSD) is defined as the development of certain symptoms following a mentally stressful event that involved actual death or the threat of death, serious injury, or a threat to oneself or others. For the person who has experienced a diagnosis of cancer, the specific trauma that triggers PTSD is unclear. It may be the actual diagnosis of a life-threatening illness, aspects of the treatment process, test results, information given about recurrence,

PDQ® Cancer Information Summary. National Cancer Institute; Bethesda, MD. Post-traumatic Stress Disorder (PDQ®) - patient. Updated 10/12/2005. Available at: http://www.cancer.gov. Accessed August 30, 2006.

or some other aspect of the cancer experience. Learning that one's child has cancer is traumatic for many parents. Because the cancer experience involves so many upsetting events, it is much more difficult to single out one event as a cause of stress than it is for other traumas, such as natural disasters or rape. The traumatic event may cause responses of extreme fear, helplessness, or horror and may trigger PTSD symptoms.

PTSD in cancer survivors may be expressed in these specific behaviors:

- Reliving the cancer experience in nightmares or flashbacks and by continuously thinking about it

- Avoiding places, events, and people connected to the cancer experience

- Being continuously overexcited, fearful, irritable, and unable to sleep

To be diagnosed as PTSD, these symptoms must last for at least one month and cause significant problems in the patient's personal relationships, employment, or other important areas of daily life. Patients who have these symptoms for less than one month often develop PTSD later.

Risk Factors, Protective Factors, and the Development of PTSD

As many as one third of people who experience an extremely upsetting event, including cancer, develop posttraumatic stress disorder (PTSD). The event alone does not explain why some people get PTSD and others don't. Although there is no clear answer as to which cancer survivors are at increased risk of developing PTSD, certain mental, physical, or social factors may make some people more likely to experience it.

Individual and Social Factors

Individual and social factors that have been associated with a higher incidence of PTSD include younger age, fewer years of formal education, and lower income.

Disease-Related Factors

Certain disease-related factors are associated with PTSD:

- In patients who received a bone marrow transplant, PTSD occurs more often when there is advanced disease and a longer hospital stay.

- In adult survivors of bone cancer and Hodgkin lymphoma, people for whom more time has passed since diagnosis and treatment tended to show fewer symptoms.

- In survivors of childhood cancer, symptoms of PTSD occur more often when there was a longer treatment time.

- Interfering thoughts occur more often in patients who experienced pain and other physical symptoms.

- Cancer that has returned has been shown to increase stress symptoms in patients.

Mental Factors

Mental factors may affect the development of PTSD in some patients:

- Previous trauma

- Previous psychological problems

- High level of general stress

- Genetic factors and biological factors (such as a hormone disorder) that affect memory and learning

- The amount of social support available

- Threat to life and body

- Having PTSD before being diagnosed with cancer

- The use of avoidance to cope with stress

Protective Factors

Certain factors may decrease a person's chance of developing PTSD. These include increased social support, accurate information about the stage of the cancer, and a satisfactory relationship with the medical staff.

How PTSD May Develop

PTSD symptoms develop by both conditioning and learning. Conditioning explains the fear responses caused by certain triggers that were first associated with the upsetting event. Neutral triggers (such as smells, sounds, and sights) that occurred at the same time as upsetting triggers (such as chemotherapy or painful treatments) later cause anxiety, stress, and fear even when they occur alone, after the trauma has ended. Once established, PTSD symptoms are continued through learning. The patient learns that avoiding the triggers prevents unpleasant feelings and thoughts, so coping by avoidance continues.

Although conditioning and learning are part of the process, many factors may explain why one person develops PTSD and another does not.

Assessment

It is important that cancer patients undergo a careful assessment for posttraumatic stress disorder (PTSD) so that early symptoms may be identified and treated. The timing of this assessment will vary with the individual patient. Cancer is an experience of repeated traumas and undetermined length. The patient may experience stress symptoms anytime from diagnosis through completion of treatment and cancer recurrence. In patients who have a history of victimization (such as Holocaust survivors) and who have PTSD or its symptoms from these experiences, symptoms can be started again by certain triggers experienced during their cancer treatment (for example, clinical procedures such as being inside MRI or CT scanners). While these patients may have problems adjusting to cancer and cancer treatment, their PTSD symptoms may vary, depending on other factors. The symptoms may become more or less prevalent during and after the cancer treatment.

Symptoms of PTSD usually begin within the first three months after the trauma, but sometimes they do not appear for months or even years afterwards. Therefore, cancer survivors and their families should be involved in long-term monitoring.

Some people who have experienced an upsetting event may show early symptoms without meeting the full diagnosis of PTSD. However, these early symptoms predict that PTSD may develop later. Early symptoms also indicate the need for repeated and long-term follow-up of cancer survivors and their families.

Diagnosing PTSD can be difficult since many of the symptoms are similar to other psychiatric problems. For example, irritability, poor concentration, increased defensiveness, excessive fear, and disturbed sleep are symptoms of both PTSD and anxiety disorder. Other symptoms are common to PTSD, phobias, and panic disorder. Some symptoms, such as loss of interest, a sense of having no future, avoidance of other people, and sleep problems may indicate the patient has PTSD or depression.

Even without PTSD or other problems, normal reactions to the cancer diagnosis and treatment of a life-threatening disease can include interfering thoughts, separating from people and the world, sleep problems, and over-excitability.

Questionnaires and interviews are used by health care providers to assess if the patient has symptoms of stress and to determine the diagnosis.

Other problems may also exist in addition to PTSD. These problems can include substance abuse, emotional problems, and other anxiety disorders, including major depression, alcohol dependence, drug dependence, social fears, or obsessive-compulsive disorder.

Treatment

Effects of posttraumatic stress disorder (PTSD) are long-lasting and serious. It may affect the patient's ability to have a normal lifestyle and may interfere with personal relationships, education, and employment. Because avoiding places and persons associated with cancer is part of PTSD, the syndrome may prevent the patient from seeking medical treatment. It is important that cancer survivors receive information about the possible psychological effects of their cancer experience and early treatment of symptoms of PTSD. Therapies used to treat PTSD are those used for other trauma victims. Treatment may involve more than one type of therapy.

The crisis intervention method tries to lessen the symptoms and return the patient to a normal level of functioning. The therapist focuses on solving problems, teaching coping skills, and providing a supportive setting for the patient.

Some patients are helped by methods that teach them to change their behaviors by changing their thinking patterns. Some of these methods include helping the patient understand symptoms, teaching coping and stress management skills (such as relaxation training), teaching the patient to reword upsetting thoughts, and helping the patient become less sensitive to upsetting triggers. Behavior therapy is used when the symptoms are avoidance of sexual activity and intimate situations.

Support groups may also help people who experience posttraumatic stress symptoms. In the group setting, patients can receive emotional support, meet others with similar experiences and symptoms, and learn coping and management skills.

For patients with severe symptoms, medications may be used. These include antidepressants, antianxiety medications, and when necessary, antipsychotic medications.

Chapter 47

Substance Abuse Concerns in Cancer Patients

People with cancer very rarely develop substance abuse problems unless they abused drugs and alcohol before cancer was diagnosed. Generally, people without a history of substance abuse can take opioids and other drugs to control cancer pain without developing substance abuse problems. People with a history of substance abuse, however, are at risk for developing problems when drugs are prescribed to control cancer symptoms.

Patients who have a history of substance abuse may find that illegal drug and alcohol use interfere with their ability to receive cancer therapy. The use of drugs may interfere with the effectiveness of anticancer therapy and may cause patients to become even sicker.

Patients with cancer who are current substance abusers, or who have been substance abusers in the past, may find it difficult to develop a trusting relationship with a network of friends and family members and with the cancer treatment team. The lack of trust may compromise cancer treatment and follow-up care and may worsen the patient's quality of life.

Prevalence among the Physically Ill

Substance abuse is very uncommon among patients with cancer. The number of known patients with cancer who are substance abusers may

PDQ® Cancer Information Summary. National Cancer Institute; Bethesda, MD. Substance Abuse Issues in Cancer (PDQ®) - Patient. Updated 09/02/2005. Available at: http:www.cancer.gov. Accessed 4/30/06.

be small because these patients do not seek medical help in hospitals, or they may not acknowledge to health care providers that they have a substance abuse problem.

Physical dependence: Physical dependence is defined as the occurrence of withdrawal symptoms when a drug is abruptly stopped, the dose is significantly reduced, or when a second drug is given that counteracts the actions of the drug to which the patient has developed a dependence. The dependence is not apparent until one of these actions occurs. When a patient with cancer is receiving an opioid drug for cancer pain, care is taken to avoid stopping the drug abruptly or prescribing other drugs that decrease or negate the effect of the opioid. Physical dependence on opioid pain medications does not seem to occur in patients with cancer. In these patients, once the pain disappears (usually through the effective treatment of the cancer), the pain medicine can be stopped without difficulty.

Tolerance: Tolerance to opioid pain medications may develop. Tolerance is the need to take increasingly larger doses of medication to relieve pain symptoms. Among patients taking opioid drugs for medical reasons, tolerance has not been shown to lead to drug addiction or drug abuse problems.

Substance abuse: Substance abuse is the use of a drug in any manner that does not conform to the physician's orders or the use of any illegal drug.

Addiction: Addiction is the use of a substance in a manner that is out of control, compulsive, used in increasing amounts, and is continued despite the risk of harm. A patient who uses opioids to relieve cancer pain may become physically dependent on the drugs, but is not described as being addicted to them.

These terms are generally used in association with people who do not have a medical illness. The terms are not entirely appropriate to use to describe medically ill people who are using drugs therapeutically.

Defining Terms for the Medically Ill

The following issues make assessing substance abuse among patients who are receiving treatment for medical illness more difficult.

Undertreatment: If cancer pain is not adequately treated, a patient may use drugs recklessly in an attempt to seek relief. Many patients may not receive effective treatment for their pain. When the prescribed treatment is adjusted and pain is controlled, the patient's need to use drugs in a manner in which they were not prescribed disappears.

People who have a history of drug abuse may revert to the use of an illegal drug when their pain is not adequately treated. Some of these patients may develop an addiction to prescribed drugs.

Sociocultural influences: Because the terminology used to describe drug abuse is not intended to include people without a history of drug abuse who are using medications therapeutically, many questions have yet to be answered. For example, while it is clear that a patient who forges a prescription, or injects a drug that was meant to be taken by mouth, is displaying deviant behavior, it is not clear if the same may be said about a patient who increases the dosage to control unrelieved pain, or takes a pain medication to fall asleep at night.

Health care professionals may make assumptions about the risk of drug abuse based on a patient's social group. If the patient belongs to a social group in which there is a high incidence of drug abuse, or if the patient has a history of drug abuse, it may be incorrectly assumed that the patient is at risk for abusing drugs prescribed for therapeutic purposes.

Disease-related factors: Substance abuse may be difficult to identify if the disease is progressing and causing the patient to have physical and mental changes. Treatment for disease may also cause these changes; radiation therapy to stop brain metastases, for example, can cause the patient to become withdrawn and experience mental changes.

To determine the cause of drug-related behaviors in patients who have advanced medical disease, the patients may be asked if the drug in question has been used at other times in the patient's life, whether drug use interfered with the patient's ability to complete treatment for the disease, and whether drug use prevented the patient from establishing a relationship with the health care team or family members.

Redefining abuse and addiction for the medically ill: The behavioral characteristics that are present in substance abusers, such as loss of control over drug use, compulsive drug use, and continued drug use despite harm, should be monitored in patients who are using drugs for medical conditions. Should a patient develop these behaviors, the health care provider should re-evaluate the patient's drug regimen.

Risk in Patients without Substance Abuse Histories

In patients who do not have a history of drug abuse, the use of opioids to control cancer pain very rarely develops into a significant abuse or addiction problem. Patients and some health care professionals continue to have unfounded fears that opioid use for controlling cancer pain may become addictive when a more significant problem is the undertreatment of pain.

At one time it was assumed that many addictions originated from the use of drugs prescribed for pain. Because cancer patients are able to use opioids for cancer pain without experiencing significant problems, the risks and benefits of long-term opioid treatment for chronic pain that is not related to cancer needs to be reassessed. Three studies of over 24,000 patients without drug addiction histories who were being treated for burn, headache, or other pain, found opioid abuse in only seven patients.

It is also suggested that the feeling of euphoria that a drug addict experiences does not happen in patients taking drugs to control pain. A patient taking opioids therapeutically more typically experiences a sense of depression rather than euphoria, thereby reducing the risk that the patient will become addicted to the drug.

The overall evidence indicates that in patients who do not have drug abuse or addiction histories, relationships with substance abusers, or psychological problems, the use of opioid therapy for control of chronic pain has a very low risk of developing into drug abuse or addiction. This is especially true for older patients who have never abused drugs.

Risk in Patients with Substance Abuse Histories

Patients who have a history of substance abuse can be treated successfully for chronic pain. Although studies have not yet been done, it is assumed that these patients may be more likely than patients without a drug history to abuse a pain medication or become addicted to it.

Treatment of Patients with Substance Abuse Histories

The following issues refer to palliative care for patients who are actively abusing alcohol or other drugs, or who are in a drug-free recovery or methadone program.

Involve a multidisciplinary team: Patients with histories of substance abuse are best treated for progressive medical illness by a team of health care providers. A team of one or more physicians, nurses, social workers and, if possible, an expert in addiction medicine, will address the many medical, psychosocial, and administrative problems that patients with drug histories and progressive illness may have.

Set realistic goals for therapy: Patients who have drug abuse and addiction problems experience periods of recovery and relapse. The risk of relapse is increased when patients have a life-threatening disease and have access to pain medication. In this situation, the goal of treatment may not be the complete prevention of relapse, but may be to provide a structure that will limit any harm done by abuse of the drugs. Some patients who have severe substance abuse and related psychological problems may never be able to use therapeutic drugs as prescribed. The health care team should monitor and revise treatment goals for these patients as often as necessary to avoid treatment that is not successful.

Treat related psychiatric disorders: Alcoholics and patients with substance abuse histories are very likely to also suffer from depression, anxiety, and personality disorders. The risk of relapse may be decreased if the patient also receives treatment for anxiety and depression.

Prevent or minimize withdrawal symptoms: Many patients with a history of drug abuse consume multiple drugs. The health care provider must be made aware of all drug use so the patient may be effectively monitored to prevent withdrawal symptoms.

The impact of tolerance: Patients who are actively abusing drugs may have developed a tolerance that limits the effectiveness of drugs prescribed for a medical condition.

Treat chronic pain: Opioid regimens used for long-term control of medical symptoms are individualized for each patient so that the dosage is large enough to control symptoms. In patients with substance abuse histories, prescribing dosages that are not large enough may result in undertreatment of the symptoms. The undertreatment does not relieve the patient's pain, and may encourage drug abuse in an effort to control the symptoms. This behavior may cause the physician to become more cautious in prescribing opioids. The physician and patient must work together closely to determine the necessary dosage and to agree on guidelines for responsible use of therapeutic drugs.

Recognize drug abuse behaviors: While all patients who are prescribed drugs that may be abused must be monitored closely, monitoring is especially important for people who have a history of substance abuse. The patient may be reassessed frequently, and the patient's significant others may be asked to provide observations about the patient's drug use. The physician may find it appropriate to test the patient's urine for illegal or unprescribed drugs. If a patient is agreeable to drug testing and monitoring and uses prescribed drugs responsibly, a trusting relationship may be established with the physician. A physician who is confident that the patient will not abuse drugs is more likely to adjust therapies to control symptoms.

Use nondrug approaches: The patient may benefit from nondrug approaches, such as learning about the complexities of the medical system, communicating with the medical staff, and learning relaxation and coping techniques.

Taking a substance abuse history: To avoid offending a patient, a health care provider may choose not to ask about drug abuse. The health care provider may assume that the patient may become offended, angry, threatened, or may not tell the truth. Such attitudes are not helpful in establishing truthful communication between health care provider and patient and may cause problems in monitoring therapy.

A patient may withhold information about his or her drug use because of negative attitudes the health care provider may have about drug users. The patient may not trust the health care provider, or the patient may fear that if his/her drug abuse history is known, inadequate medication may be prescribed to control symptoms. The physician must know the patient's drug use history in order to control symptoms and to keep the patient comfortable by prescribing adequate medication to prevent withdrawal symptoms and reduce pain. The physician needs to know which drugs the patient has taken, the length of time drugs have been used, the frequency of drug use, and the situations that cause the patient to use drugs.

Inpatient Treatment

Patients with current substance abuse problems who are scheduled to undergo surgery should, if possible, be admitted to the hospital several days early in order to stabilize drug use to prevent withdrawal and to plan treatment. To prevent the patient from obtaining illegal drugs, he or she may be given a room in a location that can be easily monitored, and he or she may be restricted to the room or the floor. Restrictions may also be placed on the patient's visitors. The patient's room as well as packages brought by visitors may be searched periodically for drugs or alcohol. The patient's urine may also undergo regular testing. The restrictions placed on the patient are necessary to ensure that medical treatment will not be jeopardized by ongoing drug use. Treatment should include frequent monitoring to prevent withdrawal and to control symptoms.

Outpatient Treatment

Ideally, outpatients who currently abuse drugs should be enrolled in a drug rehabilitation program; however, patients with advanced medical illnesses may not be able to be enrolled. The health care provider may outline for the patient the role of the treatment team, what is expected of the patient, and the consequences to the patient should he or she continue to abuse drugs while receiving treatment for medical illness. Patients must receive detailed instructions for taking prescribed drugs responsibly. They must be seen frequently so symptom control may be maintained and drug abuse may be monitored. Frequent visits also avoid the need to prescribe large amounts of drug at one time, and may help the patient stay on the treatment schedule and attend appointments with the physician. Some patients may find that a "twelve-step" program is helpful in stopping illegal drug use while they are receiving treatment.

Outpatients may be required to undergo periodic drug testing. The patient should be informed in advance of the consequences of a positive test. A urine test that indicates the patient is using illegal drugs may result in the need to visit the outpatient department more frequently, smaller quantities of prescribed drugs, referral to a drug rehabilitation program, or other restrictions.

If the patient lives with family members who are substance abusers, the family members can be encouraged to enroll in a drug treatment program to help the patient avoid illegal drugs and alcohol. The patient should also be aware that friends and family members may attempt to buy or steal the prescribed drugs. It is very helpful to identify people who will be supportive of the patient.

A treatment team that includes a specialist in addiction medicine may be able to provide more effective treatment for the outpatient with a progressive medical disease and a history of substance abuse than can a single physician.

Patients who have successfully stopped abusing drugs or alcohol may be reluctant to begin using prescribed drugs for their medical illness for fear of developing an addiction. They may fear rejection from friends and family members who will object to their use of prescribed drugs, and they may fear that others will attempt to buy or steal the drugs. The health care provider should help the patient resolve these concerns and assure the patient that use of opioids to control symptoms of progressive disease does not result in the euphoria experienced by opioid abusers who do not have a medical illness.

If the patient is very reluctant to begin opioid therapy, the physician may develop strict guidelines for use of the prescribed drug to provide the patient with a sense of control. The patient may also be provided with counseling to help identify situations in which he or she is likely to abuse drugs or alcohol, and to develop strategies for avoiding future abuse of illegal or prescribed drugs.

Part Six

Maintaining Wellness during and after Cancer Treatment

Chapter 48

Nutrition in Cancer Care

Cancer and cancer treatments may cause nutrition-related side effects. The diet is an important part of cancer treatment. Eating the right kinds of foods before, during, and after treatment can help the patient feel better and stay stronger. To ensure proper nutrition, a person has to eat and drink enough of the foods that contain key nutrients (vitamins, minerals, protein, carbohydrates, fat, and water). For many patients, however, some side effects of cancer and cancer treatments make it difficult to eat well. Symptoms that interfere with eating include anorexia, nausea, vomiting, diarrhea, constipation, mouth sores, trouble with swallowing, and pain. Appetite, taste, smell, and the ability to eat enough food or absorb the nutrients from food may be affected. Malnutrition (lack of key nutrients) can result, causing the patient to be weak, tired, and unable to resist infections or withstand cancer therapies. Eating too little protein and calories is the most common nutrition problem facing many cancer patients. Protein and calories are important for healing, fighting infection, and providing energy.

Anorexia (the loss of appetite or desire to eat) is a common symptom in people with cancer. Anorexia may occur early in the disease or later, when the tumor grows and spreads. Some patients may have anorexia when they are diagnosed with cancer. Almost all patients who have widespread cancer will develop anorexia. Anorexia is the most common cause of malnutrition in cancer patients.

Excerpted from PDQ® Cancer Information Summary. National Cancer Institute; Bethesda, MD. Nutrition in Cancer Care (PDQ®): Supportive Care - Patient. Updated 04/2006. Available at http://cancer.gov. Accessed April 30, 2006.

Cachexia is a wasting syndrome that causes weakness and a loss of weight, fat, and muscle. It commonly occurs in patients with tumors of the lung, pancreas, and upper gastrointestinal tract and less often in patients with breast cancer or lower gastrointestinal cancer. Anorexia and cachexia often occur together. Weight loss can be caused by eating fewer calories, using more calories, or a combination of the two. Cachexia can occur in people who are eating enough, but who cannot absorb the nutrients. Cachexia is not related to the tumor size, type, or extent. Cancer cachexia is not the same as starvation. A healthy person's body can adjust to starvation by slowing down its use of nutrients, but in cancer patients, the body does not make this adjustment.

Nutrition therapy can help cancer patients get the nutrients needed to maintain body weight and strength, prevent body tissue from breaking down, rebuild tissue, and fight infection. Eating guidelines for cancer patients can be very different from the usual suggestions for healthful eating. Nutrition recommendations for cancer patients are designed to help the patient cope with the effects of the cancer and its treatment. Some cancer treatments are more effective if the patient is well nourished and getting enough calories and protein in the diet. People who eat well during cancer treatment may even be able to handle higher doses of certain treatments. Being well-nourished has been linked to a better prognosis (chance of recovery).

Effect of Cancer on Nutrition

Cancer can change the way the body uses food. Tumors may produce chemicals that change the way the body uses certain nutrients. The body's use of protein, carbohydrates, and fat may be affected, especially by tumors of the stomach or intestines. A patient may appear to be eating enough, but the body may not be able to absorb all the nutrients from the food. Diets higher in protein and calories can help correct this and prevent the onset of cachexia. Drugs may also be helpful. It is important to monitor nutrition early, as cachexia is difficult to completely reverse.

Early treatment of cancer symptoms and side effects that affect eating and cause weight loss is important. Both nutrition therapy and drugs can help the patient maintain a healthy weight. The types of drugs commonly used to relieve these symptoms and side effects include the following:

- Medicines to prevent nausea and vomiting

- Medicines to prevent diarrhea
- Pancreatic enzymes
- Laxatives (to promote bowel movements)
- Medicines for mouth problems (to clean the mouth, stimulate saliva, prevent infections, relieve pain, and heal sores)
- Pain medications

Effect of Cancer Treatment on Nutrition

Effect of Surgery on Nutrition

The body needs extra energy and nutrients to heal wounds, fight infection, and recover from surgery. If the patient is malnourished before surgery, there may be complications during recovery, such as poor healing or infection. Patients with certain cancers, such as cancers of the head, neck, stomach, and intestines, may be malnourished at diagnosis. Nutrition care may therefore begin before surgery.

Nutrition-related side effects may occur as a result of surgery. More than half of cancer patients have cancer-related surgery. Surgery may include the removal of all or parts of certain organs, which may affect a patient's ability to eat and digest food. The following are nutrition problems related to specific surgeries:

- Surgery to the head and neck may cause chewing and swallowing problems. Mental stress due to the amount of tissue removed during surgery may affect appetite.

- Surgery involving cancer of organs in the digestive system may lessen the ability of the digestive system to work properly and may slow the digestion of food. Removal of part of the stomach may cause a feeling of fullness before enough food has been eaten. Stomach surgery may also cause dumping syndrome (emptying of the stomach into the intestines before food is digested). Some of the organs in the digestive system normally produce important hormones and chemicals that are necessary for digestion. If surgery affects these organs, the protein, fat, vitamins, and minerals in the diet may not be absorbed normally by the body. Levels of sugar, salt, and fluid in the body may become unbalanced.

Nutrition therapy can treat these problems and help cancer patients get the nutrients they need. Nutrition therapy may include the following:

- Nutritional supplement drinks

- Enteral nutrition (feeding liquid through a tube into the stomach or intestine)

- Parenteral nutrition (feeding through a catheter into the bloodstream)

- Medications to improve the appetite

It is common for patients to experience pain, tiredness, and loss of appetite after surgery. For a short time, some patients may not be able to eat their regular diet because of these symptoms. The following eating tips may help:

- Avoid carbonated drinks (such as sodas) and gas-producing foods (such as beans, peas, broccoli, cabbage, brussel sprouts, green peppers, radishes, and cucumbers)

- If regularity is a problem, increase fiber by small amounts and drink lots of water. Good sources of fiber include whole-grain cereals (such as oatmeal and bran), beans, vegetables, fruit, and whole grain breads.

- Choose high-protein and high-calorie foods to help wounds heal. Good choices include eggs, cheese, whole milk, ice cream, nuts, peanut butter, meat, poultry, and fish. Increase calories by frying foods and using gravies, mayonnaise, and salad dressings. Supplements high in calories and protein are available.

Effect of Chemotherapy on Nutrition

Chemotherapy is a cancer treatment that uses drugs to stop the growth of cancer cells, either by killing the cells or by stopping the cells from dividing. Because chemotherapy targets rapidly dividing cells, healthy cells that normally grow and divide rapidly may also be affected by the cancer treatments. These include cells in the mouth and digestive tract.

Side effects that interfere with eating and digestion may occur during chemotherapy. The following side effects are common:

- Anorexia

- Nausea

- Vomiting

- Diarrhea or constipation

- Inflammation and sores in the mouth
- Changes in the way food tastes
- Infections

The side effects of chemotherapy may make it difficult for a patient to obtain the nutrients needed to regain healthy blood counts between chemotherapy treatments. Nutrition therapy can treat these side effects and help chemotherapy patients get the nutrients they need to tolerate and recover from treatment, prevent weight loss, and maintain general health. Nutrition therapy may include the following:

- Supplements high in calories and protein
- Enteral nutrition (tube feedings)

Effect of Radiation Therapy on Nutrition

Radiation therapy is a cancer treatment that uses high energy x-rays or other types of radiation to kill cancer cells. There are two types of radiation therapy. External radiation therapy uses a machine outside the body to send radiation toward the cancer. Internal radiation therapy uses a radioactive substance sealed in needles, seeds, wires, or catheters that are placed directly into or near the cancer.

Healthy cells that are near the cancer may be affected by the radiation treatments, and side effects may occur. The side effects depend mostly on the radiation dose and the part of the body that is treated.

Radiation therapy to any part of the digestive system is likely to cause nutrition-related side effects. The following side effects may occur:

- Radiation therapy to the head and neck may cause anorexia, taste changes, dry mouth, inflammation of the mouth and gums, swallowing problems, jaw spasms, cavities, or infection.

- Radiation therapy to the chest may cause infection in the esophagus, swallowing problems, esophageal reflux (a backwards flow of the stomach contents into the esophagus), nausea, or vomiting.

- Radiation therapy to the abdomen or pelvis may cause diarrhea, nausea and vomiting, inflammation of the intestine or rectum, and fistula (holes) in the stomach or intestines. Long-term effects can include narrowing of the intestine, chronic inflamed intestines, poor absorption, or blockage in the stomach or intestine.

- Radiation therapy may also cause tiredness, which can lead to a decrease in appetite and a reduced desire to eat.

Nutrition therapy during radiation treatment can provide the patient with enough protein and calories to tolerate the treatment, prevent weight loss, and maintain general health. Nutrition therapy may include the following:

- Nutritional supplement drinks between meals
- Enteral nutrition (tube feedings)
- Other changes in the diet, such as eating small meals throughout the day and choosing certain kinds of foods

Effect of Immunotherapy on Nutrition

Immunotherapy is treatment that uses the patient's immune system to fight cancer. Substances made by the body or made in a laboratory are used to boost, direct, or restore the body's natural defenses against cancer. This type of cancer treatment is also called biologic therapy or biotherapy.

The following nutrition-related side effects are common during immunotherapy:

- Fever
- Nausea
- Vomiting
- Diarrhea
- Anorexia
- Tiredness

If the side effects of immunotherapy are not treated, weight loss and malnutrition may occur. These conditions can cause complications during recovery, such as poor healing or infection. Nutrition therapy can treat side effects from immunotherapy and help patients get the nutrients they need to tolerate treatment, prevent weight loss, and maintain general health.

Effect of Bone Marrow and Stem Cell Transplantation on Nutrition

Bone marrow and stem cell transplantation are methods of replacing blood-forming cells destroyed by cancer treatment with high doses of chemotherapy or radiation therapy. Stem cells (immature blood cells) are removed from the bone marrow of the patient or a donor and are frozen for storage. After the chemotherapy and radiation therapy are completed, the stored stem cells are thawed and given back to the patient through an infusion. Over a short time, these reinfused stem cells grow into (and restore) the body's blood cells.

Chemotherapy, radiation therapy, and medications used in the transplant process may cause side effects that prevent a patient from eating and digesting food as usual. These side effects include the following:

- Taste changes
- Dry mouth
- Thick saliva
- Mouth and throat sores
- Nausea and vomiting
- Diarrhea
- Constipation
- Lack of appetite
- Weight gain

Transplant patients also have a very high risk of infection. The high doses of chemotherapy and radiation therapy reduce the number of white blood cells, the cells that fight infection. Cancer patients should be especially careful to avoid infections and food-borne illnesses. Patients are advised to avoid eating certain foods that may carry harmful bacteria.

Patients undergoing the transplant process need adequate protein and calories to tolerate and recover from the treatment, prevent weight loss, fight infection, and maintain general health. Nutrition therapy is also designed to avoid possible infection from bacteria in food. Nutrition therapy during the transplant process may include the following:

- A diet of only cooked and processed foods, avoiding raw vegetables and fresh fruit
- Instruction on safe food handling
- Specific diet guidelines based on the type of transplant and the cancer site

- Parenteral nutrition (feeding through the bloodstream) during the first few weeks after the transplant is complete, to ensure the patient gets the calories, protein, vitamins, minerals and fluids needed for good health

Nutrition Suggestions for Symptom Relief

When side effects of cancer or cancer treatment interfere with normal eating, adjustments can be made to ensure the patient continues to get the necessary nutrition. Medications may be given to stimulate the appetite. Eating foods that are high in calories, protein, vitamins and minerals is usually advised. Meal planning, however, should be individualized to meet the patient's nutritional needs and tastes in food.

Anorexia

Anorexia (lack of appetite) is one of the most common problems for cancer patients. The following suggestions may help cancer patients manage anorexia:

- Eat small high-protein and high-calorie meals every one to two hours instead of three larger meals.
- Have help with preparing meals.
- Add extra calories and protein to food (such as butter, skim milk powder, honey, or brown sugar).
- Take liquid supplements (special drinks containing nutrients), soups, milk, juices, shakes, and smoothies when eating solid food is a problem.
- Eat snacks that contain plenty of calories and protein.
- Prepare and store small portions of favorite foods so they are ready to eat when hungry.
- Eat breakfasts that contain one third of the calories and protein needed for the day.
- Eat foods with odors that are appealing. Strong odors can be avoided by using boiling bags, cooking outdoors on the grill, using a kitchen fan when cooking, serving cold food instead of hot (since odors are in the rising steam), and taking off any food covers to release the odors before entering a patient's room. Small

portable fans can be used to blow food odors away from patients. Cooking odors can be avoided by ordering take-out food.

- Try new foods. Be creative with desserts. Experiment with recipes, flavorings, spices, types, and consistencies of food. Food likes and dislikes may change from day to day.

The following high-calorie, high-protein foods are recommended:

- Cheese and crackers
- Muffins
- Puddings
- Nutritional supplements
- Milkshakes
- Yogurt
- Ice cream
- Powdered milk added to foods such as pudding, milkshakes, or any recipe using milk
- Finger foods (handy for snacking) such as deviled eggs, cream cheese or peanut butter on crackers or celery, or deviled ham on crackers

Taste Changes

Changes in how foods taste may be caused by radiation treatment, dental problems, or medicines. Cancer patients often complain of changes in their sense of taste when undergoing chemotherapy, in particular a bitter taste sensation. A sudden dislike for certain foods may occur. This may result in food avoidance, weight loss, and anorexia, which can greatly reduce the patients' quality of life. Some or all of the sense of taste may return, but it may be a year after treatment ends before the sense of taste is normal again. Drinking plenty of fluids, changing the types of foods eaten and adding spices or flavorings to food may help.

The following suggestions may help cancer patients manage changes in taste:

- Rinse mouth with water before eating.
- Try citrus fruits (oranges, tangerines, lemons, grapefruit) unless mouth sores are present.

- Eat small meals and healthy snacks several times a day.
- Eat meals when hungry rather than at set mealtimes.
- Use plastic utensils if foods taste metallic.
- Try favorite foods.
- Eat with family and friends.
- Have others prepare the meal.
- Try new foods when feeling best.
- Substitute poultry, fish, eggs, and cheese for red meat.
- Find nonmeat, high-protein recipes in a vegetarian or Chinese cookbook.
- Use sugar-free lemon drops, gum, or mints if there is a metallic or bitter taste in the mouth.
- Add spices and sauces to foods.
- Eat meat with something sweet, such as cranberry sauce, jelly, or applesauce.
- Taking zinc sulfate tablets during radiation therapy to the head and neck may speed the return of normal taste after treatment.

Dry Mouth

Dry mouth is often caused by radiation therapy to the head and neck. Some medicines may also cause dry mouth. Dry mouth may affect speech, taste, ability to swallow, and the use of dentures or braces. There is also an increased risk of cavities and gum disease because less saliva is produced to wash the teeth and gums.

The main treatment for dry mouth is drinking plenty of liquids, about ½ ounce per pound of body weight per day. Other suggestions to manage dry mouth include the following:

- Eat moist foods with extra sauces, gravies, butter, or margarine.
- Suck on hard candy or chew gum.
- Eat frozen desserts (such as frozen grapes and ice pops) or ice chips.
- Clean teeth (including dentures) and rinse mouth at least four times per day (after each meal and before bedtime).
- Keep water handy at all times to moisten the mouth.
- Avoid liquids and foods that contain a lot of sugar.

- Avoid mouth rinses containing alcohol.
- Drink fruit nectar instead of juice.
- Use a straw to drink liquids.

Mouth Sores and Infections

Mouth sores can result from chemotherapy and radiation therapy. These treatments target rapidly-growing cells because cancer cells grow rapidly. Normal cells inside the mouth may be damaged by these cancer treatments because they also grow rapidly. Mouth sores may become infected and bleed, making eating difficult. By choosing certain foods and taking good care of their mouths, patients can usually make eating easier. Suggestions to help manage mouth sores and infections include the following:

- Eat soft foods that are easy to chew and swallow, such as the following:
  - Soft fruits, including bananas, applesauce, and watermelon
  - Peach, pear, and apricot nectars
  - Cottage cheese
  - Mashed potatoes
  - Macaroni and cheese
  - Custards; puddings
  - Gelatin
  - Milkshakes
  - Scrambled eggs
  - Oatmeal or other cooked cereals
- Use the blender to process vegetables (such as potatoes, peas, and carrots) and meats until smooth.
- Avoid rough, coarse, or dry foods, including raw vegetables, granola, toast, and crackers.
- Avoid foods that are spicy or salty. Avoid foods that are acidic, such as vinegar, pickles, and olives.
- Avoid citrus fruits and juices, including orange, grapefruit, and tangerine.
- Cook foods until soft and tender.

- Cut foods into small pieces.

- Use a straw to drink liquids.

- Eat foods cold or at room temperature. Hot and warm foods can irritate a tender mouth.

- Clean teeth (including dentures) and rinse mouth at least four times per day (after each meal and before bedtime).

- Add gravy, broth, or sauces to food.

- Drink high-calorie, high-protein drinks in addition to meals.

- Numb the mouth with ice chips or flavored ice pops.

- Using a mouth rinse that contains glutamine may reduce the number of mouth sores. Glutamine is a substance found in plant and animal proteins.

Nausea

Nausea caused by cancer treatment can affect the amount and kinds of food eaten. The following suggestions may help cancer patients manage nausea:

- Eat before cancer treatments.

- Avoid foods that are likely to cause nausea. For some patients, this includes spicy foods, greasy foods, and foods that have strong odors.

- Eat small meals several times a day.

- Slowly sip fluids throughout the day.

- Eat dry foods such as crackers, breadsticks, or toast throughout the day.

- Sit up or lie with the upper body raised for one hour after eating.

- Eat bland, soft, easy-to-digest foods rather than heavy meals.

- Avoid eating in a room that has cooking odors or that is overly warm. Keep the living space at a comfortable temperature and with plenty of fresh air.

- Rinse out the mouth before and after eating.

- Suck on hard candies such as peppermints or lemon drops if the mouth has a bad taste.

Diarrhea

Diarrhea may be caused by cancer treatments, surgery on the stomach or intestines, or by emotional stress. Long-term diarrhea may lead to dehydration (lack of water in the body) or low levels of salt and potassium, important minerals needed by the body.

The following suggestions may help cancer patients manage diarrhea:

- Eat broth, soups, sports drinks, bananas, and canned fruits to help replace salt and potassium lost by diarrhea.

- Avoid greasy foods, hot or cold liquids, and caffeine.

- Avoid high-fiber foods—especially dried beans and cruciferous vegetables (such as broccoli, cauliflower, and cabbage).

- Drink plenty of fluids through the day. Room temperature liquids may cause fewer problems than hot or cold liquids.

- Limit milk to two cups or eliminate milk and milk products until the source of the problem is found.

- Limit gas-forming foods and beverages such as peas, lentils, cruciferous vegetables, chewing gum, and soda.

- Limit sugar-free candies or gum made with sorbitol (sugar alcohol).

- Drink at least one cup of liquid after each loose bowel movement.

- Taking oral glutamine may help keep the intestines healthy when taking the anticancer drug fluorouracil.

Low White Blood Cell Count

Cancer patients may have a low white blood cell count for a variety of reasons, some of which include radiation therapy, chemotherapy, or the cancer itself. Patients who have a low white blood cell count are at an increased risk of infection. The following suggestions may help cancer patients prevent infections when white blood cell counts are low:

- Check dates on food and do not buy or use the food if it is out of date.

- Do not buy or use food in cans that are swollen, dented, or damaged.

- Thaw foods in the refrigerator or microwave. Never thaw foods at room temperature. Cook foods immediately after thawing.
- Refrigerate all leftovers within two hours of cooking and eat them within 24 hours.
- Keep hot foods hot and cold foods cold.
- Avoid old, moldy, or damaged fruits and vegetables.
- Avoid unpackaged tofu sold in open bins or containers.
- Cook all meat, poultry, and fish thoroughly. Avoid raw eggs or raw fish.
- Buy foods packed as single servings to avoid leftovers.
- Avoid salad bars and buffets when eating out.
- Avoid large groups of people and people who have infections.
- Wash hands often to prevent the spread of bacteria.

Hot Flashes

Hot flashes occur in most women with breast cancer and men with prostate cancer. When caused by natural or treatment-related menopause, hot flashes can be relieved with estrogen replacement. Many women, however, (including women with breast cancer), are not able to take estrogen replacement. Eating soy foods, which contain an estrogen-like substance, is sometimes suggested to relieve hot flashes in patients who cannot take estrogen replacement, but no benefit has been proven.

Fluid Intake

The body needs plenty of water to replace the fluids lost every day. Long-term diarrhea, nausea and vomiting, and pain may prevent the patient from drinking and eating enough to get the water needed by the body. One of the first signs of dehydration (lack of water in the body) is extreme tiredness. The following suggestions may help cancer patients prevent dehydration:

- Drink 8 to 12 cups of liquids a day. This can be water, juice, milk, or foods that contain a large amount of liquid such as puddings, ice cream, ice pops, flavored ices, and gelatins.
- Take a water bottle whenever leaving home. It is important to drink even if not thirsty, as thirst is not a good sign of fluid needs.

- Limit drinks that contain caffeine, such as sodas, coffee, and tea (both hot and cold).

- Drink most liquids after and between meals.

- Use medicines that help relieve nausea and vomiting.

Constipation

Constipation is defined as fewer than three bowel movements per week. It is a very common problem for cancer patients and may result from lack of water or fiber in the diet; lack of physical activity; anticancer therapies such as chemotherapy; and medications.

Prevention of constipation is a part of cancer care. The following suggestions may help cancer patients prevent constipation:

- Eat more fiber-containing foods on a regular basis. The recommended fiber intake is 25 to 35 grams per day. Increase fiber gradually and drink plenty of fluids at the same time to keep the fiber moving through the intestines.

- Drink 8 to 10 cups of fluid each day. Water, prune juice, warm juices, lemonade, and teas without caffeine can be very helpful.

- Take walks and exercise regularly. Proper footwear is important.

If constipation does occur, the following suggestions for diet, exercise, and medication may help correct it:

- Continue to eat high-fiber foods and drink plenty of fluids. Try adding wheat bran to the diet; begin with two heaping tablespoons each day for three days, then increase by one tablespoon each day until constipation is relieved. Do not exceed six tablespoons per day.

- Maintain physical activity.

- Include over-the-counter constipation treatments, if necessary. This refers to bulk-forming products (such as Citrucel, Metamucil, Fiberall, FiberCon, and Fiber-Lax); stimulants (such as Dulcolax tablets or suppositories and Senokot); stool softeners (such as Colace, Surfak, and Dialose); and osmotics (such as milk of magnesia). Cottonseed and aerosol enemas can also help relieve the problem. Lubricants such as mineral oil are not recommended because they may prevent the body's use of important nutrients.

Good food sources of fiber include the following:

4 or more grams of fiber per serving

- Legumes (½ cup, cooked)
  - Kidney beans
  - Navy beans
  - Garbanzo beans
  - Lima beans
  - Split peas
  - Pinto beans
  - Lentils
- Vegetables and fruit
  - Corn (½ cup)
  - Pears with skin (one medium-sized pear)
  - Popcorn (3 cups popped)
- Cold cereals (1 ounce)
  - Whole-grain cereals
  - Bran cereals
- Hot cereals (1/3 cup before cooking)
  - Oatmeal
  - Oat bran
  - Grits

2 or more grams of fiber per serving

- Vegetables (½ cup cooked or 1 cup raw)
  - Asparagus
  - Green beans
  - Broccoli
  - Cabbage
  - Carrots
  - Cauliflower
  - Greens
  - Onions
  - Peas

- Spinach
- Squash
- Green peppers
- Celery
- Canned tomatoes
- Fruit (½ cup serving or one medium-sized fruit)
  - Apples with the skin
  - Bananas
  - Oranges
  - Strawberries
  - Peaches
  - Blueberries
- Breads
  - Whole wheat bread (one slice)
  - Whole grain bagel (one half of medium-sized bagel)
  - Whole wheat pita (½ portion)
  - Whole grain crackers (see package for serving size)

Legumes, broccoli, and cabbage may cause gas. Over-the-counter enzyme tablets may be helpful.

Other Nutrition Issues

Advanced Cancer

Nutrition-related side effects may occur or become worse as cancer becomes more advanced. The following are the most common nutrition-related symptoms in patients who have advanced cancer:

- Cachexia (a wasting syndrome that causes weakness and a loss of weight, fat, and muscle)
- Weight loss of more than 10% of normal body weight
- Feeling too full to eat enough food
- Bloating
- Anorexia (the loss of appetite or desire to eat)
- Constipation
- Dry mouth

- Taste changes
- Nausea
- Vomiting
- Inability to swallow

The usual treatment for these problems in patients with advanced cancer is palliative care to reduce the symptoms and improve the quality of life. Palliative care includes nutrition therapy and/or drug therapy.

Eating less solid food is common in advanced cancer. Patients usually prefer soft foods and clear liquids. Those who have problems swallowing may do better with thick liquids than with thin liquids. Terminally ill patients often do not feel much hunger at all and may be satisfied with very little food.

When cancer is advanced, food should be viewed as a source of enjoyment. Eating should not just be about calories, protein, and other nutrient needs.

Dietary restriction is not usually necessary, as intake of "prohibited foods" (such as sweets for a patient with diabetes) is not enough to be of concern. Some patients, however, may need certain diet restrictions. For example, patients who have pancreatic cancer, uterine cancer, ovarian cancer, or another cancer affecting the abdominal area may need a soft diet (no raw fruits and vegetables, no nuts, no skins, no seeds) to prevent a blockage in the bowel. Diet restrictions should be considered in terms of quality of life and the patient's wishes.

The benefits and risks of nutrition support vary for each patient. Decisions about using nutrition support should be made with the following considerations:

- Will quality of life be improved?
- Do the possible benefits outweigh the risks and costs?
- Is there an advanced directive? An advanced directive is a written instruction about the provision of health care or power of attorney in the event an individual can no longer make his or her wishes known.
- What are the wishes and needs of the family?

Cancer patients and their caregivers have the right to make informed decisions. The healthcare team, with guidance from a registered dietitian, should inform patients and their caregivers about the benefits and risks of using nutrition support in advanced disease. In most cases, the risks outweigh the benefits. However, for someone who still has good quality of life but also physical barriers to achieving adequate food and water by mouth, enteral feedings may be appropriate. Parenteral support is not usually appropriate. Advantages and disadvantages of enteral nutrition include the following:

Benefits

- May improve alertness
- May provide comfort to the family
- May decrease nausea
- May decrease hopelessness and fears of abandonment

Risks

- May cause diarrhea or constipation
- May increase nausea
- Requires surgery for the placement of a tube through the abdomen
- Increases risk of choking or pneumonia
- Increases risk of infection
- Creates a greater burden on the caregiver

Guidelines for Healthy Eating

The Food Guide Pyramid: The United States Department of Agriculture (USDA) developed *Nutrition and Your Health: Dietary Guidelines for Americans* that offers diet and fitness recommendations that support good overall health. The USDA Food Guide Pyramid shows five food groups and the number of servings to be eaten each day to provide the nutrients and calories needed. The food groups shown are grains, vegetables, fruits, dairy, and meat and nonmeat protein. Small amounts of fats, oils, and sweets are advised.

Current guidelines for promoting general health and well-being include the following:

- Eat nutrient-rich foods within calorie limits.
- Maintain a healthy body weight.
- Exercise regularly.

- Eat a variety of fruits, vegetables, whole grains, and low-fat dairy products each day.

- Eat less fat and avoid trans fatty acid (trans fats).

- Choose fiber-rich fruits, vegetables, and whole grains often.

- Eat fewer foods high in salt. Choose more foods high in potassium (like bananas, spinach and potatoes).

- Those who choose to drink alcoholic beverages should do so in moderation. Certain individuals should avoid alcohol entirely.

- Keep food safety in mind when preparing, storing, and serving foods.

Cancer prevention: Healthy food choices and physical activity may help reduce the risk of cancer. The American Cancer Society and the American Institute for Cancer Research have both developed cancer prevention guidelines that are similar.

The following diet and fitness guidelines may help reduce the risk of cancer:

- Eat a plant-based diet. Eat at least 5 servings of fruit and vegetables daily. Include beans in the diet and eat grain products (such as cereals, breads, and pasta) several times daily.

- Choose foods low in fat.

- Choose foods low in salt.

- Get to and stay at a healthy weight.

- Be at least moderately active for 30 minutes on most days of the week.

- Limit alcoholic drinks.

- Prepare and store food safely.

- Do not use tobacco in any form.

Surviving Cancer and Preventing Second Cancers

Nutrition guidelines for cancer prevention may also help cancer survivors prevent the development of a second cancer. The relationship between diet and cancer continues to be studied.

Lung cancer: Study findings have shown the following associations between diet and lung cancer:

- Eating more than five servings per day of fruits and vegetables may reduce the risk of lung cancer.

- Taking beta-carotene supplements may increase the risk of lung cancer in male smokers.

Prostate cancer: Study findings have shown the following associations between diet and prostate cancer:

- Diets high in saturated fat and meat or animal fat may increase the risk of advanced prostate cancer.

- Taking daily vitamin E supplements may reduce the risk of death from prostate cancer.

- Taking daily beta-carotene supplements may reduce the chance of dying from prostate cancer. Taking beta-carotene supplements is not advised for smokers, however, as it may increase their risk of developing prostate cancer.

Breast cancer: Study findings have shown the following associations between diet and breast cancer:

- High-calorie, high-fat diets may increase the risk of recurrence.

- Drinking beer may increase the risk of recurrence and death.

- Obesity (having too much body fat) may increase the risk of recurrence.

- Lack of physical activity may increase the risk of recurrence.

- Taking vitamin C above the RDA may reduce the risk of recurrence.

- A diet high in vegetables and fruits may reduce the risk of recurrence.

- A diet rich in foods that contain beta-carotene (such as dark orange vegetables and fruits) may reduce the risk of death from breast cancer.

The effect of soy on breast cancer or breast cancer recurrence is unknown. Studies are under way.

Colon cancer: Study findings have shown that a long-term diet rich in whole grains may reduce the risk of colon cancer.

Esophageal and gastric cancer: Study findings have shown the following associations between diet and esophageal or gastric (stomach) cancer:

- A diet rich in cereal fiber may reduce the risk of gastric cancer.
- Taking daily supplements of vitamins C and E and beta-carotene may reduce the risk of esophageal cancer.

Chapter 49

Drug-Nutrient Interactions

Cancer patients may be treated with a number of drugs throughout their care. Some foods or nutritional supplements do not mix safely with certain drugs. The combination of these foods and drugs may reduce or change the effectiveness of anticancer therapy or cause life-threatening side effects. The following list provides information on some of the drug-nutrient interactions that may occur with certain anticancer drugs:

- **Targretin (bexarotene):** Grapefruit juice may increase a drug's effects.

- **Folex (methotrexate):** Alcohol may cause liver damage.

- **Rheumatrex (methotrexate):** Alcohol may cause liver damage.

- **Mithracin (plicamycin):** Supplements of calcium and vitamin D may decrease the drug's effect.

- **Matulane (procarbazine):** Alcohol may cause a reaction that includes flushing of the skin, breathing difficulty, nausea, and low blood pressure. Caffeine may raise blood pressure.

- **Temodar (temozolomide):** Food may slow or decrease the drug's effect.

Excerpted from PDQ® Cancer Information Summary. National Cancer Institute; Bethesda, MD. Nutrition in Cancer Care (PDQ®): Supportive Care - Patient. Updated 04/2006. Available at http://cancer.gov. Accessed April 30, 2006.

The combination of some herbs with certain foods and drugs may reduce or change the effectiveness of anticancer therapy or cause life-threatening side effects. The following list provides information about herbs commonly taken by cancer patients. The information provided covers known interactions only; additional side effects are possible for these herbs. A pharmacist or updated herbal supplement references may provide more information.

- **Black cohosh:** May lower blood fat or blood pressure when taken with certain drugs. May increase the effect of tamoxifen.

- **Chamomile:** May increase bleeding when used with blood-thinners. May increase the effect of certain tranquilizers.

- **Dong quai:** May increase effects of warfarin (a blood-thinner).

- **Echinacea:** May interfere with therapy that uses the immune system to fight cancer.

- **Garlic:** May increase bleeding when used with aspirin, dipyridamole, and warfarin. May increase the effects of drugs that treat high blood sugar.

- **Ginkgo biloba:** May increase bleeding when used with aspirin, dipyridamole, and warfarin. May raise blood pressure when used with certain diuretics (drugs that cause the body to lose water through the kidneys).

- **Ginseng:** May prevent the blood from clotting normally. May decrease blood sugar if taken with insulin. May interfere with drugs used to treat a mental disorder. May cause high blood pressure with long-term use of caffeine.

- **Kava:** May increase the effect of certain tranquilizers. May cause liver damage.

- **St. John's wort:** May cause life-threatening side effects when used with drugs that raise the level of serotonin in the brain, such as many antidepressants. May reduce the effect of certain drugs used for cancer, AIDS, organ transplants, heart disease, and birth control.

- **Ma huang (ephedra):** May cause high blood pressure, increased heart rate, or death if used with beta-blockers (drugs used for high blood pressure and heart conditions), monoamine oxidase inhibitors (antidepressants), caffeine, and St. John's wort.

- **Yohimbe:** Reduces the effect of St. John's wort and drugs for depression, high blood pressure, and high blood sugar.

Chapter 50

Cancer and Rehabilitation

Physical medicine and rehabilitation (PM&R) is the medical specialty principally concerned with impairments, disabilities, and handicaps that arise after acute or chronic illness.

Cancer rehabilitation can be defined as a process that assists the cancer patient to obtain maximal physical, social, psychological, and vocational functioning within the limits created by the disease and its resulting treatment.

Multidisciplinary Approach to Rehabilitation

The healthcare team must develop rehabilitation goals within the limitations of the patient's illness, environment, and social support. Goals must be objective, realistic, and attainable in a reasonable time to demonstrate gains from active participation in therapy and thereby maintain the patient's motivation.

Patients, family members, and significant others must be active participants in the rehabilitation process. Patient and family involvement assists in goal setting. Interdisciplinary rehabilitation is the collaborative effort of professional members of the team working with the patient and of an accompanying support network. The rehabilitation team must provide services to patients throughout the course of illness, during all stages. Treatment plans must be individualized to meet each patient's unique and specific needs.

Excerpted from "Cancer and Rehabilitation," by Robert J. Kaplan, MD; used with permission from eMedicine.com, Inc., © 2006.

Physicians: Professional clinicians composing the interdisciplinary team include physicians from several specialties. Primary care physicians, surgeons, radiation oncologists, and medical oncologists make active and concurrent contributions to rehabilitation efforts to manage the disease process.

The physiatrist, a specialist in PM&R, treats neuromuscular disease, musculoskeletal disease, and functional deficits, in addition to performing electrodiagnostic procedures (for example, nerve conduction studies or NCS, and electromyography or EMG). The physiatrist also prescribes treatments performed by professionals from other disciplines, such as physical, occupational, and speech therapists. The physiatrist serves as liaison among team members, providing a considerable degree of coordination, especially when rehabilitation and clinical management of the disease are simultaneous.

Care coordinator, or case manager: The clinical-care coordinator assists in organizing and managing the team. An important aspect of this role is initially evaluating patients referred to the rehabilitation team for consultation. Care coordinators may be nurses, social workers, or professionals in other rehabilitation-related fields. They must be familiar with the functions of team members from other disciplines to assess the patient's needs effectively.

Oncology or rehabilitation nurse: The role of the oncology or rehabilitation nurse is pivotal in cancer rehabilitation. The oncology or rehabilitation nurse typically functions as an extension of other members of the team because he or she frequently assists with treatment interventions that the physical, occupational, or speech therapists begins. Such interventions include assisting patients with exercises, mobility on the unit, self-care activities, and speech and swallowing techniques. Because nurses typically have extensive contact with patients and families, they may be most aware of the family's emotional stress and adjustment issues. Nurses sometimes function as counselors, providing substantial emotional support to patients and their families.

In addition to active involvement with representatives of most other disciplines participating in the treatment interventions, nurses are responsible for skin care, bowel and bladder management, and patient and family education. Cancer rehabilitation nurses are crucial in promoting the goal of maintaining optimal independent functioning.

Social worker: The role of the social worker can vary substantially, depending on the medical institution. Social workers often provide counseling to patients and families regarding emotional support, community resources, finances, lifestyle changes, and their participation in treatment. In some settings, social workers lead support groups and actively assist in discharge-planning activities, such as for arranging home-care services and for transfer to other healthcare settings.

Psychologist: Patients and their families often have a number of psychological and adjustment issues related to the illness, its treatment, and its resulting disabilities. The psychologist assesses and treats patients to help them manage their cancer-related psychological distress. As a member of the rehabilitation team, the psychologist assists other team members when psychological issues, either in patients or their family members, complicate efforts to provide effective therapy. The goal of consulting the psychologist is to maximize the benefit the patient derives from rehabilitation.

Physical therapist: The role of the physical therapist includes evaluation of the patient's muscle strength, mobility, and joint range of motion (ROM). Treatment interventions the physical therapist provides may include therapeutic exercises to maintain or increase ROM, endurance activities, and mobility training (for example, transfers, gait, and stair climbing). Physical therapists can also administer various therapeutic modalities depending on the needs of the individual patient. Examples of modalities that may be beneficial include the application of heat or cold, electrical stimulation, hydrotherapy, traction, and massage.

Occupational therapist: Occupational therapists evaluate patients' ability to carry out tasks related to self-care, including activities of daily living (ADLs), such as dressing, bathing, meal preparation, and homemaking. These professionals also assist patients to increase ability to perform ADLs, including the use of compensatory techniques and adaptive equipment. In addition, occupational therapists evaluate home environments for potential modification, and they provide instruction in driving with adaptive devices. Furthermore, they implement interventions to promote upper-extremity ROM, strength, endurance, and coordination.

Dietitian: Diet and nutrition are important factors in cancer rehabilitation. A healthy diet and adequate nutrition substantially influence the patient's ability to actively participate in an applied therapy program and are essential for radiation therapy and chemotherapy. The role of the dietitian is to evaluate the patient's current nutritional status and to provide recommendations regarding his or her specific dietary needs. Patients with cancer often require dietary supplements and alternative foods. Dietitians also assist in teaching patients and family members about the importance of appropriate diet in successful rehabilitation.

Speech therapist: The speech therapist evaluates and treats communication deficits, dysphagia, and cognitive dysfunction in patients with cancer. Speech therapists also train patients in alternative means of speech and communication, including the use of a prosthetic larynx, adaptive communication devices, laryngeal speech, and esophageal speech. The treatment of patients with oral defects or aphasia also falls within the purview of the speech therapist. This therapist also treats swallowing deficits that result from illness or treatment.

Vocational counselor: Vocational counselors assist patients in adapting to the effect of cancer and its treatment on their employment. Vocational counselors evaluate the patient's suitability for employment and for training, if needed, and they serve as liaison between patients and their employers. Healthcare professionals often overlook the effect of cancer on the patient's vocation as an area requiring possible intervention.

Others: Although the professionals mentioned above are the most common members of the cancer rehabilitation team, practitioners from many other fields also provide important and valuable advice. These include a chaplain, a dentist, an orthotist, and a prosthetist. In addition, rehabilitation programs benefit from consultative relationships with other care-providing organizations (for example, home healthcare agencies, community hospices).

After initial screening, representatives from other disciplines conduct clinical assessments based on the patient's present needs or those the care coordinator identifies.

Paradigms of Cancer Rehabilitation

A variety of approaches to rehabilitation of the patient with cancer are described below.

Preventive interventions: Preventive (or "preventative") interventions lessen the effect of expected disabilities and emphasize patient education. Preventive measures also include approaches to improving the patient's physical functioning and general health status. In addition, psychological counseling before treatment can assist with the early identification of adjustment issues to allow for prompt intervention.

Restorative interventions: Restorative interventions are procedures that attempt to return patients to previous levels of physical, psychological, social, and vocational functioning. Postoperative ROM exercises for patients undergoing mastectomy and reconstructive surgery for head and neck cancer represent this category of interventions.

Supportive interventions: Supportive rehabilitation is designed to teach patients to accommodate their disabilities and to minimize debilitating changes from ongoing disease. Supportive efforts include teaching patients how to use prosthetic devices after amputation, as well as instructing the patient on use of other devices and procedures that assist in self-management, self-care abilities, and independent functioning. Other supportive efforts include provision of emotional support associated with adjustment issues while the patient is learning to cope with physical lifestyle changes.

Palliative interventions: During the palliative phase, when increasing disability and advanced disease process may be present, interventions and goals focus on minimizing or eliminating complications and providing comfort and support. Palliative goals include pain control, prevention of contractures and pressure sores, prevention of unnecessary deterioration from inactivity, and psychological support for the patient and family members.

Purpose and Emphasis of Rehabilitation

The purpose of rehabilitation for patients with cancer is similar to that for patients with other diseases. However, the pathology of the tumor, the anticipated progression of disease, and any associated treatments must be considered carefully when goals are formed. When tumor progression and treatment causes a functional decline or when the disease causes a fluctuation in abilities, rehabilitation assumes a supportive role, and its goals are adjusted to accommodate the patient's persistent anatomic and physiologic limitation.

Thorough assessment of impairments, disabilities, and handicaps is paramount before the team proceeds with rehabilitation. Emphasis is initially placed on restoring or maximizing independence with ADLs, mobility, cognition and communication.

Chapter 51

Exercise for
Cancer Survivors

Exercise Tips

Physical activity is an essential part of good health. People who are active over a long period of time are at lower risk for cancer.

For cancer survivors, studies suggest that exercise improves long-term prospects and the quality of life. Among the quality-of-life benefits are improved fitness, enhanced self-esteem, and reduced fatigue. You might think physical activity would heighten fatigue, which is one of the most common complaints of cancer survivors. But studies show that relaxation actually increases fatigue, while a moderate exercise program reduces it. Exercise can also relieve depression and anxiety.

There are several ways in which exercise enhances the long-term prospects of cancer survivors. Physical activity improves the function of the immune system and reduces stress. Also, by helping to control weight gain and reduce the percentage of body fat, exercise can influence the risk of cancer recurrence and survival.

Here are tips to put you on the road to good health.

This chapter begins with "Exercise Tips," © 2006 American Institute for Cancer Research. Reprinted with permission. For more information from this source, visit http://www.aicr.org. Additional information is from "Vanderbilt-Ingram Cancer Center Research Earns Funding from Lance Armstrong Foundation to Study Effects of Exercise on Curbing Memory Problems Associated with Chemotherapy," © 2006 Vanderbilt-Ingram Cancer Center. Reprinted with permission.

1. Exercise guidelines for each person will vary depending on your medical condition and past fitness level. Check with your doctor about when to start and how much physical activity is right for you. Ask for advice on creating an individualized exercise program.

2. For survivors, the amount of time spent exercising depends upon your condition. Many health experts recommend that you exercise every day for 60 minutes. But do as much as you can without straining. Remember that some activity is better than none.

3. Walking is by far the most popular activity, but choose activities you enjoy. Is there a sport or active hobby you enjoyed in the past, like dancing or gardening? If you played tennis before, try it again. If you like what you are doing, you are more likely to stick with it.

4. Exercise of moderate intensity, like a brisk walk, is best. Some evidence indicates that high-intensity exercise actually undermines the immune system. To reach a moderate level, begin exercising at a relaxed pace for 10–15 minute stretches. Gradually increase the length and intensity of your activity.

5. Incorporate exercise into your daily activities. Try taking the stairs instead of the elevator, parking farther away, or doing errands by bicycle instead of by car

6. Work out in water. The buoyancy of water makes it impossible to fall. Since water supports half of your weight, this type of exercise is also gentler on your joints.

7. Consider learning tai chi, qigong, or yoga. These forms of exercise from Asia stimulate the mind/body connection. The movements can be relaxing and rewarding, both physically and mentally.

8. Have some fun with the people you care about most. With friends and family, fly a kite, throw a Frisbee, or play softball.

9. Lastly, choose a place that engages your mind and spirit. A pleasant environment, like a path through woods, will motivate you and improve your psychological health.

For more information about cancer, exercise, and other cancer survivorship issues, call the American Institute for Cancer Research (800-843-8144) or visit http://www.aicr.org.

Effects of Exercise on Curbing Memory Problems Associated with Chemotherapy

Researchers at the Vanderbilt-Ingram Cancer Center are studying whether exercise can help curb memory and cognitive problems experienced by many cancer survivors following chemotherapy, with the help of funding from the foundation established by well-known cancer survivor and athlete, Lance Armstrong.

The funding will allow Charles Matthews, Ph.D., and Laurel Brown, Ph.D., in the Departments of Medicine and Psychiatry, and a team of researchers at Vanderbilt-Ingram, to take a closer look at the chemotherapy side effect commonly referred to as "chemo brain" or "chemo fog," and determine whether starting a walking exercise program can help patients with these problems.

"A substantial number of cancer survivors who receive chemotherapy report mild to moderate cognitive impairment that persists following treatment. These impairments have been reported across a range of cancer types and chemotherapy agents," said Brown.

Participants will be asked to make three visits to Vanderbilt University Medical Center during this six-month study, and will be placed into either a walking exercise group or a control group. Study members in the exercise group will receive a personalized walking program that they can do at home, counseling to help them reach their exercise goals, and techniques to help with memory problems. People enrolled in the control group will immediately receive counseling and techniques to help with memory problems, but will only be given the exercise program at the end of the six-month study period.

All participants will be asked to complete measures of memory and cognitive function, physical activity and fitness, questionnaires, and to provide urine and blood samples. Anyone 18 and older who has received chemotherapy in the last five years, experienced persistent memory or cognitive problems since chemotherapy, does not already exercise regularly, and has no history of brain cancer, heart disease, or a serious medical condition that could be worsened by exercise, is eligible for the study.

Matthews said exercise at levels most adults can perform—such as brisk walking for 30 to 45 minutes, four to five days a week—has been shown to improve cognitive function in older adults. "A wealth of research now indicates that exercise participation preserves cognition function as we age. In addition, sedentary older adults without cancer who completed six months of exercise have been shown to improve their cognitive function. We want to see if exercise might help cancer survivors in the same way," said Matthews.

Matthews said the exercise intervention study is the first of its kind for cancer survivors. "To our knowledge this study would be the first to examine the influence of regular exercise on cancer survivors who experienced cognitive difficulties following chemotherapy."

Matthews and his research team hope to identify new tactics to help cancer survivors coping with "chemo brain" and provide substantial information to lead the way for further studies that address quality of life issues faced by cancer survivors.

Vanderbilt was one of 21 institutions across the country and in Rome, Italy, to receive cancer survivorship and testicular cancer research grants from the Lance Armstrong Foundation.

Chapter 52

The Effect of Smoking on Cancer Recurrence

This chapter briefly covers smoking as a primary risk factor for cancer, but the main focus is on the effect of smoking on cancer recurrence and diagnosis of a second primary cancer; patterns of quitting and continued smoking in cancer patients; and recommendations for cancer patients to quit smoking. Information on cancer prevention and quitting smoking in healthy people is readily available elsewhere. The information presented in this chapter is related to smoking, rather than using other forms of tobacco, such as snuff or chewing tobacco.

Smoking as a Primary Risk Factor

It has been known for almost 50 years that tobacco use can be linked to cancers of the lung and head and neck. Eighty-five percent of the cases of head and neck cancer found each year are associated with tobacco use. Long-term smoking that begins before age 30 also increases the risk for developing colorectal cancer. Smoking contributes to cancer development by causing mutations in genes, impairing lung function, and decreasing the effectiveness of the immune system.

PDQ® Cancer Information Summary. National Cancer Institute; Bethesda, MD. Smoking Cessation and Continued Risk in Cancer Patients (PDQ®): Supportive Care - Patient. Updated 08/2005. Available at http://cancer.gov. Accessed April 30, 2006.

Poorer Treatment Response in Cancer Patients

If cancer is diagnosed in a smoker, studies have found that quitting smoking will still be helpful. Even recent quitters are more likely to recover from cancer than smoking patients are. Continuing to smoke may decrease the effectiveness of treatment and may worsen treatment side effects. For example, patients who have received radiation therapy for laryngeal cancer are less likely to regain satisfactory voice quality if they continue to smoke. Also, wound healing following surgery will be more difficult if one continues to smoke.

Smoking as a Secondary Risk Factor

Whether a patient has a cancer that is smoking-related or non-smoking related, he or she is at increased risk of developing a second cancer at the same or another site if smoking is not stopped. The risk of developing a second cancer may persist for up to 20 years, even if the original cancer has been successfully treated.

Patients with oral and pharyngeal cancers who smoke also have a high rate of second primary cancers. The risk decreases significantly, however, after five years of not smoking.

Effects of a Cancer Diagnosis on Quitting Smoking and Remaining Abstinent

Most people who have a smoking-related cancer stop smoking or make serious efforts to quit when cancer is diagnosed. Patients who do not immediately stop smoking may be motivated to quit in the future. Some studies have shown that patients who have less intensive treatment are more likely to continue smoking, and if they quit, are more likely to start smoking again.

Smoking Intervention in Cancer Patients

Although smoking cessation research has been conducted in other patient groups, especially heart patients; few studies have involved cancer patients. These studies have shown the importance of involvement of physicians and other health care professionals in helping patients to stop smoking. The ASK, ADVISE, ASSIST, and ARRANGE model was developed in the late 1980s for health care providers and their patients who smoke. Using this model, the physician asks the patient about smoking status at every visit, advises the patient to stop smoking, assists the patient by setting a date to quit smoking, provides self-help materials, recommends use of nicotine replacement therapy (for example, the nicotine patch), and arranges for follow-up visits.

Not all smokers are motivated to stop smoking. Physicians should help patients become motivated to quit smoking. It is common for first time quitters to start smoking again once or many times. Quitters should be taught to anticipate stressful situations in which they will want to smoke, and to develop strategies for handling them. It may take more than a year for even motivated smokers to stop smoking.

Treatment

The drugs bupropion, fluoxetine, and lobeline have been found to be successful in helping healthy people stop smoking. They have not, however, been studied in people with cancer.

Nicotine products, such as nicotine inhalers, nicotine gum, and nicotine patches, may help with the withdrawal symptoms that one experiences when trying to stop smoking. Several precautions should be considered, and a physician should be consulted before beginning any form of treatment.

Chapter 53

What Is Normal after Cancer Treatment?

Congratulations on finishing your cancer treatment!

Ending cancer treatment can be both exciting and challenging. Most people are relieved to be finished with the demands of treatment, but many also feel sadness and worry. Many are concerned about whether the cancer will come back and what they should do after treatment.

When treatment ends, people often expect life to return to the way it was before they were diagnosed with cancer. This rarely happens. You may have permanent scars on your body, or you may not be able to do some things you once did easily. Others may think of you—or you may view yourself—as being somehow different.

Your new "normal" may include making changes in the way you eat, the activities you do, and your sources of support, all of which are discussed in this chapter.

After You've Finished Your Cancer Treatment

The information in this chapter is designed mainly for cancer survivors who have recently completed their cancer treatment, but you may find the information helpful even if you were treated a long time ago. The purpose of this chapter is to give cancer survivors and their loved ones a better idea of what to expect during the first few months after treatment ends. It covers what may happen with your medical

Excerpted from "Facing Forward Series: Life after Cancer Treatment," National Cancer Institute, April 2002.

care, your body, your mind and your feelings, your social relationships, and practical matters such as job and insurance issues.

As you'll see, this chapter talks about many concerns of those who have been through cancer treatment and offers suggestions that have helped others move forward. As you read, you may find yourself saying, "That's just how I feel."

Although this chapter describes issues that are important to many survivors, each person has a unique response to having cancer. While some of the issues covered in this chapter may reflect your experience well, other issues may not concern you. Focus on finding what works for you. The information in this chapter is not intended to be all-inclusive.

Keep in mind, in this chapter, the term cancer survivor is used to include anyone who has been diagnosed with cancer, from the time of diagnosis through the rest of his or her life. You may not like the word, or you may feel that it does not apply to you, but the word survivor helps many people think about embracing their lives beyond their illness.

Getting Medical Care after Cancer Treatment

It is natural for anyone who has finished cancer treatment to be concerned about what the future holds. Many people worry about the way they look and feel and about whether the cancer will come back. Others wonder what they can do to keep cancer from coming back. Understanding what to expect after cancer treatment can help survivors and their families plan for follow-up care, make lifestyle changes, stay hopeful, and make important decisions.

All cancer survivors should have follow-up care. But you may have a lot of questions about getting the care you need now. For example, you may want to know about such things as the following:

- Whether to tell the doctor about symptoms that worry you

- Which doctors to see after treatment

- How often to see the doctor

- What specific tests you need

- What you can do to relieve pain and other problems after treatment

- How long it will take for you to recover from treatment and feel more like yourself

Dealing with these issues can be a challenge. Yet many say that getting involved in decisions about their future medical care and lifestyle was a good way for them to regain some of the control they felt they lost during cancer treatment. Research has shown that people who feel more in control feel and function better than those who do not. Being an active partner with your doctor and getting help from other members of your health care team is the first step.

This information offers some guidance on working with the people who provide care after treatment. It describes the kinds of help you may need and provides tips for getting what you want out of your medical visits. Reading this information can also help you create a plan of action for your recovery and future health.

Follow-Up Care

The main purpose of follow-up care is to check if your cancer has returned (recurrence) or if it has spread to another part of your body (metastasis). Follow-up care can also help in finding other types of cancer and spotting side effects from treatment now or that can develop years after treatment.

Follow-up care means seeing a doctor to get regular medical check-ups. At these visits, your doctor will review your medical history and examine your body.

Your doctor may run follow-up tests:

- Imaging procedures (ways of producing pictures of areas inside the body)

- Endoscopy (the use of a thin, lighted tube to examine organs inside the body)

- Blood tests

Follow-up care can also include home care, occupational or vocational therapy, pain management, physical therapy, and support groups.

Keep in mind, if you do not have health insurance, Medicare, or Medicaid, you may feel that some of the information in this chapter will not be helpful to you. You may have already struggled just to get treated and now see getting follow-up care as another battle. It can be hard to get health care if you don't have good health insurance, but you must make sure you get the care you need—especially after treatment is over.

There may be resources in your community to help you get these services. Talk with your doctor, social worker, or the business office at your local hospital or clinic. There are also government and non-profit organizations that may be able to help with health costs.

Choosing a Doctor to See

You will need to decide which doctor will provide your cancer follow-up care and which one(s) will provide other medical care. For follow-up cancer care, this may be the same doctor who provided your cancer treatment. For other medical care, you can continue to see your family doctor or medical specialist as needed.

Depending on where you live, it may make more sense to get cancer follow-up care from your family doctor than to travel long distances to see an oncologist. No matter whom you choose as a doctor, try to find doctors you feel comfortable with.

At your first follow-up visit, ask your doctor to recommend a follow-up schedule. In general, people who have been treated for cancer return to the doctor every three to four months during the first two to three years after treatment, and once or twice a year after that for follow-up appointments. Some medical organizations also have follow-up guidelines for certain cancers and update this information as researchers develop new approaches to follow-up care.

Follow-up care will be different for each person who has been treated for cancer, depending on the type of cancer and treatment he or she had and the person's general health. Researchers are still learning about the best approaches to follow-up care. This is why it is important that your doctor help determine what follow-up care plan is right for you. Lastly, it is important to note that some insurance plans pay for follow-up care only with certain doctors and for a set number of visits. In planning your follow-up care schedule, you may want to check your health insurance plan to see what restrictions, if any, apply to your follow-up care after cancer treatment.

Keep in mind, some people may suspect that their cancer has returned, or they notice other changes in their bodies. It is important for you to be aware of any changes in your health and report any problems to your doctor. Your doctor can find out whether these problems are related to the cancer, the treatment you had, or another health problem.

Even if you learn that your cancer has returned there is no reason to lose hope. Many people live good lives for many years with cancer that has returned.

Trouble Talking to Your Doctor

It is not always easy to talk with your doctor. Sometimes, he or she uses terms you do not know. When this happens, it is important to stop and ask the doctor to explain what the words mean. You may be afraid of how you will sound to the doctor, but having questions is perfectly normal.

Talking with your doctor is important. Both of you need information to manage your care. Telling the doctor about your health and asking questions helps both of you do your "jobs" well. Here are some points to cover.

At your first follow-up visit, ask your doctor/health care team about these items:

- The tests and follow-up care you need, and how often you will need them

- The kinds of physical problems you may have from your cancer treatment and what you can do to prevent, reduce, or solve them

- The potential long-term effects of treatment and the warning signs that you might have them

- The warning signs that cancer may be coming back and what to do if you see them

- Fears you may have about follow-up care

Keep in mind, many survivors want to learn about symptoms that may indicate their cancer has come back, or recurred.

There are many types of symptoms that may show if cancer has returned, and it depends on each person, the kind of cancer she/he was treated for, and the kind of treatment he/she had.

It is for this reason that you should talk to your doctor about the signs or symptoms that you should watch for and what you should do about them.

At each visit, tell your doctor/health care team about these concerns:

- Symptoms that you think may be a sign of cancer's return

- Any pain that troubles you

- Any physical problems that get in the way of your daily life or that bother you, such as fatigue, trouble sleeping, loss of sex drive, or weight gain or loss

- Other health problems you have, such as heart disease, diabetes, or arthritis

- Any medicines, vitamins, or herbs you are taking and any other treatments you are using

- Any emotional problems you may have, and any anxiety or depression you have had in the past

- Any changes in your family medical history

- Things you want to know more about (such as new research or side effects)

Your health care team should be able to help you or refer you to someone who can help with any side effects or problems you may have. You have a right to get the help you need.

Complementary and Alternative Medicine

Complementary and alternative medicine includes many different healing approaches that people use to prevent illness, reduce stress, prevent or reduce side effects and symptoms, or control or cure disease. An approach is generally called complementary when it is used in addition to treatments prescribed by a doctor. An approach is often called alternative when it is used instead of treatments prescribed by a doctor. Research has shown that more than half of all people with cancer use one or more of these approaches.

Some common approaches include: visualization or relaxation; acupressure and massage; homeopathy; vitamins or herbal products; special diets; psychotherapy; spiritual practices; and acupuncture.

Even though you have finished your cancer treatment, if you are thinking about using these methods, discuss this decision with your doctor or nurse. Some complementary and alternative therapies may interfere or be harmful when used with treatments normally prescribed by a doctor.

Getting the Most from Your Follow-up Visits

How do you get the most from your doctor visits? Here are some ideas that have helped others deal with their follow-up care:

- Ask someone to come with you to your doctor visit. A friend or family member can help you think about and understand what was said. He or she also may think of new questions to ask.

- Bring paper or a tape recorder to make note of the answers the doctor gives you.

- Ask your most important questions first in case the doctor runs out of time.

  - Don't be afraid to ask the doctor if you can schedule more time when you set up your next appointment. Or ask the doctor to suggest a time when you could call and get answers to your questions. Ask to talk with the doctor or nurse in a private room, with the door closed.

- Express yourself clearly.

  - Describe your problem or concern briefly.

  - Tell the doctor how your problem or concern makes you feel.

  - Ask for what you want or need. Example: "I am tired most of the time each day. I've tried napping, but it does not help. My fatigue gets in the way of my daily life, which makes me upset and angry. I would like you to help me treat this problem or refer me to someone who can help."

- Tell your doctor how much you want to know.

  - Tell him/her when you've heard enough or when you want more information.

  - Ask for booklets or other materials to read at home.

- Make sure you understand the doctor's answers.

  - Repeat in your own words what you think the doctor meant.

  - Ask the doctor to explain what he or she said in terms you understand.

- If you find you cannot get answers to your questions, let your doctor know you're unhappy about it. If that does not get results, you may want to try to find a new doctor. This can be hard to do, but getting the information you need is important for your health.

- Ask your pharmacist about how to take your medicines correctly or about possible side effects.

- Keep your own set of records about the follow-up care you get.

Tell any other doctor you see about your history of cancer. The type of cancer you had and your treatment can affect decisions about your care in the future. Other doctors you see may not know about your cancer and its treatment unless you tell them.

Your Medical Records

Make sure to get a copy of your cancer treatment records or a summary. (You may be charged for these.) By keeping your records up to date, you'll have enough information to share with any new doctors you may see.

If you don't keep a copy, your records might be spread among many doctors' offices, and key facts about your cancer history could be lost.

Here are the key types of records you'll want to keep:

- The type of cancer you were treated for

- When you were diagnosed

- Details of all cancer treatment (including all surgeries; names and doses of all drugs; sites and total amounts of radiation therapy; and places and dates of treatment)

- Key lab reports, pathology reports, and x-ray reports

- Contact information for all health professionals involved in your treatment and follow-up care

- Any problems that occurred after treatment

- Information on supportive care you had (such as special medications, emotional support, and nutritional supplements)

Professional Support Services You May Need

Services to Consider

People who have had cancer agree that no one should have to go through it alone after treatment. Your friends and family can help. Ask your doctor, nurse, social worker, or local cancer organization how to find services in your area like the ones listed in Table 53.1.

Developing a Wellness Plan

After cancer treatment, many survivors want to find ways to reduce the chances of their cancer coming back. Some worry that the way they eat, the stress in their lives, or their exposure to chemicals may put them at risk. Cancer survivors also find that this is a time

Table 53.1. Professional Support Services. (*continued on next page*)

Service	How It Can Help You
Clergy; Spiritual Counseling	Some members of the clergy are trained to help you deal with cancer concerns such as feeling alone, fear of death, searching for meaning, and doubts about faith.
Couples Counseling	You and your partner can work with trained specialists who can help you talk about problems, learn about each other's needs, and find ways to cope. Counseling may include issues related to sex and intimacy.
Family Support Programs	Your whole family may be involved in the healing process. In these programs, you and your family members participate in therapy sessions with trained specialists who can help you talk about problems, learn about each other's needs, and find answers.
Genetic Counseling	Trained specialists advise on whether to have gene testing for cancer and how to deal with the results. It can be helpful for you and for family members who have concerns for their own health.
Home Care Services	State and local governments offer many services useful after cancer treatment. A nurse or physical therapist may be able to come to your home. You also may be able to get help with housework or cooking. The phone book has contact numbers under Social Services, Health Services, or Aging Services—both nonprofit and for-profit.
Individual Counseling	Trained mental health specialists help you deal with your feelings, such as anger, sadness, and concern for your future
Long-Term Follow-up Clinics	All doctors can offer follow-up care, but there are a few clinics that specialize in long-term follow-up after cancer. These clinics most often see people who are no longer being treated by an oncologist and who are considered disease-free. You may want to ask your doctor if there are follow-up cancer clinics in your area.
Nutritionists/ Dietitians	They can help you with gaining or losing weight and with healthy eating.
Occupational Therapists	They can help you regain, develop, and build skills that are important for independent living. They can help you relearn how to do daily activities such as bathing, dressing, or feeding yourself after cancer treatment.
Oncology Social Workers	These professionals are trained to counsel you about ways to cope with treatment issues and family problems related to your cancer. They can tell you about resources and connect you with services in your area.

Table 53.1. Professional Support Services. (*continued from previous page*)

Service	How It Can Help You
Pain Clinics (also called Pain and Palliative Care Services)	These are centers with professionals from many different fields who are specially trained in helping people get relief from pain.
Physical Therapists	Physical therapists are trained in the way that the body parts interact and work. They can teach you about proper exercises and body motions that can help you gain strength and mobility after treatment. They can also advise you about proper postures that help prevent injuries.
Smoking Cessation Services	Research shows that the more support you have in quitting smoking, the greater your chance for success. Many communities have "quit smoking" programs. Ask your doctor, nurse, social worker, or local hospital about what is available, or call 800-4-CANCER (800-422-6237).
Speech Therapists	Speech therapists can evaluate and treat any speech, language, or swallowing problems you may have after treatment.
Stress Management Programs	These programs teach ways to help you relax and take more control over stress. Hospitals, clinics, or local cancer organizations may offer such programs and classes.
Support Groups for Survivors	In-person and online groups enable survivors to interact with others in similar situations.
Vocational Rehabilitation Specialists	If you have disabilities or other special needs after treatment, these services can help you find suitable jobs. Such services include counseling, education and skills training, and help in obtaining and using assistive technology and tools.

when they take a good look at how they take care of themselves and their health. This is an important start to living a healthy life after cancer.

When you meet with your doctor about follow-up care, you should ask about developing a wellness plan that includes ways you can take care of your physical, emotional, social, and spiritual needs. You may not be used to talking with your doctor as a partner in planning for your health, so it may be hard for you at first, but it is very important that you do it. The more you do it, the easier it will become.

Research is just beginning to show what people can do to lower their risk of getting certain cancers. But we don't yet know why cancer comes back in some people and not others.

Making changes in the way you eat, exercise, and live your life may not prevent your cancer from coming back. However, making these changes can help you feel better and may also lower your chances of developing other health problems.

Changes you may want to think about:

- Quitting smoking. Research shows that smoking can increase the chances of developing cancer at the same site or another site.

- Cutting down on how much alcohol you drink. Research shows that drinking alcohol can increase your chances of developing certain cancers.

- Eating well and exercising.

Eating Well after Cancer Treatment

The American Cancer Society recommends these nutrition tips:

- Eat a variety of healthful foods, with an emphasis on foods from plant sources:
    - Eat five or more servings of vegetables and fruits each day.
    - Choose whole grains—rather than processed (refined) grains and sugars.
    - Limit eating red meats, especially high fat or processed meats.
    - Choose foods that help you maintain a healthy weight.
- Adopt a physically active lifestyle.
- Maintain a healthy weight throughout the rest of your life.
- Limit drinking alcohol, if you drink at all.

Exercise after Cancer Treatment

Few studies have been done to find out whether physical activity affects survival after cancer treatment. More research is needed to answer this question, but studies have shown that moderate exercise (walking, biking, swimming) for about 30 minutes every—or almost every—day can help with the following:

- Reduce anxiety and depression
- Improve mood

- Boost self-esteem

- Reduce symptoms of fatigue, nausea, pain, and diarrhea

During recovery, it is important to start an exercise program slowly and increase activity over time, working with your doctor or a specialist (such as a physical therapist) if needed. If you need to stay in bed during your recovery, even small activities—like moving your arms or legs around—can help you stay flexible, relieve muscle tension, and help you feel better. Some survivors may need to take special care in exercising. Talk with your doctor before you begin any exercise program.

Chapter 54

Cancer Survivorship: Follow-up Care Planning

There are currently 10 million Americans who are considered cancer survivors, and their ranks are growing rapidly as more than a million new cases of cancer are diagnosed each year. Unfortunately, the current U.S. health care system is failing to deliver the comprehensive and coordinated follow-up care cancer survivors deserve. Too many survivors are lost in transition once they finish treatment. They move from an orderly system of care to a "non-system" in which there are few guidelines to assist them through the next stage of their life or help them overcome the medical and psychosocial problems that may arise.

Every cancer survivor should have a comprehensive care summary and follow-up plan once they complete their primary cancer care that reflects their treatment and addresses a myriad of post-treatment needs to improve their health and quality of life.

Elements of a Survivorship Care Plan

Record of Care

Upon discharge from cancer treatment, including treatment of recurrences, every patient should be given a record of all care received and important disease characteristics. This should include, at a minimum:

- Diagnostic tests performed and results.

Reprinted with permission from *Cancer Survivorship Care Planning,* © 2005 by the National Academy of Sciences, Courtesy of the National Academies Press, Washington, D.C.

- Tumor characteristics (for example, site(s), stage and grade, hormonal status, marker information).

- Dates of treatment initiation and completion.

- Surgery, chemotherapy, radiotherapy, transplant, hormonal therapy, gene or other therapies provided, including agents used, treatment regimen, total dosage, identifying number and title of clinical trials (if any), indicators of treatment response, and toxicities experienced during treatment.

- Psychosocial, nutritional, and other supportive services provided.

- Full contact information on treating institutions and key individual providers.

- Identification of a key point of contact and coordinator of continuing care.

Standards of Care

Upon discharge from cancer treatment, every patient and their primary health care provider should receive a written follow-up care plan incorporating available evidence-based standards of care. This should include, at a minimum:

- The likely course of recovery from treatment toxicities, as well as need for ongoing health maintenance/adjuvant therapy.

- A description of recommended cancer screening and other periodic testing and examinations, and the schedule on which they should be performed (and who should provide them).

- Information on possible late and long-term effects of treatment and symptoms of such effects.

- Information on possible signs of recurrence and second tumors.

- Information on the possible effects of cancer on marital/partner relationship, sexual functioning, work, and parenting, and the potential future need for psychosocial support.

- Information on the potential insurance, employment, and financial consequences of cancer and, as necessary, referral to counseling, legal aid, and financial assistance.

- Specific recommendations for healthy behaviors (diet, exercise, healthy weight, sunscreen use, virus protection, smoking cessation, osteoporosis prevention). When appropriate, recommendations that first degree relatives be informed about their increased risk and the need for cancer screening (breast cancer, colorectal cancer, and prostate cancer).

- As appropriate, information on genetic counseling and testing to identify high risk individuals who could benefit from more comprehensive cancer surveillance, chemoprevention, or risk reducing surgery.

- As appropriate, information on known effective chemoprevention strategies for secondary prevention (for example, Tamoxifen in women at high risk for breast cancer; aspirin for colorectal cancer prevention).

- Referrals to specific follow-up care providers, support groups, or the patient's primary care provider.

- A listing of cancer-related resources and information (internet-based sources and telephone listings for major cancer support organizations).

Questions Survivors Should Ask

Like most patients, cancer survivors want to be empowered to take care of themselves and remain healthy. Once cancer treatment ends, there are some questions every patient should be asking their doctor to be informed about their care and to know what they can expect next. These include, but are not limited to the following:

What treatments and drugs have I been given?

Patients should require their doctor to provide a written record detailing the type of cancer they had, the treatments and drugs they received, and the potential side effects of these treatments.

Do I need to seek follow-up care?

Patients should be given a written cancer survivorship plan that would detail what kinds of screening or tests they should be receiving post-treatment and a schedule of when they should be following up with their primary care or oncology provider to have these performed.

Will I get cancer again?

Oncology providers should explain, both verbally and in writing, the risks of secondary cancers or recurrent cancers and what signs or symptoms to look for.

What should I do to maintain my health and well-being?

Patients should be advised on the benefits of healthy diets and routine exercise and the perils of not routinely using sunscreen or continuing to smoke. Patients also should ask their doctors, if appropriate, about whether they should inform close relatives about their increased risk of cancer and need for cancer screening.

Even though I survived cancer, will I feel differently physically?

Cancer treatment has a different effect on everyone, and for some survivors, there are serious side effects from treatment. Providers need to educate patients and make them aware of the possible short and long term effect that may arise. Radiation could affect a person's heart, stamina, or fertility. Patients may feel overly anxious or depressed about the possibility of getting cancer again. You should ask your doctor how treatment could affect your long-term health and mental functioning.

Will I have trouble getting health insurance or keeping a job because of my cancer?

Having cancer can affect access to health or life insurance, the ability to keep a job, as well as job mobility. Providers should be prepared to offer cancer patients information about what resources are available if they face employment discrimination or are unable to access or keep health and life insurance.

Are there support groups I can turn to?

Your provider should be able to provide a useful list of community or nationally based cancer-related organizations or other groups that can offer support with or information on survivorship issues and challenges.

Now that I've finished treatment, who on the cancer team will be responsible for monitoring my care?

Patients should know who will be the main point of contact working with their primary care provider to coordinate follow-up care related to their cancer treatment.

Part Seven

Information for
Friends, Family Members,
and Caregivers

Chapter 55

When Someone You Love Is Being Treated for Cancer

There Are Different Kinds of Caregivers

The information in this chapter is for you if you are helping your loved one get through cancer treatment. If this describes you, you are a "caregiver." You may not think of yourself as a caregiver. You may see what you're doing as something natural—taking care of someone you love.

There are different types of caregivers. Some are family members, while others are friends. Every situation is different. So there are different ways to give care. There isn't one way that works best.

Caregiving can mean helping with day-to-day activities such as doctor visits or preparing food. But it can also happen long-distance. You may have to coordinate care and services for your loved one by phone. Caregiving can also mean giving emotional and spiritual support. You may be helping your loved one cope and work through the many feelings that come up at this time. Talking, listening, and just being there are some of the most important things you can do.

Giving care and support during this challenging time isn't easy. The natural response of most caregivers is to put their own feelings

Excerpted from "When Someone You Love Is Being Treated for Cancer," National Cancer Institute, November 2005. The full text of this document is available online at www.cancer.gov; it can also be ordered by calling 800-4-CANCER. Note: This document uses the terms "loved one" and "patient" throughout to describe the cancer patient. In addition, for ease of reading, it alternates using the pronouns "he" and "she" when referring to the person with cancer.

and needs aside. They try to focus on the person with cancer and the many tasks of caregiving. This may be fine for a short time, but it can be hard to keep up for a long time. And it's not good for your health. If you don't take care of yourself, you won't be able to take care of others. It's important for everyone that you give care to you.

Adjusting to Being a Caregiver

Whether you're younger or older, you may find yourself in a new role as a caregiver. You may have been an active part of someone's life before cancer, but perhaps now the way you support that person is different. It may be in a way in which you haven't had much experience, or in a way that feels more intense than before. Even though caregiving may feel new to you now, many say that they learn more as they go through their loved one's cancer experience. Common situations that many caregivers describe:

- Your spouse or partner may feel comfortable with only you taking care of him.

- Your parent may have a hard time accepting help from you (their adult child) since she's always been used to caring for you.

- Your adult child with cancer may not want to rely on his parents for care.

- You may have health problems yourself, making it hard physically and emotionally to take care of someone else.

Whatever your roles are now, accepting the changes may be tough. It's very common to feel confused and stressed at this time. If you can, try to share your feelings with others or a support group. Or you may choose to seek help from a counselor or psychologist. Many caregivers say that talking with a counselor helped them. They feel they were able to say things that they weren't able to say to their loved ones.

Coping with Your Feelings

You've probably felt a range of feelings as you care for your loved one. These feelings can be quite strong and will likely come and go in strength as you go through treatment with the patient. Many caregivers describe this as "like a rollercoaster." You may feel sad, afraid, angry, and worried. There is no right or wrong way to feel or react to these feelings. Try to give yourself time to understand and work through your range of emotions.

Anger: Caregivers say that it's common to be angry with themselves, their family members, or the patient. Sometimes anger comes from feelings that are hard to show, such as fear, panic, or worry. If you can, try to avoid lashing out at others because of these emotions. Anger can be healthy if you handle it the right way. It can help motivate you to take action, find out more, or make positive changes in your life. But if these feelings persist and you remain angry at those around you, talk with a counselor or other mental health professional.

Grief: You may be mourning the loss of what you hold most dear—your loved one's health or the life you had with each other before cancer. It's important to give yourself permission to grieve these losses. It takes time to work through and accept all the changes that are occurring.

Guilt: Feeling guilty is a common reaction for caregivers. You may worry that you aren't helping enough, or that your work or distance from your loved one is getting in the way. You may even feel guilty that you are healthy. Or you may feel guilty for not acting upbeat or cheerful. But know that it's okay. You have reasons to feel upset and hiding them may keep other people from understanding your needs.

Anxiety and depression: Anxiety means you have extra worry, you can't relax, you feel tense, or you have panic attacks. Many people worry about how to pay bills, how things will affect the family, and of course, how their loved one is coping. Depression is a persistent sadness that lasts more than two weeks. If any of these symptoms start affecting your ability to function normally, talk with your health care provider. Don't think that you need to tough it out without any help. It's likely that your symptoms can be eased during this hard time.

Hope or hopelessness: You may feel hope or hopelessness to different degrees throughout your loved one's cancer treatment. And what you hope for may change over time. You may hope for a cure most of all. But you may also hope for other things, such as comfort, peace, acceptance, and joy. If you're not able to get rid of a feeling of hopelessness, talk to a trusted family member, friend, health provider, or spiritual or faith leader.

Loneliness: You can feel alone in your role as a caregiver, even if you have lots of people around you. You may feel that no one understands what you're going through. You may feel lonely because you have less time to see people and do things that you used to. Whatever your situation, you aren't alone. Other caregivers share your feelings. Here are some ways you can connect with others:

- **Look for the positive:** Caregivers say that looking for the good things in life helps them feel better. Once a day, think about something that you found rewarding about caregiving, such as gratitude you've received or extra support from a health care provider. You might also take a moment to feel good about anything else from the day that is positive—a nice sunset, a hug, or something funny that you heard or read.

- **Let yourself laugh:** It's okay to laugh, even when your loved one is in treatment. In fact, it's healthy. Laughter releases tension and makes you feel better. You can read humor columns, watch comedy shows, or talk with upbeat friends. Or just remember funny things that have happened to you in the past. Keeping your sense of humor in trying times is a good coping skill.

- **Write in a journal:** It can be a tricky balance between thinking too much about your loved one's cancer and not thinking enough about it. But research shows that writing or journaling can help relieve negative thoughts and feelings. And it may actually help improve your own health. You can write about any topic. You might write about your most stressful experiences. Or you may want to express your deepest thoughts and feelings. You can also write about things that make you feel good, such as a stress-free day or a kind coworker.

- **Be thankful:** You may feel thankful that you can be there for your loved one. You may be glad for a chance to do something positive and give to another person in a way you never knew you could. Some caregivers feel that they've been given the chance to build or strengthen a relationship. This doesn't mean that caregiving is easy or stress-free. But finding meaning in caregiving can make it easier to manage.

- **Stay active:** If you can, try to keep doing some of your regular activities. Studies show that not doing those activities increases the stress you feel. Keep it simple and stick with things you do well. If you have to, change the time of day or the length of time you normally do things.

- **Learn more about cancer:** Sometimes understanding your loved one's medical situation can make you feel more confident and in control. For example, you may want to know more about his stage of cancer. It may help you to know what to expect during treatment and what will need to be done.

Here are some other ways you can cope:

- **Let go of mistakes:** You can't be perfect. No one is. The best we can do is to learn from our mistakes and move on. Continue to do the best you can. And try not to expect too much from yourself.

- **Cry or express your feelings:** You don't have to be upbeat all the time or pretend to be cheerful. Give yourself time to cope with all the changes you are going through. It's okay to cry and show that you are sad or upset.

- **Put your energy into the things that matter to you:** Focus on the things you feel are worth your time and energy. Let the other things go for now. For example, don't fold the clothes when you're tired. Go ahead and take time to rest.

- **Understand anger:** Your loved one may get angry with you. It's very common for people to direct their feelings at those who are closest. Try not to take it personally. Sometimes patients don't realize the effect their anger has on others. So it may help to share your feelings with them when they are calm. Try to remember that the anger isn't really about you.

- **Forgive yourself:** This is one of the most important things you can do. Chances are that you are doing what you can at this moment. Each new moment and day gives you a new chance to try again.

Talking with the Health Care Team

You will be asked to do many things during your loved one's treatment. One of your main roles may be to help your loved one work with the health care team. You may be asked to go to doctor visits, among other things. A few tips are listed below.

- Keep a file or notebook of the patient's medical information. Include the dates of procedures and tests. Bring this file to doctor visits.

- Keep a list of names and doses of medicines and how often they are taken. Bring this list with you.

- Use only trusted sources if you do research for your loved one, such as government and national organizations.

- Make a list of questions and concerns. List the most important questions first.

- Call ahead of time to make sure of the following:

  - The doctor has copies of all needed test results, records, and other paperwork.

  - You have directions, transportation, and if needed, hotel information.

- If you and the patient have a lot to talk about with the doctor, ask whether:

  - You can have a longer appointment (check on fees for this).

  - You can talk to the doctor by phone if there are further questions. Or perhaps others on staff can help you. For example, a nurse may be able to answer many of your questions.

- Talk with your loved one before the visit to help prepare yourselves for the possibility that the information given could be different than what you both expect.

Asking about Pain

Although different side effects happen with cancer treatment, many caregivers say the one thing they hesitate to ask about is pain. Yet, people who have their pain managed are able to focus on healing and on enjoying life. If someone is preoccupied by pain, you may notice personality changes. These might include being distant, not being able to sleep, or not being able to focus on daily activities.

The medical team should ask regularly about pain levels, but it's up to you and your loved one to be open about any pain. The patient does not have to be in pain or discomfort. Some people assume that there will always be severe pain with cancer treatment. This is not true. Pain can be managed throughout your loved one's treatment. The key is to talk regularly with the health care team about pain and other symptoms.

Sometimes people with cancer don't want to talk to their health care team about their pain. They worry that others will think that they are complaining or that pain means the cancer is getting worse. Or they think that pain is just something they have to accept. Sometimes people get used to the pain and forget what it's like to live without it.

This is when it is important for you to encourage your loved one to speak up. Or you can speak up on his behalf. Be honest with the doctor about pain and how it is affecting the daily routine. You and your loved one may need to have talks at different times to continue to feel comfortable about the pain medicines given. These drugs can also be adjusted or changed if they aren't working or are having unpleasant side effects.

Don't be afraid to ask for stronger pain relievers or larger doses if your loved one needs them. Addiction is rarely an issue in people with cancer. Instead, drugs help patients stay as comfortable as possible.

Talking with Family and Friends

Children and teens: Children as young as 18 months begin to understand the world around them. It's important to be honest with them and explain that your loved one has cancer. Experts say that telling children the truth about cancer is better than letting them imagine the worst. (Information in this section is based on suggestions from: Harpham, W. 1997. *When A Parent Has Cancer: A Guide to Caring For Your Children*. New York, NY; HarperCollins Publishers Inc., pp. 3, 8.)

For some families, talking about serious issues is very hard. But as hard as it may be, not talking about them can be worse. Here are some things you might want to say to children of any age about your loved one's cancer:

- "Nothing you did, thought, or said caused the cancer."

- "You are not responsible for making her well. But there are ways you can help her feel better while the doctors try to make her improve."

- "You can't catch cancer from another person."

- "Just because someone has cancer doesn't mean other people in the family will get it—even later. And that includes you."

- "It is okay to be upset, angry, scared, or sad about all this. You may feel all kinds of feelings. You'll probably feel happy sometimes, too. It's fine to feel all these things."

- "No matter what happens, you will always be taken care of."

- "People may act differently around you because they're worried about you or worried about all of us."

Talking about the impact of cancer may be hard for very young children. You might try asking them to draw a picture of the person with cancer. Or have them play dolls, with one doll being the patient. Other forms of art can help older children express themselves.

Keep in mind that young children may ask the same question over and over. This is normal, and you should calmly answer the question each time. Teens may ask difficult questions or questions for which you don't have answers. Be honest with them. Remember that thinking through these issues is part of your children's process of growing up.

Be prepared for questions and concerns about death from your children. They may worry, even if your loved one's prognosis is good.

- Teach them that cancer is an illness. If your loved one's prognosis is good, let them know that the type of cancer he or she has is one the doctors feel they can treat.

- Ask them what they think about your loved one's cancer and what they worry about. Then listen patiently to their answers. Correct misinformation.

- Tell them the truth, couched in love and hopefulness. Instead of trying to convince them of a good outcome that you can't guarantee, reassure them that your loved one is getting good care, you are hoping for a recovery, and that you can live well with the uncertainty.

- Teach your children that even if the unexpected happened due to cancer or anything else, they would be taken care of and be okay. Although they would feel sad for a while and they would miss your loved one, they would also feel that love forever and learn how to be happy again.

- Remind them that your loved one is not dying now. Reassure them that you will tell them if this ever changes and dying becomes a possibility. Conclude by telling them you expect and hope your loved one to get better, and encourage them to focus on today.

Your partner with cancer: Some relationships get stronger during cancer treatment. Others are weakened. Nearly all caregivers and their partners feel more stress than usual as a couple. They often feel stress about items such as these:

- Knowing how to best support each other
- Dealing with new feelings that come up
- Figuring out how to communicate
- Making decisions
- Changing roles
- Juggling lots of roles (such as childcare, housekeeping, work, and caregiving)
- Changing their social life
- Changing their daily routine
- Not feeling connected sexually

People express their emotions differently. Some like to talk things out or focus on others. Others like to express emotions by doing things, such as washing the dishes or fixing things around the house. They may be more likely to focus inward. These differences can cause tension because each person may expect the other to act the way they would in their place. To reduce stress, it may help to remind yourself that everyone reacts differently.

Bringing up tough subjects for discussion can also be emotionally draining. You may think, for example, that your loved one needs to try a different treatment or doctor. Or she may be worrying about losing independence, being seen as weak, or about being a burden to you, but doesn't want to talk about it. Here are some tips on how to bring up hard topics:

- Practice what you'll say in advance.
- Know that your loved one may not want to hear what you have to say.
- Find a quiet time and ask if it's okay to talk.
- Be clear on what your aims are. (Let your loved one know why you are having this talk and what you hope will come from it.)
- Speak from your heart.

- Allow time for your loved one to talk. Listen and try not to interrupt.

- Don't feel the need to settle things after one talk.

- You don't have to always say, "It'll be okay."

Sometimes the best way to communicate with someone is to just listen. This is a way of showing that you are there for them. It may be one of the most valuable things you can do. And it's important to be supportive to whatever your loved one wants to say. It's her life and her cancer. People need to process their thoughts and fears in their own time and their own way. You could also ask whether she is willing to think about the issue and talk another time. Your loved one may even prefer to talk with someone else about the topic.

Some people won't start a conversation themselves, but may respond if you begin first. Here are some ways caregivers do this:

- "I know this is hard to talk about, but know that I'm ready to listen or to talk any time."

- "I feel that it would be helpful to talk about how your treatment is going so far and how we're both coping with it. Would you be willing to talk with me about that sometime this week?"

If you trouble talking about the cancer and painful issues, you could ask for help from a mental health professional. One may be able to explore issues that you didn't feel you could yourself. But if your loved one doesn't want to go with you, you can always make an appointment to go by yourself. You may pick up some ideas for how to bring up these topics, and talk about other feelings that you are coping with right now.

Issues related to intimacy can also raise concerns. You may find that you and your partner's sex life is different than it used to be. Many things could be affecting it:

- Your partner is tired, in pain, or uncomfortable because of the treatment.

- You're tired.

- Your relationship feels distant or strained.

- You or your partner may not be comfortable with the way your partner looks.

- You may be afraid of hurting your partner.

- Your partner's treatment might be affecting his or her interest in sex or ability to perform.

You can still have an intimate relationship in spite of these issues. Intimacy isn't just physical. It also involves feelings. Here are some ways to improve your intimate relationship:

- **Talk about it:** Choose a time when you and your partner can talk. Focus on just talking. Talk about how you can both renew your connection.

- **Try not to judge:** If your partner isn't performing, try not to read meaning into it. Let your partner talk—or not talk—about what he or she needs.

- **Make space:** Protect your time together. Turn off the phone and TV. If needed, find someone to take care of the kids for a few hours.

- **Take it slow:** Reconnect. Plan an hour or so to be together without being physical. For example, you may want to listen to music or take a walk. This time is about reconnecting.

- **Try new touch:** Cancer treatment or surgery can change your partner's body. Areas where touch used to feel good may now be numb or painful. Some of these changes will go away. Some will stay. For now, you can figure out together what kinds of touch feel good, such as holding, hugging, and cuddling.

- **Talk to a therapist or counselor:** There are many who deal with intimacy and sexuality issues with cancer patients.

Other family members and friends: Any problems your family may have had before the cancer diagnosis are likely to be more intense now. This is true whether you are caring for a young child, an adult child, a parent, or a spouse. Your caregiver role can often trigger feelings and role changes that affect your family in ways you never expected. And relatives you don't know very well or who live far away may be present more often, too, which may complicate things. Some people have said that they experienced the following:

- Seeing your adult child ill can trigger feelings of needing to protect or help him or her.

- Seeing your parent as someone who needs your help can be hard to accept.

- Seeing an in-law or a friend's parent worry or try to help out can feel like "too much."

Studies show that open and caring communication works best. Yet caregivers often run into the following types of issues:

- Tension from different ways of communicating

- Lack of sensitivity or understanding about appropriate ways to talk and share feelings

- People who don't know what to say, won't communicate at all, or won't be honest

Sometimes other close family and friends may not agree on what should be done. It's very common for families to argue over treatment options. Or they argue that some caregivers help more than others. While everyone may be trying to do what they think is best for your loved one, family members may disagree about what this means. People bring their own set of beliefs and values to the table, which makes decisions hard. It is often during these times that families ask their health care team to hold a family meeting.

Talk with your loved one to see if she wants a family meeting. Ask if she would like to be involved. At the meeting, all members share as much information as they can. You can ask a social worker or counselor to be there, if needed. If you need to, you can bring a list of issues to discuss. Meetings can be used to for the following purposes:

- Have the health care team explain the goals for treatment.

- Let the family state their wishes for care.

- Give everyone an open forum in which to express their feelings.

- Clarify caregiving tasks.

During these meetings, family members may want to talk about how they feel. Or you may want to decide what kind of help they can offer. Each person may have certain skills to offer.

Often, you will be the main person updating family, friends, and co-workers about how the patient is doing. Ask your loved one what he wants to share, with whom, and when. If this is a task that someone else can do, select a "point person." This person can make phone calls or send e-mail or letters to update others. It's important to let others who care know whether your loved one likes getting cards, calls, or visits.

How to Communicate when Support Is Not Helpful

If people offer help that you don't need or want, thank them for their concern. Let them know you'll contact them if you need anything. You can tell them that it always helps to send cards and letters. Or they can pray or send good thoughts.

Some people may offer unwanted parenting advice. This may come from feeling helpless to do anything, yet wanting to show their concern. Since they can't offer advice on medical care, it helps them to express their opinion on child care. While it may come from a good place, it may still seem judgmental to you.

It's your decision on how to deal with unwanted advice about your kids. You don't have to respond at all if you don't want to. If you think their concerns are valid, then talk to a counselor or teacher about what steps to take. Otherwise, thank them. And reassure them that you are taking the necessary steps to get your children through this tough time.

Life Planning

It's common to feel sad, angry, or worried that your lifestyle may change because of your loved one's cancer. You may have to make major decisions that will affect your job or your finances. Finding ways to cope with these issues can bring some peace of mind.

Facing Fertility Issues

Some people are concerned about the effects of cancer treatment on their ability to have children. If this is true for you and your loved one, talk to the doctor before starting treatment. You may want to ask about options for protecting your fertility. Or the doctor can recommend a counselor or fertility specialist. This person can discuss available options and help you and your loved one make informed choices. (For more information, call Fertile Hope at 888-994-HOPE, or go to http://www.fertilehope.org.)

Handling Money Worries

The financial challenges that people with cancer and their families face are very real. During an illness, you may find it hard to find the time or energy to review your options. Yet it's important to keep your family financially healthy.

For hospital bills, you or your loved one may want to talk with a hospital financial counselor. You may be able to work out a monthly payment plan or even get a reduced rate. You may also want to stay in touch with the insurance company to make sure certain treatment costs are covered.

You can also get the National Cancer Institute (NCI) fact sheet, "Financial Assistance for Cancer Care," at http://www.cancer.gov, by searching for the terms "financial assistance." Or call toll-free 800-4-CANCER (800-422-6237) to ask for a free copy.

Handling Work Issues

One of the greatest sources of strain for some caregivers is trying to balance work demands with providing care and support to a loved one. Caregiving can affect your work life in many ways, such as these:

- Having mood swings that leave co-workers confused or reluctant to work with you

- Being distracted or less productive

- Being late, or calling in sick because of the stress

- Feeling pressure from being the sole provider for your family if your spouse or partner is not able to work

- Feeling pressure to keep working, even though retirement may have been approaching

It's a good idea to learn more about your company's rules and policies related to a family member's illness. See if there are any support programs for employees. Many companies have employee assistance programs with work-life counselors for you to talk to. Some companies have eldercare policies or other employee benefit programs that can help support you. Your employer may let you use your paid sick leave to take care of your loved one. Or they may let you take leave without pay.

If your employer doesn't have any policies in place, you could try to arrange something informally. Examples include flex-time, shift-exchanging, adjusting your schedule, or telecommuting as needed.

The Family and Medical Leave Act may apply to your situation. Covered employers must give eligible employees up to 12 work weeks of unpaid leave during a 12-month period to care for an immediate family member with a serious health condition. Visit http://www.dol.gov/esa/whd/fmla for more information.

Looking at Living Arrangements

Sometimes treatment raises questions about living arrangements. When making these decisions, you should ask:

- What kind of help does your loved one need and for how long?

- Could you remodel the house or move to a smaller or different one?

- Is it risky for your loved one to be home alone?

You'll also need to consider how your loved one feels. She may fear losing her independence, being seen as weak or a burden to you and others, or moving to a health care or other type of assisted living facility. These are tough issues. Sometimes it's easier to consider a change in living arrangements when the advice comes from a health care professional. Social workers, doctors, nurses, home care providers, and agencies that work with older adults may be able to help.

Preparing Advance Directives

Some people prefer to let their health care team make all their cancer treatment decisions. Others want to have more input. If your loved one wants to take a more active role, urge him to complete an advance directive. Advance directives are legal papers that let your loved one decide important issues. These can include how much treatment to get and who should make decisions if he or she can't. Having an advance directive helps ensure that patients get the treatment that they want. It will also make it a lot easier for caregivers to make treatment decisions if they understand their loved one's wishes.

- A living will lets people know what kind of medical care patients want if they are unable to speak for themselves.

- A durable power of attorney for health care names a person to make medical decisions for a patient if he or she can't make them. This person, chosen by the patient, is called a health care proxy.

A lawyer does not always need to be present when you fill out these papers. However, a notary public may be needed. Each state has its own laws about advance directives. Check with a lawyer or social worker about the laws in your state.

Reflection

As a caregiver, you try to strike a balance each day. You have to care for your loved one while keeping up with the demands of family and work. Your focus tends to be on the patient's needs. But it's also up to you to try to stay in tune with yourself. Remember the things you need to maintain a healthy mind, body, and spirit. And if you can, try to find a quiet time for reflection each day. Meditating, praying, or just resting may help you keep a sense of peace at this time.

Whether good or bad, life-changing situations often give people the chance to grow, learn, and appreciate what's important to them. Many people who care for someone with cancer describe the experience as a personal journey. They say it has changed them forever. This is much like the way people with cancer describe their experience. It's not necessarily a journey that they would have chosen for themselves. But they can use their skills, strength, and talents to support their loved one while finding out more about themselves along the way.

Chapter 56

If Your Child Has Cancer

More children than ever are surviving childhood cancer. Over the last 30 years, survival into adulthood increased from 30 percent to 80 percent. There are new and better drugs and methods to help children deal with the side effects of treatment. And children who have had cancer now have a better quality of life throughout childhood and into adulthood; fewer long-term ill effects follow the treatment.

Yet, in spite of all this good news, cancer is still a serious disease. You are not alone in facing your fears; help is available. A treatment team—doctors, radiation therapists, rehabilitation specialists, dietitians, oncology nurses, and social workers, among others—can help you and your child deal with the disease. They will also help ensure that your child gets the best treatment available with as few ill effects as possible.

When Your Child Is Diagnosed

After your child's cancer has been diagnosed, a series of tests will be done to help identify your child's specific type of cancer. Called staging, this series of tests is sometimes done during diagnosis. Staging determines how much cancer is in the body and where it is located.

Excerpted from "Young People with Cancer: A Handbook for Parents," National Cancer Institute, January 2001. The full text of this document is available online at www.cancer.gov; the booklet can also be ordered by calling 800-4-CANCER.

To stage solid tumors, the doctor looks at the size of the tumor, the lymph nodes affected, and where it has spread. Staging must be done to determine the best treatment. Many different tests can be used in staging, such as x-rays, magnetic resonance imaging scans (MRIs), CT (or CAT) scans, and others.

As soon as your child is suspected to have or is diagnosed with cancer, you will face decisions about who will treat your child, whom to ask for a second opinion (if desired or if the diagnosis is not clear), and what the best treatment is. After your child's staging is complete, the treatment team develops a plan that outlines the exact type of treatment, how often your child will receive treatment, and how long it will last.

Talking with Your Child's Doctor

Your child's doctor and the treatment team will give you a lot of details about the type of cancer and possible treatments. Ask your doctor to explain the treatment choices to you. It is important for you to become a partner with your treatment team in fighting your child's cancer. One way for you to be actively involved is by asking questions. You may find it hard to concentrate on what the doctor says, remember everything you want to ask, or remember the answers to your questions. Here are some tips for talking with those who treat your child:

- Write your questions in a notebook and take it to the appointment with you. Record the answers to your questions and other important information.

- Tape record your conversations with your child's health care providers.

- Ask a friend or relative to come with you to the appointment. The friend or relative can help you ask questions and remember the answers.

Questions to Ask the Doctor and Treatment Team

- What kind of cancer does my child have?

- What is the stage, or extent, of the disease?

- Will any more tests be needed? Will they be painful? How often will they be done?

496

- What are the treatment choices? Which do you recommend for my child? Why?

- Would a clinical trial be right for my child? Why?

- Have you treated other children with this type of cancer? How many?

- What are the chances that the treatment will work?

- Where is the best place for my child to receive treatment? Are there specialists—such as surgeons, radiologists, nurses, anesthesiologists, and others—trained in pediatrics? Can my child have some or all of the treatment in our home town?

- How long will the treatment last?

- What will be the treatment schedule?

- Whom should we ask about the details of financial matters?

- Will the treatment disrupt my child's school schedule?

- What possible side effects of the treatment can occur, both right away and later?

- What can be done to help if side effects occur?

- How long will my child be in the hospital?

- Can any treatment be done at home? Will we need any special equipment?

- Does the hospital have a place where I can stay overnight during my child's treatment?

- Is there a child-life worker specialist (a professional who is responsible for making the hospital and treatment experience less scary for the child) to plan play therapy, schoolwork, and other activities?

- When can my child go back to school?

- Are there certain diseases my child cannot be around? Should I have my child and his or her siblings immunized against any diseases?

- Will my child need tutoring?

- Is information available to give to the school system about my child's needs as he or she receives treatment?

Talking with Your Child

Your first question may be, "Should I tell my child about the cancer?" You may want to protect your child, but children usually know when something is wrong. Your child may not be feeling well, may be seeing the doctor often, and may have already had some tests. Your child may notice that you are afraid. No matter how hard you try to keep information about the illness and treatment from your child, others—such as family, friends, and clinic or hospital staff—may inadvertently say things that let your child know about the cancer. In addition, it will upset your child to find out that you were not telling the truth; your child depends on you for honest answers.

Telling your child about his or her cancer is a personal matter, and family, cultural, or religious beliefs will come into play. It is important to be open and honest with your child because children who are not told about their illness often imagine things that are not true. For example, a child may think he or she has cancer as punishment for doing something wrong. Health professionals generally agree that telling children the truth about their illness leads to less stress and guilt. Children who know the truth are also more likely to cooperate with treatment. Finally, talking about cancer often helps to bring the family closer together and makes dealing with the cancer a little easier for everyone.

Parent's Questions

When should my child be told? Because you are probably the best judge of your child's personality and moods, you are the best person to decide when your child should be told. Keep in mind, though, that your child is likely to know early on that something is wrong, so you may want to tell your child soon after the diagnosis. In fact, most parents say it is easiest to tell them then. Waiting days or weeks may give your child time to imagine worse things than the truth and develop fears that may be hard to dispel later. Certainly, it would be easier for your child if he or she is told before treatment starts.

Who should tell my child? The answer to this question is personal. As a parent, you may feel that it is best for you to tell your child. Some parents, however, find it too painful to do so. Other family members or the treatment team—doctor, nurse, or social worker—may be able to help you. They may either tell your child for you or help you explain the illness.

Thinking about what you are going to say and how to say it will help you feel more relaxed. But how do you decide just what to say? Family and close friends, members of the treatment team, parents of other children who have cancer, members of support groups, and clergy members can offer ideas.

Who should be there? Your child needs love and support when hearing the diagnosis. Even if the doctor explains the illness, someone your child trusts and depends upon should be present. Having the support of other family members at this time can be very helpful.

What should my child be told? How much information and the best way to relate this information depends on your child's age and what your child can understand. Being gentle, open, and honest is usually best.

Questions Your Child May Ask

Children are naturally curious about their disease and have many questions about cancer and cancer treatment. Your child will expect you to have answers to most questions. Children may begin to ask questions right after diagnosis or may wait until later. Here are some common questions.

- Why me?
- Will I get well?
- What will happen to me?
- Why do I have to take medicine when I feel okay?

Treatment

To plan the best treatment, the doctor and treatment team will look at your child's general health, type of cancer, stage of the disease, age, and many other factors. Based on this information, the doctor will prepare a treatment plan that outlines the exact type of treatment, how often your child will receive treatment, and how long it will last. Each child with cancer has a treatment plan that is chosen just for that child; even children with the same type of cancer may receive different treatments. Depending on how your child responds to treatment, the doctor may decide to change the treatment plan or choose another plan.

Before treatment begins, your child's doctor will discuss the treatment plan with you, including the benefits, risks, and side effects. Then you and the treatment team will need to talk with your child about the treatment. After the doctor fully explains the treatment and answers your questions, you will be asked to give your written consent to go ahead with treatment. Depending on your child's age and hospital policy, your child may also be asked to give consent before treatment.

The treatment plan may seem complicated at first. But the doctor and treatment team will explain each step, and you and your child will soon become used to the routine. Many parents find it helpful to get a copy of the treatment plan to refer to as the treatment proceeds. It also helps them in arranging their own schedules. Do not be afraid to ask questions or speak up if you feel something is not going right. Your child's doctor is often the best person to answer your questions, but other members of the treatment team can give you information, too. If you feel as though you need extra time with the doctor, schedule a meeting or phone call. Remember, you are part of the treatment team and should be involved in your child's treatment.

Common Health Issues

Pain relief, nutrition, treatment for infections, immunizations, bleeding, transfusions, and dental/mouth care are all part of supportive care. The goal of supportive care is to prevent or lessen the side effects of the treatment and the disease. With this care, your child can receive the needed therapy with greater safety and comfort. You may want to talk with your child's doctor or other members of the treatment team to see how the information provided below might help your child.

Pain

Your child may have pain for a variety of reasons. Pain may be caused by the cancer itself, or it could be from the treatment, such as surgery to remove a tumor or side effects of chemotherapy. Sometimes, cancer patients have pain that has nothing to do with the cancer, such as a toothache or a headache.

- Not all children with cancer have pain. Those who do are not in pain all of the time.

- Medicine and other treatments can almost always relieve cancer pain.

- Relieving pain will not only make your child more comfortable, but also may help your child sleep and eat better.

- Parents often feel helpless when their children are in pain. This reaction is natural. Knowing what to expect and what can be done to relieve pain can help. Talk with the doctor and treatment team about whether your child is likely to have pain, what pain treatment your child can receive, or what to do for your child if pain occurs.

Managing cancer pain: The best way to relieve pain is to treat its cause. If a tumor is causing pain, the doctor may try to remove the tumor or decrease its size using surgery, radiation therapy, or chemotherapy. Other ways to relieve or control pain include use of the following techniques:

- direct pressure or cold or warm compresses
- pain medications
- physical therapy
- relaxation
- distraction
- imagery
- nerve blocks

Preventing pain from starting or getting worse is the best way to control it. Some people call this "staying on top of the pain." It may also mean that your child will need a lower dose of a pain reliever than if you wait until the pain gets bad. Different pain medicines take different lengths of time to work, from a few minutes to several hours. If your child waits too long to take pain medicine, the pain may get worse before the medicine helps.

Work closely with the treatment team in sharing information about your child. For example, if you know that your child is afraid of needles, ask the doctor if your child can be given oral medicine. In older children and adolescents, the doctor may order a self-controlled drug "pump." This method uses a portable computerized pump containing pain medicine attached to a needle that is placed in a vein or attached to the central vein catheter. When pain relief is needed, the child presses a hand-held button, and the pump injects a preset dose of medicine into the vein. Pumps are programmed to give preset doses only at preset intervals, so even if the child presses button more than once during the preset interval, he or she will not get any more pain medication than is programmed.

Pain assessment: Treating pain in children requires a special understanding of the child and of the child's age. In some cases, you may need to speak for your child, especially if your child is younger than 4 years old. For infants and very young children, you can be of great help by closely watching the expressions on your child's face and carefully listening to the way your child cries. Take note of changes in behavior, such as sadness or isolation or decreased activity. The changes may mean that your child is in pain.

Sometimes, children have pain, but they may not be able to tell you about it. They may be afraid to. It is important to ask if your child has pain. Talk with your child about where and how much pain there is. Use words that your child knows, such as "boo-boo" or "ouch." A good way to determine the amount of pain your child has is to use a pain scale. A frequently used pain scale is the Wong-Baker FACES Pain Rating Scale, which can be used with children as young as 3 years old. On this scale, each face demonstrates a level of pain, from a person who feels happy because there is no pain (hurt) or sad because there is some or a lot of pain.

Uncontrolled pain: Cancer pain almost always can be greatly lessened or relieved, but no doctor can know everything about all medical problems. If your child's doctor is unable to control your child's pain, ask to see a pain specialist. Pain specialists may be oncologists, anesthesiologists, neurosurgeons, other doctors, nurses, or pharmacists. A pain control team may also include psychologists and social workers.

Diet

Many side effects from cancer treatment may make it hard for your child to eat. Some physical side effects include loss of appetite, sore mouth, changed sense of taste, nausea, vomiting, diarrhea, constipation, and weight gain. The emotional side of cancer treatment may also affect your child's eating habits. When children are upset, worried, or afraid, they may have eating problems. Losing his or her appetite and feeling nauseated can be normal when your child is nervous or afraid. The treatment team, including the nutritionist/dietitian at the hospital where your child receives treatment, can help you plan the food to serve at home. Let the team know if you notice that your child is losing or gaining weight. Ask what has worked for other children. The good news is that even children who have trouble eating have days when eating is a pleasure. The following suggestions may help your child feel more like eating:

- Build meals around your child's favorite foods, but do not force favorite foods during nausea attacks. Forcing may cause a lasting dislike of the food.

- Try always to give high-calorie foods (for example, macaroni and cheese with real butter and cheese, or milkshakes made with ice cream). Add instant breakfast powders to all milk and milk products.

- Let your child eat whenever he or she is hungry or offer food often during the day. Have high-calorie, high-protein snacks handy. Taking just a few bites of the right foods or sips of the right liquids every hour or so can help increase your child's intake of proteins and calories. You can freeze portions of a favorite dish and serve them when your child wants them.

- Oral medicines may affect your child's appetite. Some are best given in the morning, some at midday, and some on a full stomach. Ask the doctor when and how medicines should be given. Tell the doctor if your child has no appetite or has any other side effects.

- Try changing the time, place, and surroundings of meals. A picnic, even if it is in the house, can make mealtime more fun. Watching a favorite TV show or inviting a special friend to join your child at meal or snack time also can help your child feel more like eating.

- Make mealtimes calm and relaxed. Do not hurry meals.

- Praise good eating. Try using small rewards, such as a favorite dessert or a new toy, to encourage good eating. Siblings should be considered when setting up a reward system. It is important that siblings are not left out, but be careful not to encourage healthy siblings to overeat.

- Avoid arguing, nagging, or punishing. Forcing a child to eat may make things worse.

If your child's eating becomes a serious problem, ask your child's doctor about medicines that can improve appetite.

Sometimes children gain extra weight during treatment because of the buildup of excess water in the body. Do not put your child on a diet. Instead, call the doctor. If the weight gain is due to extra water, the doctor may recommend using less salt, because salt causes the body to hold onto water. The doctor may also order medicines called diuretics to get rid of the excess water.

Children who have cancer need diets high in both calories and protein. High-calorie foods help prevent weight loss, and protein foods help the body stay strong and repair itself. To get your child to eat more protein and calories, try these tips.

- Offer liquids during the day, but not at mealtimes. Liquids are filling and take away an appetite for solid foods. Give your child a straw to make drinking easier.

- Some types of chemotherapy may change your child's sense of taste for a while. Well-seasoned foods, such as spaghetti, tacos, and pizza, may seem good at such times. Sometimes, adding extra salt or sugar, or using less, may make foods taste better.

- Avoid empty-calorie foods, such as soft drinks, chips, and candy, that can make your child's appetite worse without providing good nutrition. Milkshakes, yogurt, fruit, juices, or "instant breakfasts" provide extra calories and protein.

Infections

Infections are common in children who have cancer, especially in children who are receiving chemotherapy. Chemotherapy lowers the white blood cell count, which increases the chances of infection. You should report any sign of infection, such as a fever, to your child's doctor right away.

Infections are usually caused by bacteria or viruses. To find the cause of your child's infection, the doctor may take samples (cultures) of the throat, blood, urine, or stool. If the infection is from bacteria, your child will receive antibiotics. Antibiotics will not work against viruses. Unless a virus has been identified, however, most children are treated with antibiotics until their blood counts improve, even if bacterial infection cultures are negative. Your child may receive other medicines to help ease the symptoms. If the infection is serious, or the white blood cell count is very low, your child may need to be treated at the hospital. Your child's doctor may also stop the cancer treatment for a short time until the infection is gone.

Some viral infections, such as chickenpox, can cause major problems for a child receiving chemotherapy. Call the doctor right away if your child is exposed to chickenpox or to anyone who has recently received the chickenpox vaccine. And ask your child's teachers to let you know if a schoolmate develops chickenpox. Some families ask teachers to ask schoolmates' families to call them at once if chickenpox develops in their families.

Once children have had chickenpox, they usually do not get it again, but some children on chemotherapy who have already had chickenpox may develop shingles. Shingles is a blister-like skin rash that looks like chickenpox. Instead of appearing all over the body, however, shingles is in just one area. Call the doctor right away if you think that your child may have shingles.

Regular or red measles (also known as rubeola or 9-day measles) may also be more serious for a child on chemotherapy. If your child comes into contact with this type of measles, you should call the doctor. The doctor may give your child medicine to prevent or control the infection.

Immunizations

Most vaccines, and especially live virus vaccines (regular measles, German measles or rubella, mumps, polio, and chickenpox), should not be given to a child receiving cancer treatment, although some doctors do recommend varicella (chickenpox) vaccines for children with cancer and for their siblings. Some immunizations may be dangerous because chemotherapy cancer treatment lowers the body's ability to protect itself when given these vaccines. In addition, brothers or sisters should not receive the live polio vaccines while their sibling is having cancer treatment. You should discuss these matters in detail with both your child's oncologist and your children's primary care provider (for example, pediatrician, clinic, or family physician).

Vaccines that are not live may be safe to give during cancer treatment, including diphtheria, whooping cough, and tetanus immunizations. Flu shots are okay, but you should ask your child's doctor before any immunizations are given.

Bleeding

Platelets are blood cells that help the blood to clot. A low platelet count may cause your child to bleed more easily than usual. If your child's platelet count is low, he or she will need to avoid contact activities such as football, soccer, or skateboarding. If bleeding occurs, you may try the following:

- Apply pressure until the bleeding stops—a clean towel, handkerchief, or cloth firmly pressed to the wound will slow or stop the bleeding.

- For nosebleeds, have your child sit up; do not let your child lie down. Pinch the bridge of the nose over the bone for five minutes. The pressure must be tight on both sides to stop the bleeding.

If bleeding continues, call the doctor immediately.

Dental/Mouth Care

If possible, your child should have a complete oral exam and any needed dental work before cancer treatment begins. Dental care is important during treatment, but even checkups should be avoided when blood counts are low. Always check with the doctor before starting any dental work, and let the dentist know your child is receiving cancer treatment. Your child may need to take an antibiotic before any dental work is done to prevent possible infections. In general, a low dose of amoxicillin is given before even a routine cleaning to patients who have a central venous catheter.

Keeping the child's teeth, mouth, and gums clean to protect against decay is especially important. Make sure your child's teeth are brushed after each meal, using a soft toothbrush. After each use, rinse the brush well with cold water, shake it well, and allow it to dry. Give your child paper cups to rinse his or her mouth. Dental floss may be used if care is taken not to cut or irritate the gums.

Radiation therapy: During radiation to the head and neck, less saliva is produced, so the mouth becomes dry. This dryness can lead to tooth decay. The doctor or dentist may recommend using a fluoride mouth rinse or order a fluoride gel. Check with your doctor before buying a mouthwash—many can cause burning pain in a child with a sore mouth. All children receiving radiation should rinse their mouths often during the day. One suggested mouth rinse is a mixture of salt and baking soda (½ teaspoon of each in a cup of water). To care for infants and toddlers, wrap a soft cloth around your finger and gently wipe the teeth and gums with the mouth rinse. Soft "toothettes" can also be used to apply the rinse to the child's mouth.

When blood counts are low: When your child's blood counts are low, mouth care needs to be especially gentle; your child can get an infection or start bleeding more easily. Use very soft bristle toothbrushes, cotton or glycerin swabs, or toothettes, and avoid using water jet devices or dental floss. Call the doctor if you see any red or white patches, mouth sores, or irritated areas in the mouth.

Mouth sores: When mouth sores, bleeding areas, or irritated areas occur, use only the mouth rinse described above or one the doctor recommends. Your child should rinse the mouth out well after every meal and before bedtime. Cotton or glycerin swabs or toothettes (available in drug stores) can help remove pieces of food from the mouth. If mouth sores become painful, a local anesthetic may help. The doctor can order an anesthetic and will tell you how often to use it. To make eating easier, put the anesthetic on the sore gums before meals. For dry lips, try a lanolin lip ointment to prevent them from cracking and becoming sore.

When to Call the Doctor

If you have worried about knowing when to call the doctor, you are not alone. Parents want to watch closely for any sign that their child may need to see the doctor but may not be sure what those signs are. They also may worry about "bothering" the doctor or treatment team. The best approach is to ask the doctor when to call about any problems your child may be having. If you are unsure, this list can be used as a guide for when to call the doctor.

Call the Doctor If...

Your child shows signs of infection.

- Fever (100.4° F or 38° C) or other sign of infection, especially if your child's white count is low. (The doctor will tell you when it is low.) It is important to take your child's temperature with an accurate thermometer.

Your child has trouble eating.

- Mouth sores that keep your child from eating
- Difficulty chewing

Your child has digestive tract problems.

- Vomiting, unless you have been told that your child may vomit after the cancer treatment
- Painful urination or bowel movements
- Constipation that lasts more than two days
- Diarrhea

Your child shows changes in mobility or mood.

- Trouble walking or bending
- Trouble talking
- Dizziness
- Blurred or double vision
- Depression or a sudden change in behavior

Your child has troublesome symptoms.

- Bleeding, including nosebleeds, red or black bowel movements, pink, red, or brown urine, or many bruises
- Severe or continuing headaches
- Pain anywhere in the body
- Red or swollen areas

Your child needs treatment for other health concerns.

- Before your child receives immunizations or dental care, even scheduled vaccinations or regular dental checkups
- Before you give your child any over-the-counter medication

You are in any doubt whatsoever.

Moving on with Life

One of the challenges facing the family of a child who has cancer is going on with everyday life. Moving forward is not an easy task. It may be hardest during times of stress: when you find out your child has cancer, when your child is in the hospital, or when your child is suffering from the side effects of treatment.

Even when the treatments are going well, the cancer still affects each member of your family. When your child enters the hospital or goes for treatments, each member has to adjust in some way. Family members may be apart. Days of work may be missed. Brothers and sisters may feel left out. Everyone may be worried and tense.

Despite all this, family life goes on. Brothers and sisters have school and activities. Parents have jobs. It is hard to keep up with everyday activities and responsibilities while being with and caring for your child with cancer.

As the mother or father of a child who has cancer, remember that you are not alone. You can get help from many sources, such as the treatment team, which includes a social worker who can help you in dealing with your child's illness; other parents of children with cancer; support groups; or others. The information below may also be helpful for you, your child, the other children in your family, your extended family, and friends.

Your child: Even with a diagnosis of cancer, your child still has the same needs as other young people—going to school, having friends, and enjoying things that were a part of life before cancer. You can help meet these needs by letting your child live as normal a life as possible. Some activities, however, may need to be changed at different times during treatment. After chemotherapy or radiation therapy, your child may be very tired and, therefore, need more rest. This tiredness is to be expected. Help your child find other things to do, such as new hobbies, or ask friends to come over to draw or paint.

You: Your child's illness will bring many changes to your life. To help you cope with these changes, you may want to consider the following suggestions:

- Make time for yourself.

- Prepare yourself for a lot of waiting. Find ways to make waiting during clinic visits or while in the hospital less frustrating. Take something to read or do while your child is asleep or does not need your attention.

- Turn to treatment staff or other resources for support.

- Contact support groups.

- Share the care of your child with your partner or others close to the family.

Brothers and sisters: The lives of children who have a brother or sister who has cancer change a great deal. Siblings may have many different feelings about the brother or sister who has cancer and the extra attention the child receives. They may feel sorry for their sibling who is ill. Younger children may feel that they caused the cancer. Or they may believe that their own needs are being ignored.

When a child is in the hospital and is very ill, the focus is on that child. As a parent, you may not be able to pay as much attention to your other children as you did before. You may have to miss many of their special school or sports events. You may also use up all your energy and patience caring for your child who has cancer and not have enough energy or time to talk with your other children, play with them, or help them with their homework. It is natural, then, for siblings to be annoyed at the attention your child who has cancer is receiving.

As a result, siblings' behavior may change. They may become depressed, have headaches, or begin to have problems in school. School counselors and support groups may be able to offer you helpful advice for dealing with these issues. In addition, here are some things you can do to help your other children:

- Talk with them about their feelings. Talk with them about the special attention your child who has cancer is getting. Let them know that feeling mad is natural. Try to explain what is happening and why you may not be around as much as you were before.

- Talk with them about the cancer, the treatment, and care. Younger children's fears can be helped by knowing they couldn't have caused the illness by wishing or by spreading germs from a cold. Treatment and procedures should be explained as being helpful things and not punishments.

- Spend time with your other children. Try to spend some time with them doing the things they like.

  Encourage them to take part in outside activities. Make a point of noticing and praising what they do in these activities.

- Involve them in their brother's or sister's treatment. Let them come along with you to the clinic or hospital. Having them along will allow them to see for themselves what the hospital, clinic, and treatment are like.

- Talk with them about questions their schoolmates and friends may ask. Help them think of possible questions and answers so that they will feel comfortable talking about their brother's or sister's illness.

- Ask other family members and friends to spend time with the other children in the family. For example, an aunt or uncle might go to school events or attend important games or performances. A neighbor might help them with homework or take them on outings.

Family and friends: A diagnosis of cancer affects not only the child, parents, and siblings, but also grandparents, other relatives, and friends. These people can support and assist you during this time.

Your employers also may need to be told about your child's illness, so they will know why you are asking for extra time off from work. If needed, your child's doctor can write your employer to explain the situation.

What Does the Future Hold?

Because of better research and treatment, children who have cancer are living longer than they used to, and their quality of life is better. Although they lead normal lives, survivors of cancer have some concerns that other people may not have. For example, they must take extra-special care of their health and may have problems obtaining insurance.

Ongoing Health Care

Regular exams are very important after treatment for cancer. At these visits, your child receives both the health care needed by anyone your child's age and special care based on the type of cancer and treatments and current health.

In general, parents of children who have had cancer treatment should do the following.

- Schedule regular checkups. Children who have been treated for cancer usually return to the doctor every three to four months at first, and once or twice a year later on. Ask the doctor how often your child needs to return for follow-up exams.

- Be alert to signs of the possible return of cancer. Doctors have no way to tell for sure whether your child's cancer will return. If it does return, it could be weeks, months, or years after treatment ends. Talk with your child's doctor and treatment team about the chances of cancer returning and the signs of cancer's return.

- Be alert to signs of lasting effects of cancer treatment. Cancer treatment may cause side effects many years later. Some cancer treatments may affect your child's ability to have children in the future; affect how your child learns and grows physically; or increase your child's risk of developing a second type of cancer.

- Be tuned in to any problems your child may have in dealing with feelings about having had cancer, even years after treatment has ended. Once all the activity of treatment is over, some children suddenly fully realize what happened to them. It can be a very upsetting. At this point, they may need to talk about their feelings and may even need to see a counselor.

- Promote good health habits. Eating well and getting enough sleep and exercise will help your child feel better and be healthy.

To better understand your child's health care needs today and in the future, ask the doctor and treatment team.

You need information to continue to take care of your child's health. As your child gets older, he or she also will need this information. You may want to ask the doctor and treatment team the following questions:

- How often should my child have checkups?

- What are the signs of cancer's return or of long-term effects? How likely are they to occur?

- What changes may occur that are not danger signs?

- What kind of diet should my child follow?

- What are the choices for handling chronic pain, the return of cancer, or the long-term effects of therapy?

- What is the best way for me to talk with you about future concerns? (By phone? At a special appointment? At a regular office visit scheduled in advance to allow more time?)

- Who else is available to talk about specific problems?

Insurance Issues

Another concern of parents is what happens to health insurance coverage and costs after your child has had treatment for cancer. Your child is likely to continue to be covered under your current insurance, but you may have to pay more. If you change jobs or apply for a new policy, however, you may have trouble getting the new coverage for your child, and it may cost more. Older teenagers who may soon be leaving home and looking for a job need to pay special attention to insurance needs. Going off their parent's insurance will mean finding coverage on their own.

One key to making sure your child has insurance coverage is to ask the right questions before changing jobs and look at what your health insurance coverage will include if you change policies.

Chapter 57

When Your Parent Has Cancer

How to Use This Chapter

You may want to read this chapter from start to finish. Or maybe you'll just read those sections that interest you most. Some teens pull this information out now and again when they need it. You may want to share this information with your mom, dad, brothers, and sisters. It might help you bring up something that has been on your mind. You could ask people in your family to read a certain chapter and then talk about it together later.

You've Just Learned That Your Parent Has Cancer

You've just learned that one of the most important people in your life has cancer. Do you feel shocked, numb, angry, or afraid? Do you feel like life is unfair? One thing is certain—you don't feel good.

For now, try to focus on these facts:

- **Many people survive cancer:** There are nearly 10 million cancer survivors living in the U.S. today. That's because scientists are discovering new and better ways to find and treat cancer. During this really tough time, it will help you to have hope.

Excerpted from "When Your Parent Has Cancer: A Guide for Teens," National Cancer Institute, April 2006. The full text of this document is available online at www.cancer.gov; it can also be ordered by calling 800-4-CANCER.

- **You're not alone:** Right now it might seem that no one else in the world feels the way you do. In a way you're right. No one can feel exactly like you do. But it might help to know that many teens have a parent who has cancer. Talking to others may help you sort out your feelings. Remember, you are not alone.

- **You're not to blame:** Cancer is a disease with various causes, many of which doctors don't fully understand. None of these causes has anything to do with what you've done, thought, or said.

- **Balance is important:** Many teens feel like their parent's cancer is always on their mind. Others try to avoid it. Try to strike a balance. You can be concerned about your parent and still stay connected with people and activities that you care about.

- **Knowledge is power:** It can help to learn more about cancer and cancer treatments. Sometimes what you imagine is actually worse than the reality.

Your Feelings

As you deal with your parent's cancer, you'll probably feel all kinds of things. Many other teens who have a parent with cancer have felt the same way you do now. Some of these emotions are listed below. Think about people you can talk with about your feelings.

Scared

- My world is falling apart.
- I'm afraid that my parent might die.
- I'm afraid that someone else in my family might catch cancer. (They can't.)
- I'm afraid that something might happen to my parent at home, and I won't know what to do.

It's normal to feel scared when your parent has cancer. Some of your fears may be real. Others may be based on things that won't happen. And some fears may lessen over time.

Guilty

- I feel guilty because I'm healthy and my parent is sick.
- I feel guilty when I laugh and have fun.

You may feel bad about having fun when your parent is sick. However, having fun doesn't mean that you care any less. In fact, it will probably help your parent to see you do things you enjoy.

Angry

- I am mad that my mom or dad got sick.
- I am upset at the doctors.
- I am angry at God for letting this happen.
- I am angry at myself for feeling the way I do.

Anger often covers up other feelings that are harder to show. Try not to let your anger build up.

Neglected

- I feel left out.
- I don't get any attention any more.
- No one ever tells me what's going on.
- My family never talks anymore.

When a parent has cancer, it's common for the family's focus to change. Some people in the family may feel left out. Your parent with cancer may be using his or her energy to get better. Your well parent may be focused on helping your parent with cancer. Your parents don't mean for you to feel left out. It just happens because so much is going on.

Lonely

- No one understands what I'm going through.
- My friends don't come over anymore.
- My friends don't seem to know what to say to me anymore.

Try to remember that these feelings won't last forever.

Embarrassed

- I'm sometimes embarrassed to be out in public with my sick parent.
- I don't know how to answer people's questions.

515

Many teens who feel embarrassed about having a parent with cancer say it gets easier to deal with over time.

What You're Feeling Is Normal

There is no one "right" way to feel. And you're not alone—many other teens in your situation have felt the same way. Some have said that having a parent with cancer changes the way they look at things in life. Some even said that it made them stronger.

Dealing with Your Feelings

A lot of people are uncomfortable sharing their feelings. They ignore them and hope they'll go away. Others choose to act cheerful when they're really not. They think that by acting upbeat they won't feel sad or angry anymore. This may help for a little while, but not over the long run. Actually, holding your feelings inside can keep you from getting the help that you need.

Try these tips:

- Talk with family and friends that you feel close to. You owe it to yourself.

- Write your thoughts down in a journal.

- Join a support group to meet with other teens who are facing some of the same things you are. Or meet with a counselor.

- It is probably hard to imagine right now, but, if you let yourself, you can grow stronger as a person through this experience.

Many kids think that they need to protect their parents by not making them worry. They think that they have to be perfect and not cause any trouble because one of their parents is sick. If you feel this way, remember that no one can be perfect all the time. You need time to vent, to feel sad, and to be happy. Try to let your parents know how you feel—even if you have to start the conversation.

What Your Parent May Be Feeling

Knowing how your parent may be feeling could help you figure out how to help, or at least understand where he or she is coming from. You may be surprised to learn that they are feeling a lot of the same things you are:

- **Sad or depressed:** People with cancer sometimes can't do things they used to do. They may miss these activities and their friends. Feeling sad or down can range from a mild case of the blues to depression, which a doctor can treat.

- **Afraid:** Your parent may be afraid of how cancer will change his or her life and the lives of family members. He or she may be scared about treatment. Your parent may even be scared that he or she will die.

- **Anxious:** Your parent may be worried about a lot of things. Your mom or dad may feel stressed about going to work or paying the bills. Or he or she may be concerned about looking different because of treatment. And your mom or dad is probably very concerned about how you are doing. All these worries may upset your parent.

- **Angry:** Cancer treatment and its side effects can be difficult to go through. Anger sometimes comes from feelings that are hard to show, such as fear or frustration. Chances are your parent is angry at the disease, not at you.

- **Lonely:** People with cancer often feel lonely or distant from others. They may find that their friends have a hard time dealing with their cancer and may not visit. They may be too sick to take part in activities they used to enjoy. They may feel that no one understands what they're going through.

- **Hopeful:** There are many reasons for your parent to feel hopeful. Millions of people who have had cancer are alive today. People with cancer can lead active lives, even during treatment. Your parent's chances of surviving cancer are better today than ever before.

All these feelings are normal for people living with cancer. You might want to share this list with your mom or dad.

Changes in Your Family

Whatever your family situation, chances are that things have changed since your parent got sick. This chapter looks at some of these changes and ways that other teens have dealt with them.

Let your parents know if you feel that there is more to do than you can handle. Together you can work it out.

517

Families say that it helps to make time to talk together, even if it's only for a short time each week. Talking can help your family stay connected. Here are some things to consider when talking with brothers and sisters:

- If you are the oldest child, your brothers or sisters may look to you for support. Help them as much as you can. It's okay to let them know that you're having a tough time, too.

- If you are looking to your older brother or sister for help, tell them how you are feeling. They can help, but won't have all the answers.

Here are some things to consider when talking with your parent who is well:

- Expect your parent to feel some stress, just as you do.

- Your parent may snap at you. He or she may not always do or say the right thing.

- Lend a hand when you can.

Here are some things to consider when talking with your parent with cancer:

- Your mom or dad may be sick from the treatment or just very tired. Or maybe your parent will feel okay and want your company.

- Try talking if your mom or dad feels up to it. Let your parent know how much you love them.

Keeping Family and Friends in the Loop

Is it getting to be too much to answer the phone and tell people how your mom or dad is doing? That can be a lot for anyone. Ask others to help you share news of how your parent is doing and what help your family needs. Maybe a relative or family friend can be the contact person. Some families use telephone chains. Others use a website or e-mail listserv.

Growing Stronger as a Family

Some families can grow apart for a while when a parent has cancer. But there are ways to help your family grow stronger and closer. Teens who saw their families grow closer say that it happened because people in their family:

- Tried to put themselves in the other person's shoes and thought about how they would feel if they were the other person.

- Understood that even though people reacted differently to situations, they were all hurting. Some cried a lot. Others showed little emotion. Some used humor to get by.

- Learned to respect and talk about differences. The more they asked about how others were feeling, the more they could help each other.

Asking Others for Help

You and your family may need support from others. It can be hard to ask. Yet most of the time people really want to help you and your family. Here is a list of people that your mom, dad, or you may ask for help:

- Aunts, uncles, and grandparents
- Family friends
- Neighbors
- Teachers or coaches
- School nurses or guidance counselors
- People from your religious community
- Your friends or their parents

Some things people can do to help include the following:

- Go grocery shopping or run errands
- Make meals
- Mow the lawn
- Do chores around the house
- Keep your parent company

Other ways people can help you and your family include these suggestions:

- Give rides to school, practice, or appointments
- Help with homework
- Invite you over or on weekend outings
- Talk with and listen to you

Dealing with Stress

Stress can make you forgetful, frustrated, and more likely to catch a cold or the flu. Here are some tips that have helped other teens manage stress. Pick one or two things to do each week.

Take Care of Your Mind and Body

- Stay connected.
  - Spend some time at a friend's house.
  - Stay involved with sports or clubs.
- Relax and get enough sleep.
  - Take breaks. You'll have more energy and be in a better frame of mind.
  - Get at least 8 hours of sleep each night.
  - Pray or meditate.
  - Make or listen to music.
- Help others.
  - Join a walk against cancer.
  - Plan a bake sale or other charity event to collect money to fight cancer.
- Avoid risky behaviors.
  - Stay away from smoking, drinking, and taking drugs.
- Put your creative side to work.
  - Keep a journal to write down your thoughts and experiences.
  - Draw, paint, or take photographs.
  - Read about people who have made it through difficult experiences in life. Learn what helped them.
- Eat and drink well.
  - Drink 6–8 glasses of water a day to help prevent fatigue.
  - In the evening, switch to caffeine-free drinks that won't keep you awake.
  - Grab fresh fruit, whole-grain breads, and lean meats like chicken or turkey when you have a choice.
  - Avoid sugary foods.

- Be active.
  - Play a sport, or go for a walk or run.
  - Learn about different stretching and breathing exercises.

Take Steps to Keep Things Simple

Staying organized can also keep your stress level under control. Here are some tips to get you started.

- At home
  - Make a list of things you want to do and put the most important ones at the top.
  - Make a big calendar to help your family stay on top of things.
- At school
  - Try to get as much done in school as you can.
  - Let your teachers know what's happening at home, without using it as an excuse.
  - Talk to your teachers or a counselor if you are falling behind.

Get Help when You Feel Down

Many teens feel low or down when their parent is sick. It's normal to feel sad or "blue" during difficult times. However, if these feelings last for two weeks or more and start to interfere with things you used to enjoy, you may be depressed. The good news is that there is hope and there is help. Often, talking with a counselor can help. Below are some signs that you may need to see a counselor.

Are you:

- Feeling helpless and hopeless? Thinking that life has no meaning?
- Losing interest in being with family or friends?
- Finding that everything or everyone seems to get on your nerves?
- Feeling really angry a lot of the time?
- Thinking of hurting yourself?

Do you find that you are:

- Losing interest in the activities you used to enjoy?

- Eating too little or a lot more than usual?
- Crying easily or many times each day?
- Using drugs or alcohol to help you forget?
- Sleeping more than you used to? Less than you used to?
- Feeling tired a lot?

If you answered "yes" to any of these questions, it's important to talk to someone you trust. Consider seeing a counselor or joining a support group.

Finding Support

Don't let being afraid of the way you feel keep you from talking to your parents, a counselor, or people in a support group.

For many people, starting to talk is difficult. Some teens don't have good relationships with their parents. Others are too embarrassed to talk about personal things. It can also just be hard to make the time to talk, with all that is going on. But you and your parents really can help each other.

Tips for Talking with Your Parent

Prepare before you talk.

Step 1: Think about what you want to say and about some solutions to the problem.

Step 2: Think about how your parent might react. How will you respond to him or her?

Find a good time and place.

Step 1: Ask your mom or dad if they have a few minutes to talk.

Step 2: Find a private place—maybe in your room or on the front steps. Or maybe you can talk while taking a walk or shooting hoops.

Take things slowly.

Step 1: Don't expect to solve everything right away. Difficult problems often don't have simple solutions.

Step 2: Work together to find a way through these challenges. Some conversations will go better than others.

Keep it up.

Step 1: Don't think you have to have just one big conversation. Have lots of small ones.

Step 2: Make time to talk a little each day if you can, even if it's just for a few minutes.

Talking with a Counselor

Sometimes talking to friends is not enough. When you are having a hard time, it can be helpful to talk to a counselor or social worker.

Why go to a counselor? Teens say it can be helpful to talk with someone outside the family—someone who doesn't take sides. A counselor is a person who will listen to you. They will help you find ways to better handle the things that bother you and gain strength in your situation.

Here are some tips for finding a counselor:

- Talk with your mom, dad, or someone else that you trust. Let them know you would like to talk to a counselor. Ask for help making appointments and getting to visits. Sometimes the counselor will even let you bring a friend.

- Ask a nurse or social worker at the hospital if they know someone you can talk to.

- Ask your guidance counselor at school if you can talk to him or her.

Joining a Support Group

Another good outlet is a support group. Some groups meet in person; others meet online. Some groups go out and have fun together. In these groups you'll meet other teens going through some of the same things that you are. At first this may not sound like something you want to do. Other teens say they thought the same thing—until they went to a meeting. They were surprised that so many others felt the same way they did and had advice that really seemed to work. A doctor, nurse, or social worker can help you find a support group.

You and Your Friends

Your friends are important to you, and you're important to them. In the past, you could tell them everything. Now that your parent has cancer, it may seem like a lot is changing—even your friendships. Here are some things to think about:

- Your friends may not know what to say. It is hard for some people to know what to say. Others may think it's rude to ask questions. Try to be gentle on friends who don't ask about your parent's cancer or how you are doing. You may need to take the first step.

- Your friends may ask tough questions. You may not always feel like answering questions about your parent's cancer or treatment.

- Your friends have their own lives. It may feel like your friends don't care anymore. It might seem as though their lives are moving on, and yours isn't. It can be hard to watch them get together with others or do things without you. But try to understand that they have their own lives, too. They aren't facing the situation you are right now, so it may be hard for them to relate.

Having Fun and Making New Friends

Even though you may have a lot on your mind, you can still get together with your friends and have a good time. If you can't leave home as much, ask if your friends can come over. Take time to relax. It's good for you. Make a list of fun things you and your friends like to do together. Then do them!

New friends: A lot is happening to you right now. Sometimes old friends move on. You may not have as much in common as you used to. The good news is that you may find yourself making new friends. Kids who used to just pass you in the halls may now ask you how you are doing. Kids who you used to be friends with may enter your life again. Be open to new friendships.

Going to support groups at the hospital or clinic is a good way to meet new friends. It helps to connect with people who are going through some of the same things that you are. Try to do fun things together. The break will be good for all of you!

How You Can Help Your Parent

Here are some things that others have done to help their parent at home. Pick one or two things to try each week.

Help with Care

- Spend time with your parent. Watch a movie together. Read the paper to your parent. Ask for help with your homework. Give hugs. Say, "I love you." Or just hang out in silence.

- Lend a hand. Bring water or offer to make a snack or small meal.

Help by Being Thoughtful

- Try to be upbeat, but be "real," too. Being positive can be good for you and your whole family. But don't feel like you always have to act cheerful, especially if it's not how you really feel. It's okay to share your thoughts with your parent—and let them comfort you. Be yourself.

- Be patient. You are all under stress. If you find you are losing your cool, listen to music, read, or go outside to shoot hoops or go for a run.

- Share a laugh. You've probably heard that laughter is good medicine. Watch a comedy on TV with your parent or tell jokes if that is your thing. Also, remember that you're not responsible for making everyone happy. You can only do so much.

- Buy your parent a new scarf or hat. Your parent might enjoy a new hat or scarf if he or she has lost their hair during treatment.

Help by Staying Involved

- Keep your parent in the loop. Tell your parent what you did to-day. Try to share what is going on in your life. Ask your parent how his or her day was.

- Talk about family history. Ask your parent about the past. Talk about what you're both most proud of, your best memories, and how you both have met challenges. Tape record, write, or draw these things. Ask to see old letters or photo albums.

- Keep a journal together. Write thoughts or poems, draw, or put photos in a notebook that the two of you share. This can help you share your feelings when it might be hard to speak them aloud.

- Help with younger brothers and sisters. Play with your broth-ers and sisters to give your parent a break. Pull out games or read a book with your siblings. This will help you stay close and also give your parent time to rest.

After Treatment

When your parent is finally done with treatment, you may feel a whole range of emotions. Part of you is glad it is over. Another part of you may miss the freedom or new responsibilities you had while your parent was getting treatment. You may feel confused that your parent still looks sick and is weaker than you expected. You may be afraid the cancer will come back. You may look at life differently now. All these feelings are normal. If you and your family are still feeling that life after treatment is harder than you thought it might be, you might want to talk to a counselor to get guidance through this time.

Things may not go back to exactly how they were before cancer came into your lives. Getting back to your "old life" may take a long time—or it may not happen as you expect.

What If Treatment Doesn't Help?

If treatment doesn't help your parent, you and your family will face even more challenges. Hearing that your parent might die is very difficult. You may feel many of the same emotions you felt when you first learned that your mom or dad had cancer.

No one else can give you all the answers or tell you exactly how you will feel. But when the future is so uncertain, teens say it helps to:

Make the most of the time you have: Do special things as a family. At home, make time for your mom or dad. Call and visit as much as you can if your parent is in the hospital. Write notes and draw pictures. Say "I love you" often. If possible, try to have some special times together. If you have not gotten along in the past, you may want to let your parent know you love him or her.

Stay on track: When people get bad news, they often feel like they're living outside of themselves—that life is moving along without them. That's why it's important to keep a schedule. Get up at the same time each day. Go to school. Meet with friends.

Get help when you feel alone: Make sure you find people who can help you. In addition to your family, it may help to talk to a social worker, counselor, or people in a support group.

The Road Ahead

It can be hard to stay calm when you aren't sure what the future holds. You may be thinking—will my parent survive cancer? Will the cancer come back? Will life ever be the same? Will I laugh again?

While no one can know the future, there are things you can do to make your life a little more stable:

- Keep talking and pulling together as a family. You may find that cancer has drawn you closer together and made you appreciate each other more than ever.

- Discover your own needs. Don't let others tell you how you should feel. Allow yourself to cope at your own pace and in your own way.

- Remember that you're growing as a person. Many teens say that having a parent with cancer has made them more sympathetic, more responsible, and stronger.

- Accept people's help. Right now you may feel lonelier than you ever have in your life. But you are not alone. Family, friends, support groups, neighbors, and counselors are there to lend a helping hand, listen to you, and be there for you.

- Appreciate each day. Many teens who have a parent with cancer say that they learned to see the world more clearly. In time you may come to appreciate things you may have overlooked in the past.

Learning More on Your Own

It's great that you want to learn more. Keep in mind that cancer treatments are getting better all the time. Make sure that what you read or see is up to date and accurate. Talk with your parent or other trusted adult about what you find. Share the articles or books you've found with them. Ask them any questions you may have. You can get information from:

Your school or public library: Ask the librarian to help you find the information or support that you're looking for in books, magazines, videos, or on the internet.

The internet: Use an Internet search engine and type in general words like "parent" and "cancer" together to get started. Keep in mind that the Internet has a lot of good information. It also has a lot of poor information and false promises, so you may want to check with your parent or another trusted adult about what you find.

Your parent's hospital or clinic: Visit the patient education office at your parent's hospital, if there is one. Or, ask if you can go with your parent during their visit to the doctor—to learn more.

Chapter 58

When Your Brother or Sister Has Cancer

You've Just Learned That Your Brother or Sister Has Cancer

You've just learned that your brother or sister has cancer. You may have a lot of emotions—feeling numb, afraid, lonely, or angry. One thing is certain—you don't feel good.

For now, try to focus on these facts:

- Many kids survive cancer. You have good reason to be hopeful that your brother or sister will get better. Today, as many as 8 in 10 kids diagnosed with cancer survive their illness. Many go on to live normal lives. That's because scientists are discovering new and better ways to find and treat cancer.

- You're not alone. Right now it might seem like no one else in the world feels the way you do. In a way you're right. No one can feel exactly like you do. But it might help to know that there are other kids who have a brother or sister with cancer. Talking to others may help you sort out your feelings. Remember, you are not alone.

Excerpted from "When Your Brother or Sister Has Cancer: A Guide for Teens," National Cancer Institute, April 2006. The complete text of this document is available online at http://www.cancer.gov, or it can be ordered by calling 800-4-CANCER.

- You're not to blame. Cancer is a disease with many causes, many of which doctors don't fully understand. But your brother or sister did not get cancer because of anything you did, thought, or said.

- You can't protect, but you can give comfort. Sometimes you'll be strong for your brother or sister, and sometimes your brother or sister will be strong for you. It's okay to talk about how hard it is and even cry together.

- Knowledge is power. It can help to learn more about cancer and cancer treatments. Sometimes what you imagine is actually worse than the reality.

Your Feelings

As you deal with your sibling's cancer, you may feel lots of different emotions. Some of the emotions you may feel are listed below.

Scared

- My world is falling apart.
- I'm afraid that my brother or sister might die.
- I'm afraid that someone else in my family might catch cancer. (They can't.)

It's normal to feel scared. Some of your fears may be real. Others may be based on things that won't happen. And some fears may lessen over time.

Guilty

- I feel guilty because I'm healthy and my brother or sister is sick.
- I feel guilty when I laugh and have fun.

You might feel guilty about having fun when your sibling is sick. This shows how much you care about them. But you should know that it is both okay and important for you to do things that make you happy.

Angry

- I am mad that my brother or sister is sick.
- I am angry at God for letting this happen.

- I am angry at myself for feeling the way I do.

- I am mad because I have to do all the chores now.

Anger often covers up other feelings that are harder to show. If having cancer in your family means that you can't do what you like to do and go where you used to go, it can be hard. Even if you understand why it's happening, you don't have to like it. But, don't let anger build up inside. Try to let it out. And when you get mad, remember that it doesn't mean you're a bad person or you don't love your sibling. It just means you're mad.

Neglected

- I feel left out.

- I don't get any attention any more.

- No one ever tells me what's going on.

- My family never talks anymore.

When your brother or sister has cancer, it's common for the family's focus to change. Your parents don't mean for you to feel left out. It just happens because so much is going on. You may want to tell your parents how you feel and what you think might help. Try to remember that you are important and loved and that you deserve to feel that way, even though you might not get as much attention from your parents right now.

Lonely

- My friends don't come over anymore.

- My friends don't seem to know what to say to me anymore.

- I miss being with my brother or sister the way we used to be.

We'll look at some things that may help you deal with changes in friendships later under the headings "You and Your Friends," and at things others have done to stay close to their siblings in "How You Can Help Your Brother or Sister." For now, try to remember that these feelings won't last forever.

Embarrassed

- I'm sometimes embarrassed to be out in public with my sibling because of how they look.

- I feel silly when I don't know how to answer people's questions.

It can help to know that other teens also feel embarrassed. So do their siblings. In time it gets easier, and you will find yourself feeling more comfortable.

Jealous

- I'm feeling upset that my brother or sister is getting all the attention.

Even if you understand why you are getting less attention, it's still not easy. Others who have a brother or sister with cancer have felt the same way. Try to share your feelings with your parents and talk about what you think might help.

What You're Feeling Is Normal

There is no one "right" way to feel. And you're not alone—many other teens in your situation have felt the same way. Some have said that having a brother or sister with cancer changes the way they look at things in life. Some even said that it made them stronger.

Dealing with Your Feelings

A lot of people are uncomfortable sharing their feelings. They ignore them and hope they'll go away. Others choose to act cheerful when they're really not. They think that by acting upbeat they won't feel sad or angry anymore. This may help for awhile, but not over the long run. Actually, holding your feelings inside can keep you from getting the help that you need.

Try these tips:

- Talk with family and friends that you feel close to. You owe it to yourself.

- Write your thoughts down in a journal.

- Join a support group to meet other kids who are facing some of the same things you are. Or meet with a counselor.

It is probably hard to imagine right now, but, if you let yourself, you can grow stronger as a person through this experience.

What Your Brother or Sister May Be Feeling

Just like everyone else, your brother or sister may be worried, scared, or confused. They may also feel tired and sick because of the treatment. Some kids feel embarrassed because treatment has changed the way they look and feel. You both may be having a lot of the same feelings.

Look at the World Through Your Brother's or Sister's Eyes

Knowing how your brother or sister might be feeling could help you figure out how to help, or at least understand where they are coming from. Here are a few things young people with cancer have felt:

- **Afraid:** Depending on how old your brother or sister is and how they react to tough situations, they may be more or less afraid.

- **Sad or depressed:** People with cancer sometimes can't do things they used to do. They may miss these activities and their friends. Feeling sad or down can range from a mild case of the blues to depression, which a doctor can treat.

- **Angry:** Cancer and treatment side effects can cause your brother or sister to be mad or grumpy. Anger sometimes comes from feelings that are hard to show, like being afraid, being very sad, or feeling helpless. Chances are your sibling is angry at the disease, not at you.

- **Guilty:** Your brother or sister may feel guilty that they caused changes in your family's life. But just as you did not cause this situation to happen, neither did your brother or sister.

- **Hopeful:** There are many reasons for your brother or sister to feel hopeful. Most kids survive cancer, and treatments are getting better all the time. Hope can be an important part of your brother's or sister's recovery.

All of these feelings are normal for a person living with cancer. You might want to share this list with your sibling. Ask them how they are feeling.

Changes in Your Family

Changing Routines and Responsibilities

Your family may be going through a lot of changes. You may be the oldest, youngest, or middle child in your family. You may live with one parent or two. Whatever your family situation, chances are that things have changed since your brother or sister got sick. This section looks at some of these changes and ways that others have dealt with them.

No one can be perfect all the time. You need time to feel sad or angry, as well as time to be happy. Try to let your parents and others you trust know how you're feeling—even if you have to start the conversation.

Touching Base when Things Are Changing

Families say that it helps to make time to talk together—even if it's only for a short time each week. Talking can help your family stay connected. Here are some things to consider when talking with older brothers and sisters:

- If you are the oldest child, your younger brothers or sisters may look to you for support. Help them as much as you can. It's okay to let them know that you are having a tough time, too.

- If you are looking to your older brother or sister for help, tell them how you are feeling. They can help, but they may not have all the answers.

Here are some things to consider when talking with your parents:

- Expect your parents to feel some stress, just like you may.
  Your parents may not always do or say the right thing.

- Try to make the most of the time you do have with your parents. Let them know how much it means to you. Maybe you can go out to dinner together, or they can come to your sports game, from time to time.

- Sometimes you may have to take the first step to start a conversation. You may feel guilty for wanting to have your needs met—but you shouldn't. You are important and loved, too.

- Keep talking with your parents, even though it may be hard.

Here is something to consider when talking with your brother or sister who has cancer:

- Your brother or sister may be sick from the treatment and want to be alone. Or maybe they feel okay and want your company.
  Try saying something like this: "Want to play a game—or talk?"

Keeping the Conversation Going

If you're used to talking openly at home, you might find that your parents aren't sharing as much anymore. Maybe they're trying to protect you from bad news or unsure about what to tell you. Some teens want to know a lot, while others only want to know a little. Tell your parents how much you want to know.

Over the next few weeks or months, you may overhear parts of your parents' conversations. If what you hear confuses or scares you, talk with your parents about what you heard.

Growing Stronger as a Family

Some families can grow apart for a while when a child has cancer. But there are ways to help your family grow stronger and closer. Teens who saw their families grow closer say that it happened because people in their family:

- Tried to put themselves in the other person's shoes and thought about how they would feel if they were the other person.

- Understood that even though people reacted differently to situations, they were all hurting. Some cried a lot. Others showed little emotion. Some used humor to get by.

- Learned to respect and talk about differences. The more they asked about how others were feeling, the more they could help each other.

How You Can Help Your Brother or Sister

- Hang out together. Watch a movie together. Read or watch TV together. Decorate your brother's or sister's bedroom with pictures or drawings. Go to the activity room at the hospital and play a game or do a project together.

- Comfort one another. Just being in the same room as your brother or sister can be a big comfort. Do what feels best for the two of you. Give hugs or say "I love you." Laugh or cry together. Talk to one another. Or just hang out in silence.

- Help your brother or sister stay in touch with friends. Ask your sibling's friends to write notes, send pictures, or record messages. Help your brother or sister send messages to their friends. If your brother or sister is up for it, invite friends to hang out with them.

- Share a laugh. You've probably heard that laughter is good medicine. Watch a comedy or tell jokes together.

- Be patient. Be patient with each other. Your brother or sister may be cranky or even mean. As bad as you feel, your brother or sister is probably feeling even worse. If you find you are losing your cool, go for a run, read, or listen to music.

- Make a snack. Make a snack for the two of you to share. Make a picnic by putting a blanket on the porch or in the bedroom.

- Buy a new scarf or hat. Your brother or sister might like a new hat or scarf if they have lost their hair during treatment. Get a matching hat or scarf for yourself, too.

- Try to be upbeat, but be "real," too. Being positive can be good for you and your whole family. But don't feel like you have to act cheerful all the time if that's not how you really feel. Try to be yourself.

- Keep a journal together. Write thoughts or poems, doodle, or put photos in a notebook. Take turns with your sibling writing in a journal. This can help you both share your thoughts when it might be hard to talk about them.

- Go for a walk together. If your brother or sister feels up to it, take a walk together. Or, open a window or sit on the front porch together.

- The ideas above are for those times when you have extra energy to give. Don't forget to take care of yourself, too. You deserve it.

Taking Care of Yourself

You may be so focused on your sick brother or sister that you don't think about your own needs, or if you do, they don't seem important. But they are! Read this section to learn ways to stay balanced at a time when everything may feel up in the air.

Dealing with Stress

Here are some tips that have worked to help other teens manage stress.

- Stay connected.
  - Spend some time at a friend's house.

- Stay involved with sports or clubs.
- Relax and get enough sleep.
  - Take breaks. You'll have more energy and be in a better frame of mind.
  - Get at least 8 hours of sleep each night.
  - Pray or meditate.
  - Make or listen to music.
- Help others.
  - Join a walk against cancer.
  - Plan a bake sale or other charity event to collect money to fight cancer.
- Avoid risky behaviors: Stay away from smoking, drinking, and other risky behaviors.
- Put your creative side to work.
  - Keep a journal to write down your thoughts and experiences.
  - Draw, paint, or take photographs.
  - Read books or articles about people who have made it through difficult experiences in life. Learn what helped them.
- Eat and drink well.
  - Switch to caffeine-free drinks in the evening that won't keep you awake.
  - Grab fresh fruit, whole-grain breads, and lean meats like chicken or turkey when you have a choice.
  - Avoid foods that have a lot of sugar.
  - Drink 6–8 glasses of water a day to help prevent fatigue.
- Be active: Exercise has been proven to make you feel better. Running, swimming, or even walking at a fast pace can help improve your mood.
  - Play a sport or go for a run.
  - Take the dog for a walk.
  - Learn about different stretching and breathing exercises.

Take Steps to Keep Things Simple

Staying organized can also keep your stress level under control. Here are some tips to get you started.

- At home
  - Make a list of things you want to do. Put the most important ones at the top.
  - Make a big calendar to help your family stay on top of things.
- At school
  - Let your teachers know what's happening at home, without using it as an excuse.
  - Talk to your teachers or a counselor if you are falling behind. They can help you.

Get Help when You Feel Down

Many teens feel low or down when their brother or sister is sick. It's normal to feel sad or "blue" during difficult times. However, if these feelings last for two weeks or more and start to interfere with things you used to enjoy, you may be depressed. The good news is that there is hope and there is help. Often, talking with a counselor can help. Below are some signs that you may need to see a counselor.

Are you:

- Feeling helpless and hopeless? Thinking that life has no meaning?
- Losing interest in being with family or friends?
- Finding that everything or everyone seems to get on your nerves?
- Feeling really angry a lot of the time?
- Thinking of hurting yourself?

Do you find that you are:

- Losing interest in the activities you used to enjoy?
- Eating too little or a lot more than usual?
- Crying easily or many times each day?
- Using drugs or alcohol to help you forget?

- Sleeping more than you used to? Less than you used to?
- Feeling tired a lot?

It's important to talk to someone you trust. Going to see a counselor doesn't mean that you are crazy. In fact, it means that you have the strength and courage to recognize that you are going through a difficult time and need help.

You and Your Friends

Your friends are important to you, and you're important to them. In the past, you could tell them everything. Now that your brother or sister has cancer, it may seem like lots is changing—even your friendships. Here are some things to think about:

- Some friends may not know what to say.
  - It's hard for some people to know what to say. They may be afraid of upsetting you. Try to be gentle with friends who don't ask how you're doing or who don't talk about your brother's or sister's cancer.
  - You may need to take the first step.
  - Try saying something like this: "Talking abut what's going on is hard. I know it's not easy to ask questions. But is there anything you what to talk about or know?"

- Some friends may ask tough questions.
  - It may be hard to answer questions about what you and your family are going through. You may want to try to help your friends understand what's going on. Or sometimes you may not feel like talking at all.
  - Try saying something like this: "Thanks for asking about my family and me. Here's what the doctors are saying: (add in your own information here)."
  - If you don't feel like talking, try saying something like this: "Thanks for asking, but can we talk later?"

- Your friends have their own lives.
  - It may feel like your friends don't care anymore. It might seem as though their lives are moving on and yours is not. It can be hard to watch them get together with others or do

things without you. They aren't facing the situation you are right now, so it may be hard for them to relate.

- You might want to try saying something like this: "I miss hanging out together. I know than I've had a lot on my mind since my sister got sick. Want to hand out tomorrow?"

Dealing with Embarrassment

It may be hard to talk with your friends. You may feel embarrassed that your brother or sister has cancer, or that now your family is different. You may not want to tell anyone about it. But when someone in your family is sick, you really need friends you can talk with.

Having Fun and Making New Friends

Old friends: Even though you may have a lot on your mind, you can still get together with your friends and have a good time. If you can't leave home as much, ask if your friends can come over. Make time to relax. It's both good and important for you.

New friends: A lot is happening to you right now. Sometimes old friends move on. You may not have as much in common as you used to. The good news is that you may make new friends through this experience. Kids who used to just pass you in the halls may now ask you how you are doing. Kids who you used to be friends with may become close friends again. Be open to new friendships.

Going to support groups at the hospital or at school is a good way to meet new friends. Support groups can help connect you with other kids who can relate to you—because they're going through some of the same things that you are.

Dealing with Hurtful Remarks

Unfortunately, some kids may say mean things. Others speak before they think and before they get the facts. No matter the reason, it can hurt when kids make jokes or say hurtful things about you, cancer, or your brother or sister. What can you do?

- Ignore the comment.

- Say, "Hey, my brother/sister has cancer. It's not funny. How would you feel if it were your brother/sister?"

- Being bullied? Go to your teacher, principal, or guidance counselor right away.

Finding Support

Don't let being afraid of the way you feel keep you from talking to your parents, a counselor, or kids in a support group.

For many people, starting to talk is difficult. Some teens don't have good relationships with their parents. Others are too embarrassed to talk about personal things. It can also just be hard to make the time to talk, with all that is going on. But you and your parents really can help each other. You may think: "I can solve all my own problems." However, when faced with tough situations, both teens and adults need support from others.

Tips for Talking with Your Parents

- Prepare before you talk.

  - Think about what you want to say and about some solutions to the problem.

  - Think about how your parents might react. How will you respond to them?

- Find a good time and place.

  - Find a private place, whether it's your room or the front steps. Or maybe you can talk while taking a walk or shooting hoops.

  - Ask your parents if they have a few minutes to talk.

- Take things slowly.

  - Don't expect to solve everything right away. Difficult problems often don't have simple solutions.

  - Work together to find a way through these challenges. Some conversations will go better than others.

- Keep it up.

  - Don't think you have to have just one big conversation. Have lots of small ones.

  - Make time to talk a little each day if you can, even if it's just for a few minutes.

Talking with a Counselor

Sometimes talking to friends and your parents is not enough. When you are having a hard time, it can be helpful to talk to a counselor.

Remember—going to a counselor means you have the courage to recognize that you're going through a tough time and need some help. Simply put: talking to a counselor can help you feel better. Counselors are specially trained to help you sort out your feelings, gain new skills to deal with what's going on, and find solutions that work for you. Teens who've talked with a counselor say it helped to talk to someone outside their circle of friends and family who didn't take sides, who they could trust. Others say they learned a lot about themselves and felt better able to face life's challenges.

Joining a Support Group

A good outlet for connecting with teens that are going through the same thing that you are is a support group. Some groups meet in person; others meet online. Some groups go out and do activities together. At first this may not sound like something you want to do. Other teens have thought the same thing—until they went to a meeting. They were surprised that so many other kids felt the same way they did and had advice that really seems to work. Your parents or another trusted adult can help you find a support group.

After Treatment

When your brother or sister has finally completed treatment, you and your family may feel a whole range of emotions. Part of you is glad it is over. Another part of you may miss the freedom or new responsibilities you had while your parent was busy taking care of your sick brother or sister.

Your brother or sister may still look sick and be weaker than you expected. You may be afraid the cancer will come back. You may be looking to find more meaning in your life now. All these feelings are normal. Things may not go back to exactly how they were before cancer came into your lives. Getting back to your "old life" may take a long time—and it may not happen as you expect.

The Road Ahead

It can be hard to stay calm when you aren't sure what the future holds. You may be thinking—will my brother or sister live? Will the cancer come back? Will life ever be the same? Will I laugh again? Enjoy being with friends again?

While no one can know the future, there are things you can do to make your life a little easier:

- Keep talking and pulling together as a family. You may find that cancer has drawn you closer together and made you appreciate each other more.

- Discover your own needs. Don't let others tell you how you should feel. Allow yourself to cope at your own pace and in your own way.

- Remember that you're growing as a person. Many teens say that having a brother or sister with cancer has made them more sympathetic, more responsible, and stronger.

- Keep in mind that you aren't alone. Right now you may feel lonelier than you ever have in your life. But you are not alone. Family members, friends, neighbors, support groups, and counselors are there to lend a helping hand, listen to you, and give you good advice. Accept their help; you deserve it.

- Appreciate each day. Many teens who have a brother or sister with cancer say that they learned to see the world more clearly. In time you may come to appreciate things you may have overlooked in the past.

Unfortunately, no book or person can tell you how everything is going to work out. Cancer is tough, and your life may never be quite the same. But in the end, you will get through it. Why? You're strong. And you are capable—even if you don't always feel that way.

Learning More on Your Own

Keep in mind that cancer treatments are getting better all the time. Make sure that what you read or see is up to date and accurate. Talk with your parents or another trusted adult about what you find. Share the articles or books you've found with them. Ask them any questions you may have.

Part Eight

Additional Help and Information

Chapter 59

A Glossary of Cancer Care Terms

abdominoperineal resection: Surgery to remove the anus, the rectum, and part of the sigmoid colon through an incision made in the abdomen. The end of the intestine is attached to an opening in the surface of the abdomen and body waste is collected in a disposable bag outside of the body. This opening is called a colostomy. Lymph nodes that contain cancer may also be removed during this operation.

ablation: In medicine, the removal or destruction of a body part or tissue or its function. Ablation may be performed by surgery, hormones, drugs, radiofrequency, heat, or other methods.

action study: In cancer prevention clinical trials, a study that focuses on finding out whether actions people take can prevent cancer.

activities of daily living (ADL): The tasks of everyday life. Basic ADLs include eating, dressing, getting into or out of a bed or chair, taking a bath or shower, and using the toilet. Instrumental activities of daily living (IADL) are activities related to independent living and include preparing meals, managing money, shopping, doing housework, and using a telephone.

acupressure: The application of pressure or localized massage to specific sites on the body to control symptoms such as pain or nausea. It is a type of complementary and alternative medicine.

Excerpted from "Dictionary of Cancer Terms," National Cancer Institute (www.cancer.gov/dictionary), 2006.

acupuncture: The technique of inserting thin needles through the skin at specific points on the body to control pain and other symptoms. It is a type of complementary and alternative medicine.

acute: Symptoms or signs that begin and worsen quickly; not chronic.

adjunct therapy: Another treatment used together with the primary treatment. Its purpose is to assist the primary treatment. It is also called adjunctive therapy.

adjustment disorder: A condition in which a person responds to a stressful event (such as an illness, job loss, or divorce) with extreme emotions and actions that cause problems at work and home.

adjuvant therapy: Treatment given after the primary treatment to increase the chances of a cure. Adjuvant therapy may include chemotherapy, radiation therapy, hormone therapy, or biological therapy.

agent study: In cancer prevention clinical trials, a study that tests whether taking certain medicines, vitamins, minerals, or food supplements can prevent cancer. Also a called chemoprevention study.

allogeneic bone marrow transplantation: A procedure in which a person receives stem cells (cells from which all blood cells develop) from a genetically similar, but not identical, donor.

allogeneic stem cell transplantation: A procedure in which a person receives blood-forming stem cells (cells from which all blood cells develop) from a genetically similar, but not identical, donor. This is often a sister or brother, but could be an unrelated donor.

allopathic medicine: A system in which medical doctors and other healthcare professionals (such as nurses, pharmacists, and therapists) treat symptoms and diseases using drugs, radiation, or surgery. It is also called conventional medicine, Western medicine, mainstream medicine, orthodox medicine, and biomedicine.

anastomosis: A procedure to connect healthy sections of tubular structures in the body after the diseased portion has been surgically removed.

angiogram: An x-ray of blood vessels; the person receives an injection of dye to outline the vessels on the x-ray.

animal study: A laboratory experiment using animals to study the development and progression of diseases. Animal studies also test how safe and effective new treatments are before they are tested in people.

anti-idiotype vaccine: A vaccine made of antibodies that see other antibodies as the antigen and bind to it. Anti-idiotype vaccines can stimulate the body to produce antibodies against tumor cells.

anticarcinogenic: Having to do with preventing or delaying the development of cancer.

antioxidant: A substance that protects cells from the damage caused by free radicals (unstable molecules made by the process of oxidation during normal metabolism). Free radicals may play a part in cancer, heart disease, stroke, and other diseases of aging. Antioxidants include beta-carotene, lycopene, vitamins A, C, and E, and other natural and manufactured substances.

aromatherapy: A type of complementary and alternative medicine that uses plant oils that give off strong pleasant aromas (smells) to promote relaxation, a sense of well-being, and healing.

barium swallow: A series of x-rays of the esophagus. The x-ray pictures are taken after the person drinks a solution that contains barium. The barium coats and outlines the esophagus on the x-ray. It is also called an esophagram and upper GI series.

BCG solution: A form of biological therapy for superficial bladder cancer. A catheter is used to place the BCG solution into the bladder. The solution contains live, weakened bacteria (bacillus Calmette-Guérin) that activate the immune system. The BCG solution used for bladder cancer is not the same thing as BCG vaccine, a vaccine for tuberculosis.

benign: Not cancerous. Benign tumors may grow larger but do not spread to other parts of the body.

biofeedback: A method of learning to voluntarily control certain body functions such as heartbeat, blood pressure, and muscle tension with the help of a special machine. This method can help control pain.

biopsy: The removal of cells or tissues for examination by a pathologist. The pathologist may study the tissue under a microscope or perform other tests on the cells or tissue. When only a sample of tissue is removed, the procedure is called an incisional biopsy. When an entire lump or suspicious area is removed, the procedure is called an excisional biopsy.

blood-brain barrier disruption: The use of drugs to create openings between cells in the blood-brain barrier. The blood-brain barrier is a protective network of blood vessels and tissue that protects the brain from harmful substances, but can also prevent anticancer drugs from reaching the brain. Once the barrier is opened, anticancer drugs may be infused into an artery that goes to the brain, in order to treat brain tumors.

body mass index (BMI): A measure that relates body weight to height. BMI is sometimes used to measure total body fat and whether a person is a healthy weight. Excess body fat is linked to an increased risk of some diseases including heart disease and some cancers.

bone marrow transplantation: A procedure to replace bone marrow that has been destroyed by treatment with high doses of anticancer drugs or radiation. Transplantation may be autologous (an individual's own marrow saved before treatment), allogeneic (marrow donated by someone else), or syngeneic (marrow donated by an identical twin).

bone scan: A technique to create images of bones on a computer screen or on film. A small amount of radioactive material is injected into a blood vessel and travels through the bloodstream; it collects in the bones and is detected by a scanner.

bone-seeking radioisotope: A radioactive substance that is given through a vein, and collects in bone cells and in tumor cells that have spread to the bone. It kills cancer cells by giving off low-level radiation.

bronchoscopy: A procedure that uses a bronchoscope to examine the inside of the trachea, bronchi (air passages that lead to the lungs), and lungs. A bronchoscope is a thin, tube-like instrument with a light and a lens for viewing. It may also have a tool to remove tissue to be checked under a microscope for signs of disease. The bronchoscope is inserted through the nose or mouth. Bronchoscopy may be used to detect cancer or to perform some treatment procedures.

bypass: A surgical procedure in which the doctor creates a new pathway for the flow of body fluids.

case report: A detailed report of the diagnosis, treatment, and follow-up of an individual patient. Case reports also contain some demographic information about the patient (for example, age, gender, ethnic origin).

chemoembolization: A procedure in which the blood supply to the tumor is blocked surgically or mechanically and anticancer drugs are administered directly into the tumor. This permits a higher concentration of drug to be in contact with the tumor for a longer period of time.

chemoprevention: The use of drugs, vitamins, or other agents to try to reduce the risk of, or delay the development or recurrence of, cancer.

chemotherapy: Treatment with drugs that kill cancer cells.

chest x-ray: An x-ray of the structures inside the chest. An x-ray is a type of high-energy radiation that can go through the body and onto film, making pictures of areas inside the chest, which can be used to diagnose disease.

chronic: A disease or condition that persists or progresses over a long period of time.

clinical breast exam: An exam of the breast performed by a health care provider to check for lumps or other changes.

clinical trial: A type of research study that tests how well new medical approaches work in people. These studies test new methods of screening, prevention, diagnosis, or treatment of a disease. It is also called a clinical study.

cohort study: A research study that compares a particular outcome (such as lung cancer) in groups of individuals who are alike in many ways but differ by a certain characteristic (for example, female nurses who smoke compared with those who do not smoke).

complementary and alternative medicine (CAM): Forms of treatment that are used in addition to (complementary) or instead of (alternative) standard treatments. These practices generally are not considered standard medical approaches. Standard treatments go through a long and careful research process to prove they are safe and effective, but less is known about most types of CAM. CAM may include dietary supplements, megadose vitamins, herbal preparations, special teas, acupuncture, massage therapy, magnet therapy, spiritual healing, and meditation.

computerized axial tomography scan (CT Scan): A series of detailed pictures of areas inside the body, taken from different angles; the pictures are created by a computer linked to an x-ray machine. It is also called computed tomography (CT scan) or computerized tomography.

data safety and monitoring committee: An impartial group that oversees a clinical trial and reviews the results to see if they are acceptable. This group determines if the trial should be changed or closed.

dementia: A condition in which a person loses the ability to think, remember, learn, make decisions, and solve problems. Symptoms may also include personality changes and emotional problems. There are many causes of dementia, including Alzheimer disease, brain cancer, and brain injury. Dementia usually gets worse over time.

diagnostic mammogram: X-ray of the breasts used to check for breast cancer after a lump or other sign or symptom of breast cancer has been found.

dose-dense chemotherapy: A chemotherapy treatment plan in which drugs are given with less time between treatments than in a standard chemotherapy treatment plan.

drug resistance: The failure of cancer cells, viruses, or bacteria to respond to a drug used to kill or weaken them. The cells, viruses, or bacteria may be resistant to the drug at the beginning of treatment, or may become resistant after being exposed to the drug.

electroacupuncture: A procedure in which pulses of weak electrical current are sent through acupuncture needles into acupuncture points in the skin. This procedure is being studied in the prevention of nausea and vomiting in patients undergoing chemotherapy.

electroconvulsive therapy (ET): A treatment for severe depression and certain mental disorders. A brief seizure is induced by giving electrical stimulation to the brain through electrodes placed on the scalp. It is also called electroshock therapy.

electroporation therapy (EPT): Treatment that generates electrical pulses through an electrode placed in a tumor to enhance the ability of anticancer drugs to enter tumor cells.

endocervical curettage: A procedure in which the mucous membrane of the cervical canal is scraped using a spoon-shaped instrument called a curette.

endocrine therapy: Treatment that adds, blocks, or removes hormones. For certain conditions (such as diabetes or menopause), hormones are given to adjust low hormone levels. To slow or stop the growth of certain cancers (such as prostate and breast cancer), synthetic hormones or other drugs may be given to block the body's natural hormones.

Sometimes surgery is needed to remove the gland that makes a certain hormone. It is also called hormone therapy, hormonal therapy, or hormone treatment.

endometrial biopsy: A procedure in which a sample of tissue is taken from the endometrium (inner lining of the uterus) for examination under a microscope. A thin tube is inserted through the cervix into the uterus, and gentle scraping and suction are used to remove the sample.

endpoint: In clinical trials, an event or outcome that can be measured objectively to determine whether the intervention being studied is beneficial. The endpoints of a clinical trial are usually included in the study objectives. Some examples of endpoints are survival, improvements in quality of life, relief of symptoms, and disappearance of the tumor.

external radiation: Radiation therapy that uses a machine to aim high-energy rays at the cancer. It is also called external-beam radiation.

fluoroscope: An x-ray machine that makes it possible to see internal organs in motion.

gamma scanning: A procedure to find areas in the body where cells, such as tumor cells, are dividing rapidly. A small amount of radioactive material is injected into a vein or swallowed, and travels through the bloodstream. A machine called a scanner measures the radioactivity and produces pictures (scans) of internal parts of the body. The pictures can show abnormal changes in the area of the body containing the radioactive material. Examples of gamma scans include PET scans, gallium scans, and bone scans. It is also called radionuclide scanning.

gastroscopy: Examination of the inside of the stomach using a gastroscope passed through the mouth and esophagus. A gastroscope is a thin, tube-like instrument with a light and a lens for viewing. It may also have a tool to remove tissue to be checked under a microscope for signs of disease. It is also called upper endoscopy.

gene therapy: Treatment that alters a gene. In studies of gene therapy for cancer, researchers are trying to improve the body's natural ability to fight the disease or to make the cancer cells more sensitive to other kinds of therapy.

hepatectomy: Surgery to remove all or part of the liver.

high-dose radiation (HDR): An amount of radiation that is greater than that given in typical radiation therapy. HDR is precisely directed at the tumor to avoid damaging healthy tissue, and may kill more cancer cells in fewer treatments.

high-energy photon therapy: A type of radiation therapy that uses high-energy photons (units of light energy). High-energy photons penetrate deeply into tissues to reach tumors while giving less radiation to superficial tissues such as the skin.

historic cohort study: A research study in which the medical records of groups of individuals who are alike in many ways but differ by a certain characteristic (for example, female nurses who smoke and those who do not smoke) are compared for a particular outcome (such as lung cancer). It is also called a retrospective cohort study.

hormone replacement therapy (HRT): Hormones (estrogen, progesterone, or both) given to women after menopause to replace the hormones no longer produced by the ovaries. It is also called menopausal hormone therapy.

hospice: A program that provides special care for people who are near the end of life and for their families, either at home, in freestanding facilities, or within hospitals.

hysterectomy: Surgery to remove the uterus and, sometimes, the cervix. When the uterus and part, or all, of the cervix are removed, it is called a total hysterectomy. When only the uterus is removed, it is called a partial hysterectomy.

immunotherapy: Treatment to stimulate or restore the ability of the immune system to fight cancer, infections, and other diseases. Also used to lessen certain side effects that may be caused by cancer treatment. It is It is also called biological therapy, biotherapy, or biological response modifier (BRM) therapy.

informed consent: A process in which a person learns key facts about a clinical trial or genetic testing before deciding whether or not to take part in it. Informed consent includes information about the possible risks, benefits, and limits of the trial or genetic testing. It goes on through the entire trial or genetic testing process.

Institutional Review Board (IRB): A group of scientists, doctors, clergy, and consumers that reviews and approves the action plan for every clinical trial. There is an IRB at every health care facility that does clinical research. IRBs are designed to protect the people who take part in a clinical trial. IRBs check to see that the trial is well designed, legal, ethical, does not involve unnecessary risks, and includes safeguards for patients.

intensity-modulated radiation therapy (IMRT): A type of 3-dimensional radiation therapy that uses computer-generated images to show the size and shape of the tumor. Thin beams of radiation of different intensities are aimed at the tumor from many angles. This type of radiation therapy reduces the damage to healthy tissue near the tumor.

internal radiation: A procedure in which radioactive material sealed in needles, seeds, wires, or catheters is placed directly into or near a tumor. It is It is also called brachytherapy, implant radiation, or interstitial radiation therapy.

intrathecal chemotherapy: Treatment in which anticancer drugs are injected into the fluid-filled space between the thin layers of tissue that cover the brain and spinal cord.

intravenous pyelogram (IVP): A series of x-rays of the kidneys, ureters, and bladder. The x-rays are taken after a dye is injected into a blood vessel. The dye is concentrated in the urine, which outlines the kidneys, ureters, and bladder on the x-rays.

investigational drug: A substance that has been tested in a laboratory and has gotten approval from the U.S. Food and Drug Administration (FDA) to be tested in people. A drug may be approved by the FDA for use in one disease or condition but be considered investigational in other diseases or conditions. It is also called an experimental drug.

laboratory test: A medical procedure that involves testing a sample of blood, urine, or other substance from the body. Tests can help determine a diagnosis, plan treatment, check to see if treatment is working, or monitor the disease over time.

laparoscopy: A procedure that uses a laparoscope, inserted through the abdominal wall, to examine the inside of the abdomen. A laparoscope is a thin, tube-like instrument with a light and a lens for viewing. It may also have a tool to remove tissue to be checked under a microscope for signs of disease.

light-emitting diode therapy (LED therapy): Treatment with drugs that become active and may kill cancer cells when exposed to light. LED therapy is type of photodynamic therapy which uses a special type of light to activate the drug.

local therapy: Treatment that affects cells in the tumor and the area close to it.

lymph node dissection: A surgical procedure in which the lymph nodes are removed and examined to see whether they contain cancer. For a regional lymph node dissection, some of the lymph nodes in the tumor area are removed; for a radical lymph node dissection, most or all of the lymph nodes in the tumor area are removed. It is also called lymphadenectomy.

magnetic resonance imaging (MRI): A procedure in which radio waves and a powerful magnet linked to a computer are used to create detailed pictures of areas inside the body. These pictures can show the difference between normal and diseased tissue. MRI makes better images of organs and soft tissue than other scanning techniques, such as CT or x-ray. MRI is especially useful for imaging the brain, spine, the soft tissue of joints, and the inside of bones. It is also called nuclear magnetic resonance imaging.

maintenance therapy: Treatment that is given to help a primary (original) treatment keep working. Maintenance therapy is often given to help keep cancer in remission.

massage therapy: A treatment in which the soft tissues of the body are kneaded, rubbed, tapped, and stroked. Massage therapy may help people relax, relieve stress and pain, lower blood pressure, and improve circulation. It is being studied in the treatment of cancer symptoms such as lack of energy, pain, swelling, and depression.

microwave therapy: A type of treatment in which body tissue is exposed to high temperatures to damage and kill cancer cells or to make cancer cells more sensitive to the effects of radiation and certain anticancer drugs. It is also called microwave thermotherapy.

needle biopsy: The removal of tissue or fluid with a needle for examination under a microscope. It is also called fine-needle aspiration.

ointment: A substance used on the skin to soothe or heal wounds, burns, rashes, scrapes, or other skin problems. It is also called unguent.

oophorectomy: Surgery to remove one or both ovaries.

open colectomy: An operation to remove all or part of the colon through a long incision made in the wall of the abdomen. When only part of the colon is removed, it is called a partial colectomy.

open label study: A type of study in which both the health providers and the patients are aware of the drug or treatment being given.

operable: Describes a condition that can be treated by surgery.

outpatient: A patient who visits a health care facility for diagnosis or treatment without spending the night. Sometimes called a day patient.

over-the-counter (OTC): A medicine that can be bought without a prescription (doctor's order). Examples include analgesics (pain relievers) such as aspirin and acetaminophen. It is also called nonprescription.

pain threshold: The point at which a person becomes aware of pain.

palliation: Relief of symptoms and suffering caused by cancer and other life-threatening diseases. Palliation helps a patient feel more comfortable and improves the quality of life, but does not cure the disease.

palliative therapy: Treatment given to relieve the symptoms and reduce the suffering caused by cancer and other life-threatening diseases. Palliative cancer therapies are given together with other cancer treatments, from the time of diagnosis, through treatment, survivorship, recurrent or advanced disease, and at the end of life.

Pap smear: A procedure in which cells are scraped from the cervix for examination under a microscope. It is used to detect cancer and changes that may lead to cancer. A Pap smear can also show noncancerous conditions, such as infection or inflammation. It is also called a Pap test.

pelvic examination: A physical examination in which the health care professional will feel for lumps or changes in the shape of the vagina, cervix, uterus, fallopian tubes, ovaries, and rectum. The health care professional will also use a speculum to open the vagina to look at the cervix and take samples for a Pap test. It is also called an internal examination.

phase I trial: The first step in testing a new treatment in humans. These studies test the best way to give a new treatment (for example, by mouth, intravenous infusion, or injection) and the best dose. The dose is usually increased a little at a time in order to find the highest dose that does not cause harmful side effects. Because little is known about the possible risks and benefits of the treatments being tested, phase I trials usually include only a small number of patients who have not been helped by other treatments.

phase I/II trial: A trial to study the safety, dosage levels, and response to a new treatment.

phase II trial: A study to test whether a new treatment has an anti-cancer effect (for example, whether it shrinks a tumor or improves blood test results) and whether it works against a certain type of cancer.

phase II/III trial: A trial to study response to a new treatment and the effectiveness of the treatment compared with the standard treatment regimen.

phase III trial: A study to compare the results of people taking a new treatment with the results of people taking the standard treatment (for example, which group has better survival rates or fewer side effects). In most cases, studies move into phase III only after a treatment seems to work in phases I and II. Phase III trials may include hundreds of people.

phase IV trial: After a treatment has been approved and is being marketed, it is studied in a phase IV trial to evaluate side effects that were not apparent in the phase III trial. Thousands of people are involved in a phase IV trial.

physical therapy: The use of exercises and physical activities to help condition muscles and restore strength and movement. For example, physical therapy can be used to restore arm and shoulder movement and build back strength after breast cancer surgery.

placebo: An inactive substance or treatment that looks the same as, and is given the same way as, an active drug or treatment being tested. The effects of the active drug or treatment are compared to the effects of the placebo.

positron emission tomography scan (PET scan): A procedure in which a small amount of radioactive glucose (sugar) is injected into a vein, and a scanner is used to make detailed, computerized pictures of areas inside the body where the glucose is used. Because cancer cells often use more glucose than normal cells, the pictures can be used to find cancer cells in the body.

quality of life: The overall enjoyment of life. Many clinical trials assess the effects of cancer and its treatment on the quality of life. These studies measure aspects of an individual's sense of well-being and ability to carry out various activities.

radiation surgery: A radiation therapy procedure that uses special equipment to position the patient and precisely deliver a large radiation dose to a tumor and not to normal tissue. This procedure does not use surgery. It is used to treat brain tumors and other brain disorders. It is also being studied in the treatment of other types of cancer, such as lung cancer. It is also called radiosurgery, stereotactic external-beam radiation, stereotactic radiation therapy, stereotactic radiosurgery, and stereotaxic radiosurgery.

radioimmunotherapy: Treatment with a radioactive substance that is linked to an antibody that will attach to the tumor when injected into the body.

recurrent cancer: Cancer that has returned after a period of time during which the cancer could not be detected. The cancer may come back to the same place as the original (primary) tumor or to another place in the body. It is also called recurrence.

remission: A decrease in or disappearance of signs and symptoms of cancer. In partial remission, some, but not all, signs and symptoms of cancer have disappeared. In complete remission, all signs and symptoms of cancer have disappeared, although cancer still may be in the body.

single blind study: A type of clinical trial in which only the doctor knows whether a patient is taking the standard treatment or the new treatment being tested. This helps prevent bias in treatment studies.

spinal tap: A procedure in which a needle is put into the lower part of the spinal column to collect cerebrospinal fluid or to give drugs. It is also called a lumbar puncture.

stem cell transplantation: A method of replacing immature blood-forming cells that were destroyed by cancer treatment. The stem cells are given to the person after treatment to help the bone marrow recover and continue producing healthy blood cells.

supportive care: Care given to improve the quality of life of patients who have a serious or life-threatening disease. The goal of supportive care is to prevent or treat as early as possible the symptoms of the disease, side effects caused by treatment of the disease, and psychological, social, and spiritual problems related to the disease or its treatment. It is also called palliative care, comfort care, and symptom management.

survivorship: In cancer, survivorship covers the physical, psychosocial, and economic issues of cancer, from diagnosis until the end of life. It includes issues related to the ability to get health care and follow up treatment, late effects of treatment, second cancers, and quality of life.

transperineal biopsy: A procedure in which a sample of tissue is removed from the prostate for examination under a microscope. The sample is removed with a thin needle that is inserted through the skin between the scrotum and rectum and into the prostate.

ultrasound: A procedure in which high-energy sound waves (ultrasound) are bounced off internal tissues or organs and make echoes. The echo patterns are shown on the screen of an ultrasound machine, forming a picture of body tissues called a sonogram. It is also called ultrasonography.

vaccine therapy: A type of treatment that uses a substance or group of substances to stimulate the immune system to destroy a tumor or infectious microorganisms such as bacteria or viruses.

Chapter 60

Terms to Help You Understand Your Medical Bill and Health Insurance

access: The right or ability to obtain health care services. Often determined by location of facilities, transportation, hours of operation, cost of care and availability.

activities of daily living (ADLs): Daily routine of self-care activities such as dressing, bathing, and eating.

allowed expenses: The maximum amount a plan pays for a covered service.

ambulatory care: Medical services provided on an outpatient (non-hospitalized) basis.

ancillary services: Health care services provided by professionals other than primary care physicians.

average length of stay: Average number of inpatient days spent in a hospital or other health care facility per admission or discharge. Calculated by total number of days in the facility for all admissions occurring during a period divided by the number of admission during the same period. This varies and is measured for patients based on age, specific diagnoses or sources of payment.

"Glossary of Financial and Medical Terms," by Maggie Hampshire, RN, BSN, reprinted with permission from www.oncolink.com. Copyright © 2001 by the Trustees of the University of Pennsylvania. All rights reserved.

balance billing: The practice of billing patients for all charges over the physician rate paid by insurers. Many managed care plans prohibit this practice.

benefits: These are medical services for which your insurance plan will pay, in full or in part.

capitation: Method of payment for health services in which a physician or hospital is paid a fixed amount for each enrollee regardless of the actual amount or type of services provided to each person. The provider is responsible for delivering or arranging for the delivery of all health services required by the covered person under the conditions of the provider contract.

case management: A planned approach to manage services or treatments to an individual with specific health care needs. The goal is to contain costs and promote more effective intervention to meet patient needs and achieve optimum patient outcome.

case manager: An experienced health care professional (nurse, social worker, doctor or pharmacist) who works with patients, providers, and insurers to coordinate all necessary aspects of health care. Case managers evaluate necessity, appropriateness, and efficiency of services and drugs provided to individual patients.

claim: A notice to the insurance company that a person received care covered by the plan. A claim is also a request for payment.

co-insurance: A term that describes a shared payment between an insurance company and an insured individual. It's usually described in percentages; for example, the insurance company agrees to pay 80% of covered charges and the individual picks up 20%.

co-payment: The insured individual's portion of the cost of their care, usually a flat dollar amount, like $10 per office visit. Under many plans, co-payments are made at the time of the service and the health plan pays for the remainder of the fee.

coverage: What services the health plan does and does not pay for.

covered expenses: What the insurance company will consider paying for as defined in the contract. For example, under some plans generic prescriptions are covered expenses while brand name prescriptions are not.

customary charge: A fee is considered "Customary" if it is within the range of fees that most physicians who practice in the area charge.

deductible: A portion of the covered expenses (typically $100, $200 or $500) that an insured individual must pay before insurance coverage with co-insurance goes into effect. Deductibles are standard in many policies, and are usually based on a calendar year.

diagnosis related groups (DRGs): The hospital classification and reimbursement system that groups patients by diagnosis, surgical procedures, age, sex, and presence of complications. This is a financing mechanism used to reimburse hospital and selected other providers for services rendered.

exclusive provider organization (EPO): Arrangement consisting of a group of providers who have a contract with an insurer, employer, third party administrator or other sponsoring group. Criteria for provider participation may be the same of those in PPOs but have a more restrictive provider selection and credentialing process.

experimental procedures: Any health care services, that are determined by the insurance plan to be either; not generally accepted by informed health care professionals in the United States as effective in treating the condition, illness or diagnosis for which their use is proposed; or not proven by scientific evidence to be effective in treating the condition for which it is proposed.

fee-for-service: A traditional health care payment system in which physicians and other providers receive payment based on each billed charge for a visit or service rendered.

health maintenance organization (HMO): An organization that provides, offers or arranges for a wide range of covered health care services for a specified group of enrollees for a fixed, periodic prepayment. Models include: group model, individual practice association, network model, mixed model, and staff model. Under the Federal HMO Act, an entity must have three characteristics to call itself an HMO:

1. An organized system for providing health care or otherwise assuring health care delivery in a geographic area.

2. An agreed upon set of basic and supplemental health maintenance and treatment services.

3. A voluntarily enrolled group of people.

inpatient care: The type of treatment you receive when you are an overnight patient at a hospital or treatment center.

managed care: A system that integrates financing, delivery, and measurement of appropriate medical care through:

1. contracts with selected physicians, hospitals, and pharmacy benefit networks to furnish a comprehensive set of health care services to enrolled members, usually for a predetermined monthly premium,

2. utilization and quality controls that contracting providers agree to accept,

3. financial incentives for patients to use providers and facilities associated with the plan, and

4. in some cases an assumption of some financial risk by physicians. The goal is to provide value through a system that provides people access to quality, cost-effective health care.

managed care plan: A term that typically refers to an HMO, Point of Service, or PPO, but technically means any health plan with specific requirements, like pre-authorization or second opinions which enable your primary care physician to coordinate or manage all aspects of your medical care.

maximum out-of-pocket: The most money you can expect to pay for covered expenses. The maximum limit varies from plan to plan. Once the maximum out-of-pocket has been met, the health plan will pay 100% of certain covered expenses.

Medicaid: A program of health insurance provided by the state and federal government for the poor, elderly and disabled.

Medicare: Health insurance provided by the federal government for the elderly and disabled.

open enrollment: A specified period of time in which employees may change insurance plans and medical groups offered by their employer and have the new insurance effective at a later date.

outpatient care: Treatment in a doctor's office or clinic.

participating provider: A provider who has contracted with the health plan to deliver medical services to covered persons. The provider may be a hospital, pharmacy, or other facility or a physician who has contractually accepted the terms and conditions as set forth by the health plan.

physician hospital organization (PHO): An arrangement between a hospital and physicians to pursue managed care contracts. A PHO fosters mutual interests while allowing for some autonomy. In a physician hospital organization, physicians retain ownership of their practices.

point of service (POS) plan: Managed care product that offers enrollees a choice among options when they need medical services, rather than when they enroll in the plan. Enrollees may use providers outside the managed care network, but usually at higher cost. (This should not be confused with POS as used in retail pharmacy, where it stands for point of sale.)

preauthorization: An insurance plan requirement in which you or your primary care physician need to notify your insurance company in advance about certain medical procedures (like outpatient surgery) in order for those procedures to be considered a covered expense.

preexisting conditions: Illnesses or problems a patient had before obtaining an insurance policy. Some insurance companies may refuse to issue a policy or not pay for care for the preexisting or may not pay for that condition for a set period of time.

preferred provider organization: A program in which contracts are established with providers of medical care. Usually the benefit contract provides significantly better benefits (few co-payments) for services received from preferred providers, thus encouraging covered persons to use these providers. Covered persons generally are allowed benefits for non-participating providers services, usually on an indemnity basis with significant co-payments. A PPO arrangement can be insured or self-funded. Providers may be, but are not necessarily, paid on a discounted fee-for-service.

premium: The amount paid for any insurance policy.

primary care physician: (PCP) A PCP is the doctor responsible for coordinating all of your care. Any specialist referrals you'll need must first be approved by your PCP in order to be considered a covered expense.

private insurance: Traditional health care coverage purchased from an insurance company. Gives you free choice of physicians, hospitals, and other health care facilities.

provider: The supplier of health care services. This could be a physician, a hospital, or a physical therapist.

reasonable charge: A fee is considered "reasonable" if it is both usual and customary or if it is justified because there is a complex problem involved.

referral: Approval or consent by a primary care physician for patient referral to ancillary services and specialists.

second opinion: An opinion obtained from an additional health care professional prior to the performance of a medical service or a surgical procedure. May refer to a formalized process, voluntary or mandatory, which is used to help educate a patient regarding treatment alternatives or to determine medical necessity.

single-payer: Government-paid health care (often called "socialized medicine") using tax dollars.

specialist: A physician who practices medicine in a specialty area. Cardiologists, orthopedists, and gynecologists are all examples of specialists. Under most health plans, family practice physicians, pediatricians, and internal medicine physicians are not specialists.

subscriber: The person responsible for payment of premiums or whose employment is the basis for eligibility for membership in an HMO or other health plan.

subsidies: Government assistance to help low-income patients pay for basic services like health care.

tertiary care: Health care services provided by highly specialized providers such as neurosurgeons, thoracic surgeons, and intensive care units. These services often require highly sophisticated technologies and facilities.

usual charge: A fee is considered "Usual" if it is the amount that most physicians in the area charge for this same service.

utilization review: Programs designed to reduce unnecessary medical services, both inpatient and outpatient. Utilization reviews may be prospective, retrospective, concurrent, or in relation to discharge planning.

viatical settlement: An option which involves selling the ill person's life insurance policy for a percentage of the total face value. By selling it while the person is still alive, the insured person can receive a sizable sum of money, to be used entirely at the person's own discretion.

References

Encyclopedia of Practice and Financial Management, Second Edition, Edited By Lawrence Farber, Medical Economics Books, 1988, Page 250, 7:2:1.

HealthNet Customer Service Glossary: Copyright © Mid America Health Network, Inc., 1997.

The HMO Page: Copyright © 1996 by Physicians Who Care. All Rights Reserved.

Chapter 61

Resources for Cancer Patients

To make specific information easier to find, the resources in this chapter are listed alphabetically under the following headings:

- Resources for Finding and Evaluating Cancer Treatments and Healthcare Providers
- Resources for Locating Clinical Trials for Cancer Care
- National Organizations That Offer Services to People with Cancer and Their Families

Resources for Finding and Evaluating Cancer Treatments and Healthcare Providers

Agency for Healthcare Research and Quality
Publications Clearinghouse:
800-358-9295
Website: http://www.ahrq.gov

American Board of Medical Specialties
1007 Church Street, Suite 404
Evanston, IL 60201-5913
Website: http://www.abms.org

This chapter includes excerpts from "National Organizations That Offer Services to People with Cancer and Their Families," National Cancer Institute (http://www.cancer.gov) and information from other sources deemed reliable. Inclusion does not constitute endorsement and omission does not imply disapproval. All contact information was updated and verified in October 2006.

569

American College of Surgeons
633 North Saint Clair Street
Chicago, IL 60611-3211
Phone: 312-202-5000
Website: http://web.facs.org

American Society for Laser Medicine and Surgery
2100 Stewart Ave., Suite 240
Wausau, WI 54401
Phone: 715-845-9283
Fax: 715-848-2493
Website: http://www.aslms.org
E-mail: information@aslms.org

American Society of Clinical Oncology
1900 Duke Street, Suite 200
Alexandria, VA 22314
Toll-Free: 888-651-3038
Phone: 703-299-0150
Website: http://www.asco.org

Association of Community Cancer Centers
11600 Nebel Street, Suite 201
Rockville, MD 20852-2557
Phone: 301-984-9496
Fax: 301-770-1949
Website: http://
www.accc-cancer.org

Blood and Marrow Transplant Information Network
2900 Skokie Valley Road, Suite B
Highland Park, IL 60035
Toll-Free: 888-597-7674
Phone: 847-433-3313
Fax: 847-433-4599
Website: http://bmtinfonet.org
E-mail: help@bmtinfonet.org

Cancer Trials Support Unit
CTSU Data Operations Center
1441 W. Montgomery Ave.
Rockville, MD 20850-2062
Toll-Free: 888-823-5923
Toll-Free Fax: 888-691-8039
Website: www.ctsu.org
E-mail:
CTSUcontact@westat.com

CancerGuide
Website: http://cancerguide.org

CureSearch
4600 East West Highway
Suite 600
Bethesda, MD 20814-3457
Toll-Free: 800-458-6223
Website: http://
www.curesearch.org
E-mail: info@curesearch.org

Dana Farber Cancer Institute
44 Binney Street
Boston, MA 02115
Toll-free: 866-408-3324
Phone: 617-632-6366
Spanish: 617-632-3673
TDD: 617-632-5330
Website: www.dana-farber.org
E-mail: Dana-FarberContactUs
@dfci.Harvard.edu

Federal Trade Commission
Consumer Response Center
CRC-240
Washington, DC 20580
Toll-Free: 877-FTC-HELP
TTY: 202-326-2502
Website: http://www.ftc.gov

International Cancer Information Service Group
National Cancer Institute Public Inquiries Office
Cancer Information Service, Room 3036A
Website: http://www.icisg.org
E-mail: info@icisq.org

Joint Commission on Accreditation of Healthcare Organizations
One Renaissance Boulevard
Oakbrook Terrace, IL 60181-4294
Phone: 630-792-5800
Website: http://
www.jointcommision.org

National Association for Proton Therapy
1301 Highland Drive
Silver Spring, MD 20910
Phone: 301-587-6100
Website: http://
www.proton-therapy.org

National Cancer Institute (NCI)
Public Inquiries Office
Suite 3036A
6116 Executive Boulevard, MSC8322
Bethesda, MD 20892-8322
Toll-Free: 800-4-CANCER
(800-422-6237)
TTY: 800-332-8615
Website: http://www.cancer.gov

National Center for Complementary and Alternative Medicine
NCCAM Clearinghouse
Post Office Box 7923
Gaithersburg, MD 20898-7923
Toll-Free: 888-644-6226
International: 301-519-3153
TTY: 1-866-464-3615
Fax-on-Demand: 888-644-6226
Website: http://nccam.nih.gov
E-mail: info@nccam.nih.gov

National Comprehensive Cancer Network
Toll-Free: 888-909-6226
Website: http://www.nccn.org

Pediatric Oncology Branch
National Cancer Institute
Toll-Free: 877-624-4878
Phone: 301-496-4256
Website: http://home.ccr.cancer
.gov/oncology/pediatric

U.S. Food and Drug Administration (FDA)
5600 Fishers Lane
Rockville, MD 20857
Toll-Free: 888-463-6332
Website: http://www.fda.gov
Dietary Supplements Web page:
http://www.cfsan.fda.gov/~dms/
supplmnt.html

Resources for Locating Clinical Trials for Cancer Care

Acurian
Website: http://www.acurian.com

Cancer411
Website: http://
www.cancer411.com

CancerConsultants
411 6th Street
Ketchum, ID 83340
Website: http://www
.patient.cancerconsultants.com

**Centerwatch Clinical
Trials Listing Service**
22 Thompson Place, 36T1
Boston, MA 02210-1212
Toll-Free: 800-765-9647
Phone: 617-856-5900
Fax: 617-856-5901
Website: www.centerwatch.com
E-mail:
cw.trialwatch@centerwatch.com

ClinicalTrialsSearch.org
Website: http://
www.clinicaltrialssearch.org

EmergingMed
Website: http://
www.emergingmed.com

**National Cancer Institute
Cancer Trials**
NCI Public Inquiries Office
6116 Executive Blvd., MSC8322
Suite 3036A
Toll-free: 800-4-CANCER
(800-422-6237)
TTY: 800-332-8615
Website: www.cancer.gov/
clinicaltrials

TrialCheck
Coalition of National Cancer
Cooperative Groups
Website: http://
www.trialcheck.org

**U.S. National Library of
Medicine**
Website: http://
www.clinicaltrials.gov

Veritas Medicine
Website: http://
www.veritasmedicine.com

National Organizations That Offer Services to People with Cancer and Their Families

American Cancer Society
13599 Clifton Road, NE
Atlanta, GA 30329-4251
Toll-Free: 800-227-2345
Phone: 404-320-3333
Website: http://www.cancer.org

The ACS is a voluntary organization that offers a variety of services to patients and their families. The ACS also supports research, provides printed materials, and conducts educational programs. Staff can accept calls and distribute publications in Spanish. A local ACS unit may be listed in the white pages of the telephone directory under "American Cancer Society."

Armstrong (Lance) Foundation (LAF)
P.O. Box 161150
Austin, TX 78716-1150
Phone: 512-236-8820
Website: http://www.laf.org

The LAF, a nonprofit organization founded by cancer survivor and cyclist Lance Armstrong, provides resources and support services to people diagnosed with cancer and their families. The LAF's services include Cycle of Hope, a national cancer education campaign for people with cancer and those at risk for developing the disease, and the Cancer Profiler, a free interactive treatment decision support tool. The LAF also provides scientific and research grants for the better understanding of cancer and cancer survivorship.

Bloch Cancer Foundation, Inc.
4400 Main Street
Kansas City, MO 64111
Toll-Free: 800-433-0464
Phone: 816-854-5050
E-mail: hotline@hrblock.com
Website: http://www.blochcancer.org

The R. A. Bloch Cancer Foundation matches newly diagnosed cancer patients with trained, home-based volunteers who have been treated for the same type of cancer. They also distribute informational materials, including a multidisciplinary list of institutions that offer second opinions. Information is available in Spanish.

Cancer Hope Network
Two North Road
Chester, NJ 07930
Toll-Free: 877-467-3638
Website: http://www.cancerhopenetwork.org
E-mail: info@cancerhopenetwork.org

Cancer Hope Network provides individual support to cancer patients and their families by matching them with trained volunteers who have undergone and recovered from a similar cancer experience. Such matches are based on the type and stage of cancer, treatments used, side effects experienced, and other factors.

Cancer Information and Counseling Line
1600 Pierce Street
Denver, CO 80214
Toll-Free: 800-525-3777

The CICL, part of the Psychosocial Program of the AMC Cancer Research Center, is a toll-free telephone service for cancer patients, their family members and friends, cancer survivors, and the general public. Professional counselors provide up-to-date medical information, emotional support through short-term counseling, and resource referrals to callers nationwide between the hours of 8:30 A.M. and 5:00 P.M. Mountain Standard Time, Monday through Friday. Individuals may also submit questions about cancer and request resources via e-mail.

CancerCare, Inc.
National Office
275 Seventh Avenue
New York, NY 10001
Toll-Free: 800-813-4673; Phone: 212-712-8400
Website: http://www.cancercare.org
E-mail: info@cancercare.org

CancerCare is a national nonprofit agency that offers free support, information, financial assistance, and practical help to people with cancer and their loved ones. Services are provided by oncology social workers and are available in person, over the telephone, and through the agency's website.

Candlelighters® Childhood Cancer Foundation
P.O. Box 498
Kensington, MD 20895-0498
Toll-Free: 800-366-2223
Phone: 301-962-3520
Website: http://www.candlelighters.org
E-mail: info@candlelighters.org

The CCCF is a nonprofit organization that provides information, peer support, and advocacy through publications, an information clearinghouse, and a network of local support groups. A financial aid list is available that lists organizations to which eligible families may apply for assistance.

ENCOREPlus®
YWCA of the USA
Office of Women's Health Advocacy
015 18th Street, NW
Suite 1100
Washington, DC 20036
Toll-Free: 800-953-7587 (800-95E-PLUS)
Phone: 202-467-0801
E-mail: ywca.@info.org
Website: http://www.ywca.org

ENCOREPlus is the YWCA's discussion and exercise program for women who have had breast cancer surgery. It is designed to help restore physical strength and emotional well-being. A local branch of the YWCA, listed in the telephone directory, can provide more information about ENCOREPlus.

Fertile Hope
P.O. Box 624
New York, NY 10014
Toll-Free: 888-994-4673
Phone: 212-242-6798
E-mail: info@fertilehope.org
Website: http://www.fertilehope.org

Fertile Hope is a national organization that provides reproductive information, support, and hope to cancer patients whose medical treatments present the risk of infertility. They also offer fertility preservation financial assistance options for patients.

Gilda's Club® Worldwide

322 Eighth Avenue, Suite 1402
New York, NY 10001
Toll-Free: 888-445-3248
Website: http://www.gildasclub.org
E-mail: info@gildasclub.org

Gilda's Club Worldwide works with communities to start and maintain local Gilda's Clubs, which provide social and emotional support to cancer patients, their families, and friends. Lectures, workshops, support and networking groups, special events, and children's programs are offered. Services are available in Spanish.

International Association of Laryngectomees

P.O. Box 691060
Stockton, CA 95269-1060
Website: http://www.larynxlink.com
E-mail: ialhq@larynxlink.com

The IAL assists people who have lost their voice as a result of cancer. It provides information on the skills needed by laryngectomees and works toward total rehabilitation of patients.

KidsCope

2045 Peachtree Road, Suite 150
Atlanta, GA 30309
Phone: 404-892-1437
Website: http://www.kidscope.org

This website provides information for children of cancer patients.

Living Beyond Breast Cancer

10 East Athens Avenue, Suite 204
Ardmore, PA 19003
Toll-Free: 888-753-5222 (Survivors' Helpline); Phone: 610-645-4567
E-mail: mail@lbbc.org
Website: http://www.lbbc.org

The LBBC is an educational organization that aims to empower women living with breast cancer to live as long as possible with the best quality of life. The LBBC offers an interactive message board and information about upcoming conferences and teleconferences on its website. In addition, the organization has a toll-free Survivors' Helpline, a Young Survivors' Network for women diagnosed with breast cancer who are age 45 or younger, and outreach programs for medically underserved communities. The LBBC also offers a quarterly educational newsletter and a book for African American women living with breast cancer.

National Asian Women's Health Organization
250 Montgomery Street, Suite 900
San Francisco, CA 94104
E-mail: nawho@nawho.org
Website: http://www.nawho.org

The NAWHO is working to improve the health status of Asian women and families through research, education, leadership, and public policy programs. They have resources for Asian women in English, Cantonese, Laotian, Vietnamese, and Korean. Publications on subjects such as reproductive rights, breast and cervical cancer, and tobacco control are available.

National Bone Marrow Transplant Link
20411 West 12 Mile Road, Suite 108
Southfield, MI 48076
Toll-Free: 800-546-5268
Website: http://www.nbmtlink.org
E-mail: info@nbmtlink.org

The nbmtLink motto is "A second chance at life is our first priority." The nbmtLink operates a 24-hour, toll-free number and provides peer support to bone marrow transplant (BMT) patients and their families. It serves as an information center for prospective BMT patients as well as a resource for health professionals. Educational publications, brochures, and videos are available. Staff can respond to calls in Spanish.

National Childhood Cancer Foundation
440 East Huntington Drive
Arcadia, CA 91006-6012
Toll-Free: 800-458-6223; Phone: 626-447-1674
Fax: 626-447-6359

The NCCF supports research conducted by a network of institutions, each of which has a team of doctors, scientists, and other specialists with the special skills required for the diagnosis, treatment, supportive care, and research on the cancers of infants, children, and young adults. Advocating for children with cancer and the centers that treat them is also a focus of the NCCF.

577

National Children's Cancer Society

1015 Locust, Suite 600
St. Louis, MO 63101
Toll-Free: 800-532-6459; Phone: 314-241-1600
Fax: 314-241-1996
Program Services Fax: 314-241-6949
Website: http://www.children-cancer.org

The NCCS helps children with cancer get the care and support they deserve. They provide emotional support, advocacy, education and financial assistance. The website contains links to organizations which provide scholarships for survivors.

National Coalition for Cancer Survivorship

1010 Wayne Avenue, Suite 770
Silver Spring, MD 20910-5600
Toll-Free: 877-622-7937
Phone: 301-650-9127
Website: http://www.canceradvocacy.org
E-mail: info@canceradvocacy.org

The NCCS is a network of groups and individuals that offer support to cancer survivors and their loved ones. It provides information and resources on cancer support, advocacy, and quality-of-life issues. A section of the NCCS website and a limited selection of publications are available in Spanish.

National Lymphedema Network

1611 Telegraph Avenue, Suite 1111
Oakland, CA 94612-2138
Toll-Free: 800-541-3259; Phone: 510-208-3200
Website: http://www.lymphnet.org
E-mail: nln@lymphnet.org

The NLN provides education and guidance to lymphedema patients, health care professionals, and the general public by disseminating information on the prevention and management of primary and secondary lymphedema. They provide a toll-free support hotline, a referral service to lymphedema treatment centers and health care professionals, a quarterly newsletter with information about medical and scientific developments, support groups, pen pals, educational courses for health care professionals and patients, and a computer database. Some Spanish-language materials are available.

National Marrow Donor Program®
3001 Broadway Street, NE, Suite 500
Minneapolis, MN 55413-1753
Toll-Free: 800-526-7809; Phone: 612-627-5800
Office of Patient Advocacy: 888-999-6743
Website: http://www.marrow.org

The NMDP, which is funded by the federal government, was created to improve the effectiveness of the search for bone marrow donors. It keeps a registry of potential bone marrow donors and provides free information on bone marrow transplantation, peripheral blood stem cell transplant, and unrelated donor stem cell transplant, including the use of umbilical cord blood. The NMDP's Office of Patient Advocacy assists transplant patients and their physicians through the donor search and transplant process by providing information, referrals, support, and advocacy.

Office of Cancer Survivorship
Website: http://dccps.nci.nih.gov/ocs

The National Cancer Institute's Office of Cancer Survivorship provides information on new and innovative research in cancer survivorship.

Patient Advocate Foundation
753 Thimble Shoals Boulevard, Suite B
Newport News, VA 23606
Toll-Free: 800-532-5274; Phone: 757-873-6668
Website: http://www.patientadvocate.org
E-mail: help@patientadvocate.org

The PAF provides education, legal counseling, and referrals to cancer patients and survivors concerning managed care, insurance, financial issues, job discrimination, and debt crisis matters.

People Living With Cancer
American Society of Clinical Oncology
1900 Duke Street, Suite 200
Alexandria, VA 22314
Phone: 703-797-1914; Fax: 703-299-1044
Website: http://www.plwc.org
E-mail: contactus@plwc.org

PLWC is a website for patients provided by the American Society of Clinical Oncology. It provides general cancer information, a guide to comprehensive information about different types of cancers and related syndromes, facts about cancer diagnosis and treatment options. The site also provides information about cancer survivorship and practical suggestions for coping with cancer's physical effects.

Sisters Network®, Inc.
8787 Woodway Drive, Suite 4206
Houston, TX 77063
Toll-Free: 866-781-1808; Phone: 713-781-0255
Website: http://www.sistersnetworkinc.org
E-mail: infonet@sisternetworkinc.org

Sisters Network seeks to increase local and national attention to the impact that breast cancer has in the African American community. All chapters are run by breast cancer survivors and receive volunteer assistance from community leaders and associate members. The services provided by Sisters Network include individual/group support, community education, advocacy, and research. The national headquarters serves as a resource and referral base for survivors, clinical trials, and private/government agencies. Teleconferences are held to update chapters with the latest information and share new ideas. An educational brochure designed for underserved women is available. In addition, a national African American breast cancer survivors' newsletter is distributed to survivors, medical facilities, government agencies, organizations, and churches nationwide.

Starlight Starbright Children's Foundation
5757 Wilshire Boulevard, Suite M100
Los Angeles, CA 90036
Toll-Free: 800-315-2580; Phone: 310-479-1212
Website: http://www.starlight.org

In July 2004, the Starlight Children's Foundation and the STARBRIGHT Foundation merged to form the Starlight Starbright Children's Foundation. Starlight Starbright is an international nonprofit organization designed to help seriously ill children and adolescents cope with the psychosocial and medical challenges they face. Starlight Starbright offers in-hospital, outpatient, school, and home-based programs and services free of charge to children, adolescents, and their families during the course of an illness and during recovery. Staff can respond to calls in Spanish, and some of the programs are offered in Spanish.

Support for People with Oral and Head and Neck Cancer
P.O. Box 53
Locust Valley, NY 11560-0053
Toll-Free: 800-377-0928
Website: http://www.spohnc.org
E-mail: info@spohnc.org

The SPOHNC is a self-help organization that serves oral and head and neck cancer patients, survivors, and their families. The organization offers support group meetings, information, newsletters, and teleconferences. The SPOHNC also offers a "Survivor to Survivor" network which pairs survivors or their family members with volunteers who have had a similar diagnosis and treatment program.

Teens Living with Cancer
Website: http://www.teenslivingwithcancer.org

This site, which is written for adolescent cancer patients, includes basic information about cancer, facts about specific cancers, and descriptions of cancer treatments.

United Ostomy Association
19772 MacArthur Boulevard, Suite 200
Irvine, CA 92612-2405
Toll-Free: 800-826-0826
Website: http://www.uoa.org

The United Ostomy Association helps ostomy patients through mutual aid and emotional support. It provides information to patients and the public and sends volunteers to visit with new ostomy patients.

US® TOO! International, Inc.
5003 Fairview Avenue
Downers Grove, IL 60515
Toll-Free: 800-808-7866
Phone: 630-795-1002
E-mail: ustoo@ustoo.org
Website: http://www.ustoo.org

US TOO is a prostate cancer support group organization. Goals of US TOO are to increase awareness of prostate cancer in the community, educate men newly diagnosed with prostate cancer, offer support groups, and provide the latest information about treatment for this disease.

Vital Options® International TeleSupport® Cancer Network
15821 Ventura Boulevard, Suite 645
Encino, CA 91436-2946
Toll-Free: 800-477-7666
Phone: 818-788-5225
E-mail: info@vitaloptions.org
Website: http://www.vitaloptions.org

The mission of Vital Options is to use communications technology to reach people dealing with cancer. This organization holds a weekly syndicated call-in cancer radio talk show called "The Group Room®," which provides a forum for patients, long-term survivors, family members, physicians, and therapists to discuss cancer issues. Listeners can participate in the show during its broadcast every Sunday from 4 PM to 6 PM. Eastern time by calling the toll-free telephone number. A live Web simulcast of "The Group Room" can be heard by logging onto the Vital Options Web site.

Wellness Community®
919 18th Street, NW, Suite 54
Washington, DC 20006
Toll-Free: 888-793-9355
Phone: 202-659-9709
Website: http://www.thewellnesscommunity.org
E-mail: help@thewellnesscommunity.org

The Wellness Community provides free psychological and emotional support to cancer patients and their families. They offer support groups facilitated by licensed therapists, stress reduction and cancer education workshops, nutrition guidance, exercise sessions, and social events.

Chapter 62

The National Cancer Institute Cancer Centers Program

The Cancer Centers Program of the National Cancer Institute (NCI) supports major academic and research institutions throughout the United States to sustain broad-based, coordinated, interdisciplinary programs in cancer research. These institutions are characterized by scientific excellence and the capability to integrate a diversity of research approaches to focus on the problem of cancer. The NCI and its Cancer Centers Program are dedicated to the advancement of cancer research to ultimately impact on the reduction of cancer incidence, morbidity, and mortality.

Several cancer centers existed in the late 1960s, but it was the National Cancer Act of 1971 that strengthened the program by authorizing the establishment of 15 new cancer centers while continuing to support existing ones. The passage of the Act also dramatically transformed the structure of the centers and broadened the scope of their mission to include all aspects of basic, clinical, and cancer control research. Today, 60 NCI-designated cancer centers continue to work toward creating new and innovative approaches to cancer research. Through interdisciplinary efforts, cancer centers can effectively move this research from the laboratory into clinical trials (research studies) and finally into clinical practice.

An NCI-designated cancer center may be a freestanding operation, a center within an academic institution, or a formal consortium

"The National Cancer Institute Cancer Centers Program," National Cancer Institute (www.cancer.gov), reviewed April 2006. All contact information was verified and updated in January 2007.

under centralized leadership. But all NCI-designated cancer centers must meet the same scientific, organizational, and administrative criteria.

Cancer centers seeking NCI-designation must first apply for an NCI cancer center support grant. Application for NCI-designation is voluntary and is awarded through a peer-review process. Institutes that are awarded the grant are then recognized as NCI-designated. All NCI-designated cancer centers receive substantial financial support from NCI grants and are reevaluated each time their cancer center support grant comes up for renewal (generally every three to five years).

The NCI recognizes two types of centers: Cancer Centers and Comprehensive Cancer Centers. Each type of center has special characteristics and capabilities for organizing new programs of research that can take advantage of important new findings and address timely research questions. It is important to note, however, that the terms NCI-designated Comprehensive Cancer Center and NCI-designated Cancer Center do not denote a difference in the quality of care they provide to patients.

Facilities designated Cancer Centers generally conduct a combination of basic, population sciences, and clinical research, and are encouraged to stimulate collaborative research involving more than one field of study. Several of these centers conduct only laboratory research and do not provide patient care. The NCI-designated Cancer Centers that do provide patient care are also expected to conduct early-phase, innovative clinical trials and to participate in the NCI Cooperative Group Program. (More information about the Institute's Cooperative Group Program can be found in the NCI fact sheet NCI's Clinical Trials Cooperative Group Program, which is available at http://www.cancer.gov/cancertopics/factsheet/NCI/clinical-trials-cooperative-group on the internet.)

NCI-designated Comprehensive Cancer Centers conduct research and provide services directly to cancer patients. These facilities must demonstrate expertise in each of three areas: laboratory, clinical, and behavioral and population-based research. Comprehensive Cancer Centers are expected to initiate and conduct early-phase, innovative clinical trials, and to participate in the NCI's cooperative groups by providing leadership and recruiting patients for trials. Comprehensive Cancer Centers must also conduct activities in outreach and education, and provide information on advances in health care for both health care professionals and the public.

Included is a list of the NCI-designated cancer centers. Additional information about the Cancer Centers Program can be found on the Cancer Centers Branch website at http://www3.cancer.gov/cancercenters/ on the internet.

Key

* * Comprehensive Cancer Centers supported by NCI
* ** Cancer Centers supported by NCI
* ° denotes facilities that are strictly laboratories and do not provide patient services

Information about referral procedures, treatment costs, and services available to patients can be obtained by contacting the individual cancer centers listed below.

Alabama

University of Alabama at Birmingham Comprehensive Cancer Center*
1824 Sixth Avenue South
Birmingham, AL 35294-3300
Toll-Free: 800-822-0933 (800-UAB-0933)
Phone: 205-975-8222
Website: http://www3.ccc.uab.edu

Arizona

Arizona Cancer Center*
University of Arizona
1515 North Campbell Avenue
Tucson, AZ 85724
Toll-Free: 800-622-2673
Phone: 520-694-2873
Website: http://
www.arizonacancercenter.org

Mayo Clinic Cancer Center—Scottsdale*
13400 East Shea Boulevard
Scottsdale, AZ 85259
Phone: 480-301-8484
Appointment Office: 480-301-1735
Website: http://www
.mayoclinic.org/cancercenter

California

Burnham Institute**°
10901 North Torrey Pines Road
La Jolla, CA 92037
Phone: 858-646-3100
Website: http://
www.burnhaminstitute.org
E-mail: info@burnham.org

Chao Family Comprehensive Cancer Center*
University of California, Irvine
101 The City Drive
Building 23, Route 81
Orange, CA 92868
Phone: 714-456-8200
Building 23: 714-456-8000
Website: http://
www.ucihs.uci.edu/cancer

City of Hope*
Cancer Center and Beckman Research Institute
1500 East Duarte Road
Duarte, CA 91010-3000
Toll-Free: 800-826-4673 (800-826-HOPE)
Phone: 626-256-4673 (626-256-HOPE)
Website: http://
www.cityofhope.org

Jonsson Comprehensive Cancer
Center at UCLA*
8-684 Factor Building
UCLA Box 951781
Los Angeles, CA 90095-1781
Phone: 310-825-5268
Website: http://
www.cancer.mednet.ucla.edu
E-mail:
jcccinfo@mednet.ucla.edu

Rebecca and John Moores
University of California, San
Diego Cancer Center*
3855 Health Sciences Drive
La Jolla, CA 92093-0658
Phone: 858-534-7600
Cancer Information: 858-822-
6146
Fax: 858-534-7628
Website: http://cancer.ucsd.edu

Salk Institute for Biological
Studies** °
10010 North Torrey Pines Road
La Jolla, CA 92037
Phone: 858-453-4100
Website: http://www.salk.edu

UC Davis Cancer Center**
University of California, Davis
4501 X Street
Sacramento, CA 95817
Toll-Free: 800-362-5566 (patient
referral)
Phone: 916-734-5900
Website: http://
cancer.ucdmc.ucdavis.edu

University of California, San
Francisco Comprehensive
Cancer Center*
1600 Divisadero Street
San Francisco, CA 94143-0128
Toll-Free Cancer Referral Line:
800-888-8664
Phone: 515-353-9888
Website: http://cancer.ucsf.edu
E-mail: referral.center
@ucsfmedicalcenter.org

USC/Norris Comprehensive
Cancer Center*
1441 Eastlake Avenue
Los Angeles, CA 90033
Phone: 323-865-3000
Toll-Free: 800-872-2273
(800-USC-CARE)
Website: http://ccnt.hsc.usc.edu

Colorado

University of Colorado Cancer
Center*
Anschutz Cancer Pavilion
1665 North Ursula Street
Aurora, CO 80045
Toll-Free Cancer Referral Line:
800-473-2288
Phone: 720-848-0300
Website: http://www.uccc.info

Connecticut

Yale Cancer Center*
Yale University School of
Medicine
333 Cedar Street
Post Office Box 208032
New Haven, CT 06520-8032
Phone: 203-785-4191
Website: http://
www.info.med.yale.edu/ycc

District of Columbia

Lombardi Comprehensive
Cancer Center*
Georgetown University Medical
Center
3800 Reservoir Road, NW
Washington, DC 20007
Phone: 202-444-4000
Website: http://
lombardi.georgetown.edu

Florida

Mayo Clinic Cancer Center—
Jacksonville*
4500 San Pablo Road
Jacksonville, FL 32224
Phone: 904-953-2000
TTD: 904-953-2300
Website: http://www
.mayoclinic.org/cancercenter

H. Lee Moffitt Cancer Center &
Research Institute at the
University of South Florida*
12902 Magnolia Drive
Tampa, FL 33612-9497
Phone: 813-745-4673
Toll-Free: 800-456-3434
Website: http://www.moffitt.org

Hawaii

Cancer Research Center of
Hawaii**
1236 Lauhala Street
Honolulu, HI 96813
Phone: 808-586-3010
Website: http://www.crch.org

Illinois

Robert H. Lurie Comprehensive
Cancer Center*
Northwestern University
Galter Pavilion
675 N. St. Clair, 21st Floor
Chicago, IL 60611
Phone: 312-908-5250
Toll-Free Appointment Line:
866-587-4322 (866-LURIE-CC)
Website: http://cancer
.northwestern.edu/home/index
.cfm
E-mail:
cancer@northwestern.edu

University of Chicago Cancer
Research Center**
5841 South Maryland Avenue
Mail Code 1140
Chicago, IL 60637-1470
Toll-Free New Patient Line:
888-824-0200
Phone: 773-702-6180
Website: http://
uccrc.uchicago.edu

Indiana

Indiana University Cancer
Center**
535 Barnhill Drive
Indianapolis, IN 46202-5289
Phone: 317-278-4822
Toll-Free: 888-600-4822
Website: http://cancer.iu.edu

Iowa

Holden Comprehensive Cancer
Center at The University of
Iowa*
4802 JPP
200 Hawkins Drive
Iowa City, IA 52242-1009
Toll-Free: 800-237-1225
Website: http://
www.uihealthcare.com/depts/
cancercenter
E-mail: Cancer-info@uiowa.edu

Maine

Jackson Laboratory** °
600 Main Street
Bar Harbor, ME 04609-0800
Phone: 207-288-6000 (main)
Phone: 207-288-6051 (public
information)
Website: http://www.jax.org
E-mail: pubinfo@jax.org

Maryland

Sidney Kimmel Comprehensive
Cancer Center at Johns
Hopkins*
Harry and Jeanette Weinberg
Building
401 North Broadway, Suite 1100
Baltimore, MD 21231-2410
Phone: 410-955-8964 (patient
referral)
Phone: 410-955-8804 (clinical
trials)
Website: http://www
.hopkinskimmelcancercenter.org

Massachusetts

Dana-Farber Cancer Institute*
44 Binney Street
Boston, MA 02115
Toll-Free: 866-408-3324 (866-
408-DFCI)
Website: http://www.dana-farber
.org

MIT Center for Cancer
Research** °
Massachusetts Institute of
Technology
77 Massachusetts Avenue
Room E17-110
Cambridge, MA 02139-4307
Phone: 617-253-8511
Website: http://web.mit.edu/ccr

Michigan

Barbara Ann Karmanos Cancer Institute*
Operating the Meyer L. Prentis Comprehensive Cancer Center of Metropolitan Detroit
Wertz Clinical Cancer Center
4100 John R Street
Detroit, MI 48201-1379
Toll-Free: 800-527-6266 (800-KARMANOS)
Website: http://www.karmanos.org
E-mail: info@karmanos.org

University of Michigan Comprehensive Cancer Center*
1500 East Medical Center Drive
Ann Arbor, MI 48109-0944
Toll-Free Cancer Answer Line: 800-865-1125
Website: http://www.mcancer.org
E-mail: www.cancer@umich.edu

Minnesota

Mayo Clinic Cancer Center*
200 First Street, SW.
Rochester, MN 55905
Phone: 507-266-9288
Website: http://www.mayoclinic.org/cancercenter

University of Minnesota Cancer Center*
Mayo Mail Code 806
420 Delaware Street, SE.
Minneapolis, MN 55455
Phone: 612-624-8484
Website: http://www.cancer.umn.edu
E-mail: info@cancer.umn.edu

Missouri

Siteman Cancer Center*
Barnes-Jewish Hospital and Washington University School of Medicine Cancer Information Center
4921 Parkview Place
Mail Stop 90-35-703
St. Louis, MO 63110
Toll-Free: 800-600-3606
Phone: 314-362-07844
Website: http://www.siteman.wustl.edu

Nebraska

UNMC Eppley Cancer Center**
University of Nebraska Medical Center
986805 Nebraska Medical Center
Omaha, NE 68198-6805
Phone: 402-559-4238
or 402-553-4090
Website: http://www.unmc.edu/cancercenter

New Hampshire

Norris Cotton Cancer Center*
Dartmouth-Hitchcock Medical Center
One Medical Center Drive
Lebanon, NH 03756-0002
Toll-Free Cancer Helpline: 800-639-6918
Phone: 603-653-9000
Website: http://www.cancer.dartmouth.edu
E-mail: cancerhelp@dartmouth.edu

New Jersey

Cancer Institute of New Jersey*
195 Little Albany Street
New Brunswick, NJ 08903-2681
Phone: 732-235-2465 (732-235-CINJ)
Website: http://www.cinj.org

New Mexico

UNM Cancer Research and
Treatment Center **
University of New Mexico
Health Sciences Center
MSC 08 4630
900 Camino de Salud NE
Albuquerque, NM 87131-0001
Toll-Free: 800-432-6806
Phone: 505-272-4946
Website: http://cancer.unm.edu

New York

Cold Spring Harbor
Laboratory**°
Post Office Box 100
One Bungtown Road
Cold Spring Harbor, NY 11724
Phone: 516-367-8397
or 516-367-8800
Website: http://www.cshl.org

Albert Einstein Cancer Center**
Albert Einstein College of
Medicine
1300 Morris Park Avenue
Bronx, NY 10461
Phone: 718-430-2302
Website: http://
www.aecom.yu.edu/cancer
E-mail: aecc@aecom.yu.edu

Herbert Irving Comprehensive
Cancer Center*
New York-Presbyterian Hospital
Columbia University Medical
Center
PH 18, Room 200
622 West 168th Street
New York, NY 10032
Toll-Free: 877-697-9355
(877-NYP-WELL)
Toll-Free Physician Referral
Line: 800-227-2762
Website: www.nyp.org

Memorial Sloan-Kettering
Cancer Center*
1275 York Avenue
New York, NY 10021
Toll-Free: 800-525-2225
Phone: 212-639-2000
Website: http://www.mskcc.org

NYU Cancer Institute**
New York University Cancer
Institute
550 First Avenue
New York, NY 10016
Phone: 212-263-6485
Website: http://
www.nyucancerinstitute.org

Roswell Park Cancer Institute*
Elm and Carlton Streets
Buffalo, NY 14263-0001
Toll-Free: 800-767-9355
(800-ROSWELL)
Website: http://
www.roswellpark.org

North Carolina

Comprehensive Cancer Center
of Wake Forest University*
Wake Forest University Baptist
Medical Center
Medical Center Boulevard
Winston-Salem, NC 27157
Phone: 336-716-2255
Toll-Free: 800-446-2255
Website: http://
www1.wfubmc.edu/cancer

Duke Comprehensive Cancer
Center*
Duke University Medical Center
2424 Erwin Rd.
Durham, NC 27705
Toll-Free Consultation and
Referral: 888-275-3853 (888-
ASK-DUKE)
Phone: 919-684-3377
Website: http://
www.cancer.duke.edu

UNC Lineberger Comprehensive
Cancer Center*
School of Medicine
University of North Carolina at
Chapel Hill
Campus Box 7295
Chapel Hill, NC 27599-7295
Phone: 919-966-3036
Website: http://
cancer.med.unc.edu
E-mail: dgs@med.unc.edu

Ohio

Ireland Cancer Center*
University Hospitals Health
System
11100 Euclid Avenue
Cleveland, OH 44106-5065
Toll-Free: 800-641-2422
Phone: 216-844-5432
Website: http://
www.irelandcancercenter.org

Ohio State University
Comprehensive Cancer Center*
Arthur G. James Cancer
Hospital and Richard J. Solove
Research Institute
300 West 10th Avenue, Suite 519
Columbus, OH 43210-1240
Toll-Free: 800-293-5066
Website: http://
www.jamesline.com

Oregon

OHSU Cancer Institute**
Oregon Health Sciences
University Cancer Institute
3181 Southwest Sam Jackson
Park Road
CR145
Portland, OR 97239-3098
Toll-Free: 800-494-1234
Phone: 503-494-1617
Website: http://
www.ohsucancer.com
E-mail: cancer@ohsu.edu

Pennsylvania

Abramson Cancer Center of the University of Pennsylvania*
15th Floor, Penn Tower
3400 Spruce Street
Philadelphia, PA 19104-4283
Toll-Free for Referrals and Appointments: 800-789-7366 (800-789-PENN)
Phone: 215-662-4000
Website: http://www.penncancer.org

Fox Chase Cancer Center*
333 Cottman Avenue
Philadelphia, PA 19111-2497
Toll-Free: 888-369-2427 (888-FOX CHASE)
Phone: 215-728-2570 (appointments)
Website: http://www.fccc.edu

Kimmel Cancer Center**
Thomas Jefferson University
Bluemle Life Sciences Building
233 South 10th Street
Philadelphia, PA 19107-5541
Toll-Free: 888-955-1212
Toll-Free Jefferson Cancer Network: 800-533-3669 (800-JEFF-NOW)
Website: http://www.kimmelcancercenter.org

University of Pittsburgh Cancer Institute*
5150 Centre Avenue
Pittsburgh, PA 15232
Phone: 412-647-2811
Website: http://www.upci.upmc.edu
E-mail: PCI-INFO@upmc.edu

Wistar Institute** °
3601 Spruce Street
Philadelphia, PA 19104
Phone: 215-898-3700
Website: http://www.wistar.org

Tennessee

St. Jude Children's Research Hospital**
332 North Lauderdale Street
Memphis, TN 38105-2794
Phone: 901-495-3300
Website: http://www.stjude.org

Vanderbilt-Ingram Cancer Center*
Vanderbilt University
691 Preston Building
Nashville, TN 37232-6838
Toll-Free: 800-811-8480 (clinical trial or treatment option information)
Toll-Free: 888-488-4089 (all other calls)
Phone: 615-936-1782
or 615-936-5847
Website: http://www.vicc.org

Texas

San Antonio Cancer Institute**
7703 Floyd Curl Drive
San Antonio, TX 78229
Suite DTL 5.210S
Phone: 210-567-2710
Website: http://saci.uthscsa.edu

University of Texas M. D. Anderson Cancer Center*
1515 Holcombe Boulevard
Houston, TX 77030
Toll-Free: 800-392-1611
Toll-Free: 877-632-6788
(877-MDA-6788)
Website: http://www.mdanderson.org

Utah

Huntsman Cancer Institute**
University of Utah
2000 Circle of Hope
Salt Lake City, UT 84112
Toll-Free: 877-585-0303
Phone: 801-585-0303
Website: http://www.hci.utah.edu

Vermont

Vermont Cancer Center*
University of Vermont
Given Building
Room E231
89 Beaumont Avenue
Burlington, VT 05405
Phone: 802-656-4414
Website: http://www.vermontcancer.org
E-mail: vcc@uvm.edu

Virginia

Cancer Center at The University of Virginia**
University of Virginia Health System
Post Office Box 800334
Charlottesville, VA 22908
Toll-Free: 800-223-9173
Phone: 434-924-9333
Website: http://www.healthsystem.virginia.edu

Massey Cancer Center**
Virginia Commonwealth University
401 College Street
Post Office Box 980037
Richmond, VA 23298-0037
Phone: 804-828-0450
Website: http://www.massey.vcu.edu

Washington

Fred Hutchinson Cancer Research Center*
1100 Fairview Avenue North
Seattle, WA 98109-1024
Toll-Free for Referrals and Appointments: 800-804-8824
(Seattle Cancer Care Alliance)
Phone: 206-667-5000 and 206-288-1000
Website: http://www.fhcrc.org
E-mail: hutchdoc@seattlecca.org
(patient information)

Wisconsin

University of Wisconsin
Comprehensive Cancer Center*
600 Highland Avenue, K5/601
Madison, WI 53792-6164
Toll-Free Cancer Connect:
800-622-8922
Phone: 608-263-8600
Phone: 608-262-5223 (Cancer
Connect)
Website: http://
www.cancer.wisc.edu
E-mail: uwccc@uwcc.wisc.edu

Chapter 63

Financial Assistance for Cancer Care

Cancer imposes heavy economic burdens on both patients and their families. For many people, a portion of medical expenses is paid by their health insurance plan. For individuals who do not have health insurance or who need financial assistance to cover health care costs, resources are available, including government-sponsored programs and services supported by voluntary organizations.

Cancer patients and their families should discuss any concerns they may have about health care costs with their physician, medical social worker, or the business office of their hospital or clinic.

In addition to the organizations listed below, community voluntary agencies and service organizations such as the Salvation Army, Lutheran Social Services, Jewish Social Services, Catholic Charities, and the Lions Club may offer help. These organizations are listed in your local phone directory. Some churches and synagogues may provide financial help or services to their members.

Fund-raising is another mechanism to consider. Some patients find that friends, family, and community members are willing to contribute financially if they are aware of a difficult situation. Contact your local library for information about how to organize fund-raising efforts.

Information in this chapter was compiled from many sources deemed reliable, including "Financial Assistance for Cancer Care," and "National Organizations That Offer Services to People With Cancer and Their Families," National Cancer Institute (http://www.cancer.gov). Inclusion does not constitute endorsement and omission does not imply disapproval. All contact information was updated and verified in October 2006.

Air Care Alliance
Website: www.aircareall.org

The Air Care Alliance site can link you organizations that provide charitable transportation for patients who must travel for health care.

BBB Wise Giving Alliance
4200 Wilson Boulevard, Suite 800
Arlington, VA 22203-1838
Phone: 703-276-0100; Fax: 703-525-8277
Website: http://www.give.org
E-mail: bnd@bbb.org

Local Better Business Bureaus (BBBs) report on local fund-raising organizations. The address for the office nearest you is available in your telephone directory.

Candlelighters® Childhood Cancer Foundation
P.O. Box 498
Kensington, MD 20895-0498
Toll-Free: 800-366-2223; Phone: 301-962-3520
Website: http://www.candlelighters.org
E-mail: info@candlelighters.org

The CCCF, nonprofit organization, maintains a list of organizations to which eligible families may apply for assistance.

Centers for Medicare and Medicaid Services (CMS)
7500 Security Boulevard
Baltimore, MD 21244-1850
Medicare Hotline: 800-633-4227
TTY: 877-486-2048
Website: http://www.medicare.gov

Medicare is a health insurance program for the elderly or disabled that is administered by the Centers for Medicare and Medicaid Services (CMS). Medicare may offer reimbursement for some home care services. Cancer patients who qualify for Medicare may also be eligible for coverage of hospice services if they are accepted into a Medicare-certified hospice program. Medicaid, a jointly funded, federal-state health insurance program for people who need financial assistance for medical expenses, is also coordinated by CMS. Medicaid coverage includes part-time nursing, home care aide services, and medical supplies and equipment. Information about coverage is available from local state welfare offices, state health departments, state social services agencies, or the state Medicaid office. The phone number for the state Medicaid office can be found in the blue pages of government listings in the phone book, under the state health department heading. A list of state Medicaid phone numbers is also available on the CMS website at http://cms.hhs.gov/medicaid/mcontact.asp.

Corporate Angel Network
Website: www.corpangelnetwork.org

This nonprofit organization provides air transportation for cancer patients by using empty seats on corporate aircrafts.

Department of Veterans Affairs
1722 I Street NW
Washington, DC 20421
Toll-Free: 877-222-8387
Website: http://www.va.gov/health_benefits

Veterans who are disabled as a result of military service can receive home care services from the Department of Veterans Affairs (VA).

CancerCare, Inc.
National Office
275 Seventh Avenue
New York, NY 10001
Toll-Free: 800-813-4673; Phone: 212-712-8080, 212-712-8400
Website: http://www.cancercare.org
E-mail: info@cancercare.org

CancerCare operates the AVONCares Program for Medically Underserved Women, which provides financial assistance to low-income, under- and uninsured, underserved women throughout the country who need supportive services (transportation, child care, and home care) related to the treatment of breast and cervical cancers.

Hill-Burton
5600 Fishers Lane
Rockville, MD 20857
Toll-Free: 800-638-0742
Website: http://www.hrsa.gov

Hill-Burton is the program through which hospitals receive construction funds from the federal government. Hospitals that receive

Hill-Burton funds are required by law to provide some services to people who cannot afford to pay for their hospitalization.

Internal Revenue Service (IRS)
1111 Constitution Ave., NW
Washington, DC 20224
Toll-Free: 800-829-1040
Website: http://www.irs.gov

Medical costs not covered by insurance policies can sometimes be deducted from annual income before taxes. Examples of tax-deductible expenses can include mileage for trips to medical appointments and out-of-pocket costs for treatment, prescription drugs, or equipment. The local IRS office, tax consultants, or certified public accountants can determine what medical costs are tax-deductible. These telephone numbers can be found in the local phone book.

Leukemia and Lymphoma Society
1311 Mamaroneck Avenue
White Plains, NY 10605-5221
Toll-Free: 800-955-4572
Website: http://www.leukemia-lymphoma.org
E-mail: infocenter@leukemia-lymphoma.org

LLS provides information and financial aid to patients who have leukemia, non-Hodgkin lymphoma, Hodgkin disease, or multiple myeloma. Callers may request a booklet describing LLS' Patient Aid Program or the telephone number for their local LLS office.

National Association of Area Agencies on Aging
1730 Rhode Island Ave., NW, Suite 1200
Washington, DC 20036
Eldercare Locator: 800-677-1116
Phone: 202-872-0888
Fax: 202-872-0057

The Older Americans Act provides federal funds for state and local social service programs that help frail and disabled people age 60 and older remain independent. This funding covers home care aide, personal care, escort, meal delivery, and shopping services. Older persons, their caregivers, or anyone concerned about the welfare of an older person can contact their local Area Agency on Aging (AAA) for information and referrals to services and benefits in the community.

AAAs are usually listed in the white pages of the phone book under the city or county government headings. A nationwide toll-free hotline operated by the Administration on Aging, the Eldercare Locator, provides information about AAAs and other assistance for older people.

National Association of Hospital Hospitality Houses, Inc.
Website: www.nahhh.org

Programs served by organizations who are members of National Association of Hospital Hospitality Houses, Inc. meet the needs of hospital patients' family members who require lodging.

National Children's Cancer Society
1015 Locust, Suite 600
St. Louis, MO 63101
Toll-Free: 800-532-6459
Phone: 314-241-1600; Fax: 314-241-1996
Program Services Fax: 314-241-6949
Website: http://www.children-cancer.org

The NCCS helps children with cancer. Among their other services, they provide financial assistance and links to organizations which provide scholarships for cancer survivors.

National Foundation for Credit Counseling
801 Roeder Road, Suite 900
Silver Spring, MD 20910
Toll-Free: 800-388-2227 (National Crisis Hotline)
Phone: 301-589-5600
Fax: 301-495-5623
Website: http://www.nfcc.org

NFCC is a national nonprofit network designed to provide assistance to people dealing with stressful financial situations. You can find nonprofit consumer credit counseling services in your area. If you cannot find one in the phone book, the National Foundation for Consumer Credit, Inc., can direct you to a certified consumer credit counselor in your area.

National Foundation for Transplants
Website: www.transplants.org

The National Foundation for Transplants helps patients who need bone marrow, stem cell, cord blood, or solid organ transplants.

National Patient Travel Center
4620 Haygood Road, Suite One
Virginia Beach, VA 23455
Toll-Free: 800-296-1217
Website: http://www.patienttravel.org
E-mail: mercymedical@erols.com

The NPTC provides the National Patient Travel Helpline, a telephone service that facilitates patient access to charitable medical air transportation resources in the United States. The NPTC also offers information about discounted airline ticket programs for patients and patient escorts, operates Special-Lift and Child-Lift programs, and brings ambulatory outpatients to the United States from many overseas locations.

NeedyMeds
Website: http://www.needymeds.com

Most of the large drug companies have what is called an "Indigent Patient Program." These programs help provide medications to people who cannot afford them. NeedyMeds, an internet website, lists medicine assistance programs available from drug companies. Usually, patients cannot apply directly for these programs. You can ask your doctor, nurse, or social worker to contact them.

Patient Assistance Program
c/o Patient Advocate Foundation
700 Thimble Shoals Boulevard, Suite 200
Newport News, VA 23606
Toll-Free: 866-512-3861; Phone: 757-873-6668
Website: http://www.patientadvocate.org
E-mail: info@patientadvocate.org

The Patient Assistance Program is a subsidiary of the Patient Advocate Foundation. It provides financial assistance to patients who meet certain qualifications.

Pharmaceutical Research and Manufacturers of America (PhRMA)
Toll-Free: 800-762-4636
Website: http://www.phrma.org

To make it easier for physicians to identify the growing number of programs available for needy patients, PhRMA created a *Directory of Prescription Drug Patient Assistance Programs*. It lists programs that provide drugs to physicians whose patients could not otherwise afford them. The *Directory* is available on the internet or can be requested over the phone.

Social Security Administration (SSA)
Office of Public Inquiries
Windsor Park Building
6401 Security Blvd.
Baltimore, MD 21235
Toll-Free: 800-772-1213; Toll-Free TTY: 800-325-0778
Website: www.ssa.gov

The Social Security Administration (SSA) is a government agency that provides income for eligible elderly and disabled individuals. Contact the SSA for information about eligibility.

State Children's Health Insurance Program
U.S. Department of Health and Human Services
P.O. Box 30412
Lansing MI, 48909
Toll-Free: 877-543-7669
Website: www.insurekidsnow.gov

SCHIP is a federal-state partnership that offers low-cost or free health insurance coverage to uninsured children of low-wage, working parents. Callers will be referred to the SCHIP program in their state for further information about what the program covers, who is eligible, and the minimum qualifications.

State Prescription Drug Assistance Programs
Medicare Hotline: 800-MEDICARE
Website: http://www.medicare.gov

Some states have a pharmaceutical assistance program that will help pay for needed medicines. For a listing of Prescription Drug Assistance Programs in your state, call or visit the Medicare website. You can also ask your doctor or social worker about programs for which you may be eligible.

U.S. Department of Labor (DOL)
Pension and Welfare Benefits Administration
Office of Public Affairs
200 Constitution Avenue, NW, Room N-5656
Washington, DC 20210

Toll-Free: 866-275-7922
TTY: 877-889-5627
Website: http://www.dol.gov/dol/pwba

For information about health insurance and your legal rights, contact the DOL Pension and Welfare Benefits Administration. They can help you find out about or confirm your rights under COBRA and ERISA (Federal laws about pensions and keeping insurance coverage when you change jobs).

Index

Index

Page numbers followed by 'n' indicate a footnote. Page numbers in *italics* indicate a table or illustration.

Health Reference Series

COMPLETE CATALOG

List price $87 per volume. **School and library price $78 per volume.**

Adolescent Health Sourcebook, 2nd Edition

Basic Consumer Health Information about the Physical, Mental, and Emotional Growth and Development of Adolescents, Including Medical Care, Nutritional and Physical Activity Requirements, Puberty, Sexual Activity, Acne, Tanning, Body Piercing, Common Physical Illnesses and Disorders, Eating Disorders, Attention Deficit Hyperactivity Disorder, Depression, Bullying, Hazing, and Adolescent Injuries Related to Sports, Driving, and Work

Along with Substance Abuse Information about Nicotine, Alcohol, and Drug Use, a Glossary, and Directory of Additional Resources

Edited by Joyce Brennfleck Shannon. 683 pages. 2006. 978-0-7808-0943-7.

"It is written in clear, nontechnical language aimed at general readers. . . . Recommended for public libraries, community colleges, and other agencies serving health care consumers."
— *American Reference Books Annual, 2003*

"Recommended for school and public libraries. Parents and professionals dealing with teens will appreciate the easy-to-follow format and the clearly written text. This could become a 'must have' for every high school teacher." — *E-Streams, Jan '03*

"A good starting point for information related to common medical, mental, and emotional concerns of adolescents." — *School Library Journal, Nov '02*

"This book provides accurate information in an easy to access format. It addresses topics that parents and caregivers might not be aware of and provides practical, useable information."
— *Doody's Health Sciences Book Review Journal, Sep-Oct '02*

"Recommended reference source."
— *Booklist, American Library Association, Sep '02*

AIDS Sourcebook, 3rd Edition

Basic Consumer Health Information about Acquired Immune Deficiency Syndrome (AIDS) and Human Immunodeficiency Virus (HIV) Infection, Including Facts about Transmission, Prevention, Diagnosis, Treatment, Opportunistic Infections, and Other Complications, with a Section for Women and Children, Including Details about Associated Gynecological Concerns, Pregnancy, and Pediatric Care

Along with Updated Statistical Information, Reports on Current Research Initiatives, a Glossary, and Directories of Internet, Hotline, and Other Resources

Edited by Dawn D. Matthews. 664 pages. 2003. 978-0-7808-0631-3.

"The 3rd edition of the *AIDS Sourcebook*, part of Omnigraphics' *Health Reference Series*, is a welcome update. . . . This resource is highly recommended for academic and public libraries."
— *American Reference Books Annual, 2004*

"Excellent sourcebook. This continues to be a highly recommended book. There is no other book that provides as much information as this book provides."
— *AIDS Book Review Journal, Dec-Jan '00*

"Recommended reference source."
— *Booklist, American Library Association, Dec '99*

Alcoholism Sourcebook, 2nd Edition

Basic Consumer Health Information about Alcohol Use, Abuse, and Dependence, Featuring Facts about the Physical, Mental, and Social Health Effects of Alcohol Addiction, Including Alcoholic Liver Disease, Pancreatic Disease, Cardiovascular Disease, Neurological Disorders, and the Effects of Drinking during Pregnancy

Along with Information about Alcohol Treatment, Medications, and Recovery Programs, in Addition to Tips for Reducing the Prevalence of Underage Drinking, Statistics about Alcohol Use, a Glossary of Related Terms, and Directories of Resources for More Help and Information

Edited by Amy L. Sutton. 653 pages. 2006. 978-0-7808-0942-0.

"This title is one of the few reference works on alcoholism for general readers. For some readers this will be a welcome complement to the many self-help books on the market. Recommended for collections serving general readers and consumer health collections."
— *E-Streams, Mar '01*

"This book is an excellent choice for public and academic libraries."
— *American Reference Books Annual, 2001*

"Recommended reference source."
— *Booklist, American Library Association, Dec '00*

"Presents a wealth of information on alcohol use and abuse and its effects on the body and mind, treatment, and prevention." — *SciTech Book News, Dec '00*

"Important new health guide which packs in the latest consumer information about the problems of alcoholism." — *Reviewer's Bookwatch, Nov '00*

SEE ALSO *Drug Abuse Sourcebook*

Allergies Sourcebook, 3rd Edition

Basic Consumer Health Information about Allergic Disorders, Such as Anaphylaxis, Hives, Eczema, Rhinitis, Sinusitis, and Conjunctivitis, and Their Triggers, Including Pollen, Mold, Dust Mites, Animal Dander, Insects, Chemicals, Food, Food Additives, and Medications;

Along with Advice about the Diagnosis and Treatment of Allergy Symptoms, a Glossary of Related Terms, a Directory of Resources for Help and Information, and Suggestions for Additional Reading

Edited by Amy L. Sutton. 598 pages. 2007. 978-0-7808-0950-5.

"This book brings a great deal of useful material together. . . . This is an excellent addition to public and consumer health library collections."
— *American Reference Books Annual, 2003*

"This second edition would be useful to laypersons with little or advanced knowledge of the subject matter. This book would also serve as a resource for nursing and other health care professions students. It would be useful in public, academic, and hospital libraries with consumer health collections."
— *E-Streams, Jul '02*

■

Alternative Medicine Sourcebook

SEE Complementary & Alternative Medicine Sourcebook

■

Alzheimer's Disease Sourcebook, 3rd Edition

Basic Consumer Health Information about Alzheimer's Disease, Other Dementias, and Related Disorders, Including Multi-Infarct Dementia, AIDS Dementia Complex, Dementia with Lewy Bodies, Huntington's Disease, Wernicke-Korsakoff Syndrome (Alcohol-Related Dementia), Delirium, and Confusional States

Along with Information for People Newly Diagnosed with Alzheimer's Disease and Caregivers, Reports Detailing Current Research Efforts in Prevention, Diagnosis, and Treatment, Facts about Long-Term Care Issues, and Listings of Sources for Additional Information

Edited by Karen Bellenir. 645 pages. 2003. 978-0-7808-0666-5.

"This very informative and valuable tool will be a great addition to any library serving consumers, students and health care workers."
— *American Reference Books Annual, 2004*

"This is a valuable resource for people affected by dementias such as Alzheimer's. It is easy to navigate and includes important information and resources."
— *Doody's Review Service, Feb '04*

"Recommended reference source."
— *Booklist, American Library Association, Oct '99*

SEE ALSO *Brain Disorders Sourcebook*

Arthritis Sourcebook, 2nd Edition

Basic Consumer Health Information about Osteoarthritis, Rheumatoid Arthritis, Other Rheumatic Disorders, Infectious Forms of Arthritis, and Diseases with Symptoms Linked to Arthritis, Featuring Facts about Diagnosis, Pain Management, and Surgical Therapies

Along with Coping Strategies, Research Updates, a Glossary, and Resources for Additional Help and Information

Edited by Amy L. Sutton. 593 pages. 2004. 978-0-7808-0667-2.

"This easy-to-read volume is recommended for consumer health collections within public or academic libraries."
— *E-Streams, May '05*

"As expected, this updated edition continues the excellent reputation of this series in providing sound, usable health information. . . . Highly recommended."
— *American Reference Books Annual, 2005*

"Excellent reference."
— *The Bookwatch, Jan '05*

■

Asthma Sourcebook, 2nd Edition

Basic Consumer Health Information about the Causes, Symptoms, Diagnosis, and Treatment of Asthma in Infants, Children, Teenagers, and Adults, Including Facts about Different Types of Asthma, Common Co-Occurring Conditions, Asthma Management Plans, Triggers, Medications, and Medication Delivery Devices

Along with Asthma Statistics, Research Updates, a Glossary, a Directory of Asthma-Related Resources, and More

Edited by Karen Bellenir. 609 pages. 2006. 978-0-7808-0866-9.

"A worthwhile reference acquisition for public libraries and academic medical libraries whose readers desire a quick introduction to the wide range of asthma information."
— *Choice, Association of College & Research Libraries, Jun '01*

"Recommended reference source."
— *Booklist, American Library Association, Feb '01*

"Highly recommended."
— *The Bookwatch, Jan '01*

"There is much good information for patients and their families who deal with asthma daily."
— *American Medical Writers Association Journal, Winter '01*

"This informative text is recommended for consumer health collections in public, secondary school, and community college libraries and the libraries of universities with a large undergraduate population."
— *American Reference Books Annual, 2001*

■

Attention Deficit Disorder Sourcebook

Basic Consumer Health Information about Attention Deficit/Hyperactivity Disorder in Children and Adults,

636

Including Facts about Causes, Symptoms, Diagnostic Criteria, and Treatment Options Such as Medications, Behavior Therapy, Coaching, and Homeopathy

Along with Reports on Current Research Initiatives, Legal Issues, and Government Regulations, and Featuring a Glossary of Related Terms, Internet Resources, and a List of Additional Reading Material

Edited by Dawn D. Matthews. 470 pages. 2002. 978-0-7808-0624-5.

"Recommended reference source."
— Booklist, American Library Association, Jan '03

"This book is recommended for all school libraries and the reference or consumer health sections of public libraries." — American Reference Books Annual, 2003

■

Back & Neck Sourcebook, 2nd Edition

Basic Consumer Health Information about Spinal Pain, Spinal Cord Injuries, and Related Disorders, Such as Degenerative Disk Disease, Osteoarthritis, Scoliosis, Sciatica, Spina Bifida, and Spinal Stenosis, and Featuring Facts about Maintaining Spinal Health, Self-Care, Pain Management, Rehabilitative Care, Chiropractic Care, Spinal Surgeries, and Complementary Therapies

Along with Suggestions for Preventing Back and Neck Pain, a Glossary of Related Terms, and a Directory of Resources

Edited by Amy L. Sutton. 633 pages. 2004. 978-0-7808-0738-9.

"Recommended . . . an easy to use, comprehensive medical reference book." — E-Streams, Sep '05

"The strength of this work is its basic, easy-to-read format. Recommended." — Reference and User Services Quarterly, American Library Association, Winter '97

■

Blood & Circulatory Disorders Sourcebook, 2nd Edition

Basic Consumer Health Information about the Blood and Circulatory System and Related Disorders, Such as Anemia and Other Hemoglobin Diseases, Cancer of the Blood and Associated Bone Marrow Disorders, Clotting and Bleeding Problems, and Conditions That Affect the Veins, Blood Vessels, and Arteries, Including Facts about the Donation and Transplantation of Bone Marrow, Stem Cells, and Blood and Tips for Keeping the Blood and Circulatory System Healthy

Along with a Glossary of Related Terms and Resources for Additional Help and Information

Edited by Amy L. Sutton. 659 pages. 2005. 978-0-7808-0746-4.

"Highly recommended pick for basic consumer health reference holdings at all levels."
— The Bookwatch, Aug '05

"Recommended reference source."
— Booklist, American Library Association, Feb '99

"An important reference sourcebook written in simple language for everyday, non-technical users. "
— Reviewer's Bookwatch, Jan '99

■

Brain Disorders Sourcebook, 2nd Edition

Basic Consumer Health Information about Acquired and Traumatic Brain Injuries, Infections of the Brain, Epilepsy and Seizure Disorders, Cerebral Palsy, and Degenerative Neurological Disorders, Including Amyotrophic Lateral Sclerosis (ALS), Dementias, Multiple Sclerosis, and More

Along with Information on the Brain's Structure and Function, Treatment and Rehabilitation Options, Reports on Current Research Initiatives, a Glossary of Terms Related to Brain Disorders and Injuries, and a Directory of Sources for Further Help and Information

Edited by Sandra J. Judd. 625 pages. 2005. 978-0-7808-0744-0.

"Highly recommended pick for basic consumer health reference holdings at all levels."
— The Bookwatch, Aug '05

"Belongs on the shelves of any library with a consumer health collection." — E-Streams, Mar '00

"Recommended reference source."
— Booklist, American Library Association, Oct '99

SEE ALSO Alzheimer's Disease Sourcebook

■

Breast Cancer Sourcebook, 2nd Edition

Basic Consumer Health Information about Breast Cancer, Including Facts about Risk Factors, Prevention, Screening and Diagnostic Methods, Treatment Options, Complementary and Alternative Therapies, Post-Treatment Concerns, Clinical Trials, Special Risk Populations, and New Developments in Breast Cancer Research

Along with Breast Cancer Statistics, a Glossary of Related Terms, and a Directory of Resources for Additional Help and Information

Edited by Sandra J. Judd. 595 pages. 2004. 978-0-7808-0668-9.

"This book will be an excellent addition to public, community college, medical, and academic libraries."
— American Reference Books Annual, 2006

"It would be a useful reference book in a library or on loan to women in a support group."
— Cancer Forum, Mar '03

"Recommended reference source."
— Booklist, American Library Association, Jan '02

"This reference source is highly recommended. It is quite informative, comprehensive and detailed in nature, and yet it offers practical advice in easy-to-read language. It could be thought of as the 'bible' of breast cancer for the consumer." — *E-Streams, Jan '02*

"From the pros and cons of different screening methods and results to treatment options, *Breast Cancer Sourcebook* provides the latest information on the subject." — *Library Bookwatch, Dec '01*

"This thoroughgoing, very readable reference covers all aspects of breast health and cancer. . . . Readers will find much to consider here. Recommended for all public and patient health collections." — *Library Journal, Sep '01*

SEE ALSO Cancer Sourcebook for Women, Women's Health Concerns Sourcebook

■

Breastfeeding Sourcebook

Basic Consumer Health Information about the Benefits of Breastmilk, Preparing to Breastfeed, Breastfeeding as a Baby Grows, Nutrition, and More, Including Information on Special Situations and Concerns Such as Mastitis, Illness, Medications, Allergies, Multiple Births, Prematurity, Special Needs, and Adoption

Along with a Glossary and Resources for Additional Help and Information

Edited by Jenni Lynn Colson. 388 pages. 2002. 978-0-7808-0332-9.

"Particularly useful is the information about professional lactation services and chapters on breastfeeding when returning to work. . . . *Breastfeeding Sourcebook* will be useful for public libraries, consumer health libraries, and technical schools offering nurse assistant training, especially in areas where Internet access is problematic." — *American Reference Books Annual, 2003*

SEE ALSO Pregnancy & Birth Sourcebook

■

Burns Sourcebook

Basic Consumer Health Information about Various Types of Burns and Scalds, Including Flame, Heat, Cold, Electrical, Chemical, and Sun Burns

Along with Information on Short-Term and Long-Term Treatments, Tissue Reconstruction, Plastic Surgery, Prevention Suggestions, and First Aid

Edited by Allan R. Cook. 604 pages. 1999. 978-0-7808-0204-9.

"This is an exceptional addition to the series and is highly recommended for all consumer health collections, hospital libraries, and academic medical centers." — *E-Streams, Mar '00*

"This key reference guide is an invaluable addition to all health care and public libraries in confronting this ongoing health issue." — *American Reference Books Annual, 2000*

"Recommended reference source." — *Booklist, American Library Association, Dec '99*

SEE ALSO Dermatological Disorders Sourcebook

Cancer Sourcebook, 5th Edition

Basic Consumer Health Information about Major Forms and Stages of Cancer, Featuring Facts about Head and Neck Cancers, Lung Cancers, Gastrointestinal Cancers, Genitourinary Cancers, Lymphomas, Blood Cell Cancers, Endocrine Cancers, Skin Cancers, Bone Cancers, Metastatic Cancers, and More

Along with Facts about Cancer Treatments, Cancer Risks and Prevention, a Glossary of Related Terms, Statistical Data, and a Directory of Resources for Additional Information

Edited by Karen Bellenir. 1,133 pages. 2007. 978-0-7808-0947-5.

"With cancer being the second leading cause of death for Americans, a prodigious work such as this one, which locates centrally so much cancer-related information, is clearly an asset to this nation's citizens and others." — *Journal of the National Medical Association, 2004*

"This title is recommended for health sciences and public libraries with consumer health collections." — *E-Streams, Feb '01*

". . . can be effectively used by cancer patients and their families who are looking for answers in a language they can understand. Public and hospital libraries should have it on their shelves." — *American Reference Books Annual, 2001*

"Recommended reference source." — *Booklist, American Library Association, Dec '00*

SEE ALSO Breast Cancer Sourcebook, Cancer Sourcebook for Women, Pediatric Cancer Sourcebook, Prostate Cancer Sourcebook

■

Cancer Sourcebook for Women, 3rd Edition

Basic Consumer Health Information about Leading Causes of Cancer in Women, Featuring Facts about Gynecologic Cancers and Related Concerns, Such as Breast Cancer, Cervical Cancer, Endometrial Cancer, Uterine Sarcoma, Vaginal Cancer, Vulvar Cancer, and Common Non-Cancerous Gynecologic Conditions, in Addition to Facts about Lung Cancer, Colorectal Cancer, and Thyroid Cancer in Women

Along with Information about Cancer Risk Factors, Screening and Prevention, Treatment Options, and Tips on Coping with Life after Cancer Treatment, a Glossary of Cancer Terms, and a Directory of Resources for Additional Help and Information

Edited by Amy L. Sutton. 715 pages. 2006. 978-0-7808-0867-6.

"An excellent addition to collections in public, consumer health, and women's health libraries." — *American Reference Books Annual, 2003*

"Overall, the information is excellent, and complex topics are clearly explained. As a reference book for the consumer it is a valuable resource to assist them to make informed decisions about cancer and its treatments." — *Cancer Forum, Nov '02*

Cancer Survivorship Sourcebook

Basic Consumer Health Information about the Physical, Educational, Emotional, Social, and Financial Needs of Cancer Patients from Diagnosis, through Cancer Treatment, and Beyond, Including Facts about Researching Specific Types of Cancer and Learning about Clinical Trials and Treatment Options, and Featuring Tips for Coping with the Side Effects of Cancer Treatments and Adjusting to Life after Cancer Treatment Concludes

Along with Suggestions for Caregivers, Friends, and Family Members of Cancer Patients, a Glossary of Cancer Care Terms, and Directories of Related Resources

Edited by Karen Bellenir. 6561 pages. 2007. 978-0-7808-0985-7.

Cardiovascular Diseases & Disorders Sourcebook, 3rd Edition

Basic Consumer Health Information about Heart and Vascular Diseases and Disorders, Such as Angina, Heart Attacks, Arrhythmias, Cardiomyopathy, Valve Disease, Atherosclerosis, and Aneurysms, with Information about Managing Cardiovascular Risk Factors and Maintaining Heart Health, Medications and Procedures Used to Treat Cardiovascular Disorders, and Concerns of Special Significance to Women

Along with Reports on Current Research Initiatives, a Glossary of Related Medical Terms, and a Directory of Sources for Further Help and Information

Edited by Sandra J. Judd. 713 pages. 2005. 978-0-7808-0739-6.

Caregiving Sourcebook

Basic Consumer Health Information for Caregivers, Including a Profile of Caregivers, Caregiving Responsibilities and Concerns, Tips for Specific Conditions, Care Environments, and the Effects of Caregiving

Along with Facts about Legal Issues, Financial Information, and Future Planning, a Glossary, and a Listing of Additional Resources

Edited by Joyce Brennfleck Shannon. 600 pages. 2001. 978-0-7808-0331-2.

Child Abuse Sourcebook

Basic Consumer Health Information about the Physical, Sexual, and Emotional Abuse of Children, with Additional Facts about Neglect, Munchausen Syndrome by Proxy (MSBP), Shaken Baby Syndrome, and Controversial Issues Related to Child Abuse, Such as Withholding Medical Care, Corporal Punishment, and Child Maltreatment in Youth Sports, and Featuring Facts about Child Protective Services, Foster Care, Adoption, Parenting Challenges, and Other Abuse Prevention Efforts

Along with a Glossary of Related Terms and Resources for Additional Help and Information

Edited by Dawn D. Matthews. 620 pages. 2004. 978-0-7808-0705-1.

SEE ALSO: *Domestic Violence Sourcebook*

Childhood Diseases & Disorders Sourcebook

Basic Consumer Health Information about Medical Problems Often Encountered in Pre-Adolescent Children, Including Respiratory Tract Ailments, Ear Infections, Sore Throats, Disorders of the Skin and Scalp, Digestive and Genitourinary Diseases, Infectious Diseases, Inflammatory Disorders, Chronic Physical and Developmental Disorders, Allergies, and More

Along with Information about Diagnostic Tests, Common Childhood Surgeries, and Frequently Used Medications, with a Glossary of Important Terms and Resource Directory

Edited by Chad T. Kimball. 662 pages. 2003. 978-0-7808-0458-6.

"This is an excellent book for new parents and should be included in all health care and public libraries."
—American Reference Books Annual, 2004

SEE ALSO: Healthy Children Sourcebook

Colds, Flu & Other Common Ailments Sourcebook

Basic Consumer Health Information about Common Ailments and Injuries, Including Colds, Coughs, the Flu, Sinus Problems, Headaches, Fever, Nausea and Vomiting, Menstrual Cramps, Diarrhea, Constipation, Hemorrhoids, Back Pain, Dandruff, Dry and Itchy Skin, Cuts, Scrapes, Sprains, Bruises, and More

Along with Information about Prevention, Self-Care, Choosing a Doctor, Over-the-Counter Medications, Folk Remedies, and Alternative Therapies, and Including a Glossary of Important Terms and a Directory of Resources for Further Help and Information

Edited by Chad T. Kimball. 638 pages. 2001. 978-0-7808-0435-7.

"A good starting point for research on common illnesses. It will be a useful addition to public and consumer health library collections."
—American Reference Books Annual, 2002

"Will prove valuable to any library seeking to maintain a current, comprehensive reference collection of health resources. . . . Excellent reference."
—The Bookwatch, Aug '01

"Recommended reference source."
—Booklist, American Library Association, Jul '01

Communication Disorders Sourcebook

Basic Information about Deafness and Hearing Loss, Speech and Language Disorders, Voice Disorders, Balance and Vestibular Disorders, and Disorders of Smell, Taste, and Touch

Edited by Linda M. Ross. 533 pages. 1996. 978-0-7808-0077-9.

"This is skillfully edited and is a welcome resource for the layperson. It should be found in every public and medical library."
—Booklist Health Sciences Supplement, American Library Association, Oct '97

Complementary & Alternative Medicine Sourcebook, 3rd Edition

Basic Consumer Health Information about Complementary and Alternative Medical Therapies, Including Acupuncture, Ayurveda, Traditional Chinese Medicine, Herbal Medicine, Homeopathy, Naturopathy, Biofeedback, Hypnotherapy, Yoga, Art Therapy, Aromatherapy, Clinical Nutrition, Vitamin and Mineral Supplements, Chiropractic, Massage, Reflexology, Crystal Therapy, Therapeutic Touch, and More

Along with Facts about Alternative and Complementary Treatments for Specific Conditions Such as Cancer, Diabetes, Osteoarthritis, Chronic Pain, Menopause, Gastrointestinal Disorders, Headaches, and Mental Illness, a Glossary, and a Resource List for Additional Help and Information

Edited by Sandra J. Judd. 657 pages. 2006. 978-0-7808-0864-5.

"Recommended for public, high school, and academic libraries that have consumer health collections. Hospital libraries that also serve the public will find this to be a useful resource."
—E-Streams, Feb '03

"Recommended reference source."
—Booklist, American Library Association, Jan '03

"An important alternate health reference."
—MBR Bookwatch, Oct '02

"A great addition to the reference collection of every type of library."
—American Reference Books Annual, 2000

Congenital Disorders Sourcebook, 2nd Edition

Basic Consumer Health Information about Non-hereditary Birth Defects and Disorders Related to Prematurity, Gestational Injuries, Congenital Infections, and Birth Complications, Including Heart Defects, Hydrocephalus, Spina Bifida, Cleft Lip and Palate, Cerebral Palsy, and More

Along with Facts about the Prevention of Birth Defects, Fetal Surgery and Other Treatment Options, Research Initiatives, a Glossary of Related Terms, and Resources for Additional Information and Support

Edited by Sandra J. Judd. 647 pages. 2006. 978-0-7808-0945-1.

"Recommended reference source."
—Booklist, American Library Association, Oct '97

SEE ALSO Pregnancy & Birth Sourcebook

Contagious Diseases Sourcebook

Basic Consumer Health Information about Infectious Diseases Spread by Person-to-Person Contact through

Direct Touch, Airborne Transmission, Sexual Contact, or Contact with Blood or Other Body Fluids, Including Hepatitis, Herpes, Influenza, Lice, Measles, Mumps, Pinworm, Ringworm, Severe Acute Respiratory Syndrome (SARS), Streptococcal Infections, Tuberculosis, and Others

Along with Facts about Disease Transmission, Antimicrobial Resistance, and Vaccines, with a Glossary and Directories of Resources for More Information

Edited by Karen Bellenir. 643 pages. 2004. 978-0-7808-0736-5.

"This easy-to-read volume is recommended for consumer health collections within public or academic libraries." —E-Streams, May '05

"This informative book is highly recommended for public libraries, consumer health collections, and secondary schools and undergraduate libraries." —American Reference Books Annual, 2005

"Excellent reference." —The Bookwatch, Jan '05

Death & Dying Sourcebook, 2nd Edition

Basic Consumer Health Information about End-of-Life Care and Related Perspectives and Ethical Issues, Including End-of-Life Symptoms and Treatments, Pain Management, Quality-of-Life Concerns, the Use of Life Support, Patients' Rights and Privacy Issues, Advance Directives, Physician-Assisted Suicide, Caregiving, Organ and Tissue Donation, Autopsies, Funeral Arrangements, and Grief

Along with Statistical Data, Information about the Leading Causes of Death, a Glossary, and Directories of Support Groups and Other Resources

Edited by Joyce Brennfleck Shannon. 653 pages. 2006. 978-0-7808-0871-3.

"Public libraries, medical libraries, and academic libraries will all find this sourcebook a useful addition to their collections." —American Reference Books Annual, 2001

"An extremely useful resource for those concerned with death and dying in the United States." —Respiratory Care, Nov '00

"Recommended reference source." —Booklist, American Library Association, Aug '00

"This book is a definite must for all those involved in end-of-life care." —Doody's Review Service, 2000

Dental Care & Oral Health Sourcebook, 2nd Edition

Basic Consumer Health Information about Dental Care, Including Oral Hygiene, Dental Visits, Pain Management, Cavities, Crowns, Bridges, Dental Implants, and Fillings, and Other Oral Health Concerns, Such as Gum Disease, Bad Breath, Dry Mouth, Genetic and Developmental Abnormalities, Oral Cancers, Orthodontics, and Temporomandibular Disorders

Along with Updates on Current Research in Oral Health, a Glossary, a Directory of Dental and Oral Health Organizations, and Resources for People with Dental and Oral Health Disorders

Edited by Amy L. Sutton. 609 pages. 2003. 978-0-7808-0634-4.

"This book could serve as a turning point in the battle to educate consumers in issues concerning oral health." —American Reference Books Annual, 2004

"Unique source which will fill a gap in dental sources for patients and the lay public. A valuable reference tool even in a library with thousands of books on dentistry. Comprehensive, clear, inexpensive, and easy to read and use. It fills an enormous gap in the health care literature." —Reference & User Services Quarterly, American Library Association, Summer '98

"Recommended reference source." —Booklist, American Library Association, Dec '97

Depression Sourcebook

Basic Consumer Health Information about Unipolar Depression, Bipolar Disorder, Postpartum Depression, Seasonal Affective Disorder, and Other Types of Depression in Children, Adolescents, Women, Men, the Elderly, and Other Selected Populations

Along with Facts about Causes, Risk Factors, Diagnostic Criteria, Treatment Options, Coping Strategies, Suicide Prevention, a Glossary, and a Directory of Sources for Additional Help and Information

Edited by Karen Bellenir. 602 pages. 2002. 978-0-7808-0611-5.

"Depression Sourcebook is of a very high standard. Its purpose, which is to serve as a reference source to the lay reader, is very well served." —Journal of the National Medical Association, 2004

"Invaluable reference for public and school library collections alike." —Library Bookwatch, Apr '03

"Recommended for purchase." —American Reference Books Annual, 2003

Dermatological Disorders Sourcebook, 2nd Edition

Basic Consumer Health Information about Conditions and Disorders Affecting the Skin, Hair, and Nails, Such as Acne, Rosacea, Rashes, Dermatitis, Pigmentation Disorders, Birthmarks, Skin Cancer, Skin Injuries, Psoriasis, Scleroderma, and Hair Loss, Including Facts about Medications and Treatments for Dermatological Disorders and Tips for Maintaining Healthy Skin, Hair, and Nails

Along with Information about How Aging Affects the Skin, a Glossary of Related Terms, and a Directory of Resources for Additional Help and Information

Edited by Amy L. Sutton. 645 pages. 2005. 978-0-7808-0795-2.

641

"... comprehensive, easily read reference book."
— *Doody's Health Sciences Book Reviews*, Oct '97

SEE ALSO Burns Sourcebook

■

Diabetes Sourcebook, 3rd Edition

Basic Consumer Health Information about Type 1 Diabetes (Insulin-Dependent or Juvenile-Onset Diabetes), Type 2 Diabetes (Noninsulin-Dependent or Adult-Onset Diabetes), Gestational Diabetes, Impaired Glucose Tolerance (IGT), and Related Complications, Such as Amputation, Eye Disease, Gum Disease, Nerve Damage, and End-Stage Renal Disease, Including Facts about Insulin, Oral Diabetes Medications, Blood Sugar Testing, and the Role of Exercise and Nutrition in the Control of Diabetes

Along with a Glossary and Resources for Further Help and Information

Edited by Dawn D. Matthews. 622 pages. 2003. 978-0-7808-0629-0.

"This edition is even more helpful than earlier versions. . . . It is a truly valuable tool for anyone seeking readable and authoritative information on diabetes."
— *American Reference Books Annual*, 2004

"An invaluable reference." — *Library Journal*, May '00

Selected as one of the 250 "Best Health Sciences Books of 1999." — *Doody's Rating Service*, Mar-Apr '00

"Provides useful information for the general public."
— *Healthlines, University of Michigan Health Management Research Center*, Sep/Oct '99

"... provides reliable mainstream medical information ... belongs on the shelves of any library with a consumer health collection." — *E-Streams*, Sep '99

"Recommended reference source."
— *Booklist, American Library Association*, Feb '99

■

Diet & Nutrition Sourcebook, 3rd Edition

Basic Consumer Health Information about Dietary Guidelines and the Food Guidance System, Recommended Daily Nutrient Intakes, Serving Proportions, Weight Control, Vitamins and Supplements, Nutrition Issues for Different Life Stages and Lifestyles, and the Needs of People with Specific Medical Concerns, Including Cancer, Celiac Disease, Diabetes, Eating Disorders, Food Allergies, and Cardiovascular Disease

Along with Facts about Federal Nutrition Support Programs, a Glossary of Nutrition and Dietary Terms, and Directories of Additional Resources for More Information about Nutrition

Edited by Joyce Brennfleck Shannon. 633 pages. 2006. 978-0-7808-0800-3.

"This book is an excellent source of basic diet and nutrition information." — *Booklist Health Sciences Supplement, American Library Association*, Dec '00

"This reference document should be in any public library, but it would be a very good guide for beginning students in the health sciences. If the other books in this publisher's series are as good as this, they should all be in the health sciences collections."
— *American Reference Books Annual*, 2000

"This book is an excellent general nutrition reference for consumers who desire to take an active role in their health care for prevention. Consumers of all ages who select this book can feel confident they are receiving current and accurate information." — *Journal of Nutrition for the Elderly*, Vol. 19, No. 4, 2000

SEE ALSO Digestive Diseases & Disorders Sourcebook, Eating Disorders Sourcebook, Gastrointestinal Diseases & Disorders Sourcebook, Vegetarian Sourcebook

■

Digestive Diseases & Disorders Sourcebook

Basic Consumer Health Information about Diseases and Disorders that Impact the Upper and Lower Digestive System, Including Celiac Disease, Constipation, Crohn's Disease, Cyclic Vomiting Syndrome, Diarrhea, Diverticulosis and Diverticulitis, Gallstones, Heartburn, Hemorrhoids, Hernias, Indigestion (Dyspepsia), Irritable Bowel Syndrome, Lactose Intolerance, Ulcers, and More

Along with Information about Medications and Other Treatments, Tips for Maintaining a Healthy Digestive Tract, a Glossary, and Directory of Digestive Diseases Organizations

Edited by Karen Bellenir. 335 pages. 2000. 978-0-7808-0327-5.

"This title would be an excellent addition to all public or patient-research libraries."
— *American Reference Books Annual*, 2001

"This title is recommended for public, hospital, and health sciences libraries with consumer health collections." — *E-Streams*, Jul-Aug '00

"Recommended reference source."
— *Booklist, American Library Association*, May '00

SEE ALSO Eating Disorders Sourcebook, Gastrointestinal Diseases & Disorders Sourcebook

■

Disabilities Sourcebook

Basic Consumer Health Information about Physical and Psychiatric Disabilities, Including Descriptions of Major Causes of Disability, Assistive and Adaptive Aids, Workplace Issues, and Accessibility Concerns

Along with Information about the Americans with Disabilities Act, a Glossary, and Resources for Additional Help and Information

Edited by Dawn D. Matthews. 616 pages. 2000. 978-0-7808-0389-3.

"It is a must for libraries with a consumer health section." — *American Reference Books Annual*, 2002

"A much needed addition to the Omnigraphics *Health Reference Series*. A current reference work to provide people with disabilities, their families, caregivers or those who work with them, a broad range of information in one volume, has not been available until now. . . . It is recommended for all public and academic library reference collections." —*E-Streams, May '01*

"An excellent source book in easy-to-read format covering many current topics; highly recommended for all libraries." —*Choice, Association of College & Research Libraries, Jan '01*

"Recommended reference source." —*Booklist, American Library Association, Jul '00*

■

Domestic Violence Sourcebook, 2nd Edition

Basic Consumer Health Information about the Causes and Consequences of Abusive Relationships, Including Physical Violence, Sexual Assault, Battery, Stalking, and Emotional Abuse, and Facts about the Effects of Violence on Women, Men, Young Adults, and the Elderly, with Reports about Domestic Violence in Selected Populations, and Featuring Facts about Medical Care, Victim Assistance and Protection, Prevention Strategies, Mental Health Services, and Legal Issues

Along with a Glossary of Related Terms and Resources for Additional Help and Information

Edited by Dawn D. Matthews. 628 pages. 2004. 978-0-7808-0669-6.

"Educators, clergy, medical professionals, police, and victims and their families will benefit from this realistic and easy-to-understand resource." —*American Reference Books Annual, 2005*

"Recommended for all collections supporting consumer health information. It should also be considered for any collection needing general, readable information on domestic violence." —*E-Streams, Jan '05*

"This sourcebook complements other books in its field, providing a one-stop resource . . . Recommended." —*Choice, Association of College & Research Libraries, Jan '05*

"Interested lay persons should find the book extremely beneficial. . . . A copy of *Domestic Violence and Child Abuse Sourcebook* should be in every public library in the United States." —*Social Science & Medicine, No. 56, 2003*

"This is important information. The Web has many resources but this sourcebook fills an important societal need. I am not aware of any other resources of this type." —*Doody's Review Service, Sep '01*

"Recommended reference source." —*Booklist, American Library Association, Apr '01*

"Important pick for college-level health reference libraries." —*The Bookwatch, Mar '01*

"Because this problem is so widespread and because this book includes a lot of issues within one volume, this work is recommended for all public libraries." —*American Reference Books Annual, 2001*

SEE ALSO *Child Abuse Sourcebook*

■

Drug Abuse Sourcebook, 2nd Edition

Basic Consumer Health Information about Illicit Substances of Abuse and the Misuse of Prescription and Over-the-Counter Medications, Including Depressants, Hallucinogens, Inhalants, Marijuana, Stimulants, and Anabolic Steroids

Along with Facts about Related Health Risks, Treatment Programs, Prevention Programs, a Glossary of Abuse and Addiction Terms, a Glossary of Drug-Related Street Terms, and a Directory of Resources for More Information

Edited by Catherine Ginther. 607 pages. 2004. 978-0-7808-0740-2.

"Commendable for organizing useful, normally scattered government and association-produced data into a logical sequence." —*American Reference Books Annual, 2006*

"This easy-to-read volume is recommended for consumer health collections within public or academic libraries." —*E-Streams, Sep '05*

"An excellent library reference." —*The Bookwatch, May '05*

"Containing a wealth of information, this book will be useful to the college student just beginning to explore the topic of substance abuse. This resource belongs in libraries that serve a lower-division undergraduate or community college clientele as well as the general public." —*Choice, Association of College & Research Libraries, Jun '01*

"Recommended reference source." —*Booklist, American Library Association, Feb '01*

SEE ALSO *Alcoholism Sourcebook*

■

Ear, Nose & Throat Disorders Sourcebook, 2nd Edition

Basic Consumer Health Information about Disorders of the Ears, Hearing Loss, Vestibular Disorders, Nasal and Sinus Problems, Throat and Vocal Cord Disorders, and Otolaryngologic Cancers, Including Facts about Ear Infections and Injuries, Genetic and Congenital Deafness, Sensorineural Hearing Disorders, Tinnitus, Vertigo, Ménière Disease, Rhinitis, Sinusitis, Snoring, Sore Throats, Hoarseness, and More

Along with Reports on Current Research Initiatives, a Glossary of Related Medical Terms, and a Directory of Sources for Further Help and Information

Edited by Sandra J. Judd. 659 pages. 2006. 978-0-7808-0872-0.

"Overall, this sourcebook is helpful for the consumer seeking information on ENT issues. It is recommended for public libraries."
— *American Reference Books Annual, 1999*

"Recommended reference source."
— *Booklist, American Library Association, Dec '98*

■

Eating Disorders Sourcebook, 2nd Edition

Basic Consumer Health Information about Anorexia Nervosa, Bulimia Nervosa, Binge Eating, Compulsive Exercise, Female Athlete Triad, and Other Eating Disorders, Including Facts about Body Image and Other Cultural and Age-Related Risk Factors, Prevention Efforts, Adverse Health Effects, Treatment Options, and the Recovery Process

Along with Guidelines for Healthy Weight Control, a Glossary, and Directories of Additional Resources

Edited by Joyce Brennfleck Shannon. 585 pages. 2007. 978-0-7808-0948-2.

"Recommended for health science libraries that are open to the public, as well as hospital libraries. This book is a good resource for the consumer who is concerned about eating disorders." — *E-Streams, Mar '02*

"This volume is another convenient collection of excerpted articles. Recommended for school and public library patrons; lower-division undergraduates; and two-year technical program students."
— *Choice, Association of College & Research Libraries, Jan '02*

"Recommended reference source."
— *Booklist, American Library Association, Oct '01*

SEE ALSO *Diet & Nutrition Sourcebook, Digestive Diseases & Disorders Sourcebook, Gastrointestinal Diseases & Disorders Sourcebook*

■

Emergency Medical Services Sourcebook

Basic Consumer Health Information about Preventing, Preparing for, and Managing Emergency Situations, When and Who to Call for Help, What to Expect in the Emergency Room, the Emergency Medical Team, Patient Issues, and Current Topics in Emergency Medicine

Along with Statistical Data, a Glossary, and Sources of Additional Help and Information

Edited by Jenni Lynn Colson. 494 pages. 2002. 978-0-7808-0420-3.

"Handy and convenient for home, public, school, and college libraries. Recommended."
— *Choice, Association of College & Research Libraries, Apr '03*

"This reference can provide the consumer with answers to most questions about emergency care in the United States, or it will direct them to a resource where the answer can be found."
— *American Reference Books Annual, 2003*

"Recommended reference source."
— *Booklist, American Library Association, Feb '03*

■

Endocrine & Metabolic Disorders Sourcebook

Basic Information for the Layperson about Pancreatic and Insulin-Related Disorders Such as Pancreatitis, Diabetes, and Hypoglycemia; Adrenal Gland Disorders Such as Cushing's Syndrome, Addison's Disease, and Congenital Adrenal Hyperplasia; Pituitary Gland Disorders Such as Growth Hormone Deficiency, Acromegaly, and Pituitary Tumors; Thyroid Disorders Such as Hypothyroidism, Graves' Disease, Hashimoto's Disease, and Goiter; Hyperparathyroidism; and Other Diseases and Syndromes of Hormone Imbalance or Metabolic Dysfunction

Along with Reports on Current Research Initiatives

Edited by Linda M. Shin. 574 pages. 1998. 978-0-7808-0207-0.

"Omnigraphics has produced another needed resource for health information consumers."
— *American Reference Books Annual, 2000*

"Recommended reference source."
— *Booklist, American Library Association, Dec '98*

■

Environmental Health Sourcebook, 2nd Edition

Basic Consumer Health Information about the Environment and Its Effect on Human Health, Including the Effects of Air Pollution, Water Pollution, Hazardous Chemicals, Food Hazards, Radiation Hazards, Biological Agents, Household Hazards, Such as Radon, Asbestos, Carbon Monoxide, and Mold, and Information about Associated Diseases and Disorders, Including Cancer, Allergies, Respiratory Problems, and Skin Disorders

Along with Information about Environmental Concerns for Specific Populations, a Glossary of Related Terms, and Resources for Further Help and Information

Edited by Dawn D. Matthews. 673 pages. 2003. 978-0-7808-0632-0.

"This recently updated edition continues the level of quality and the reputation of the numerous other volumes in Omnigraphics' *Health Reference Series.*"
— *American Reference Books Annual, 2004*

"An excellent updated edition."
— *The Bookwatch, Oct '03*

"Recommended reference source."
— *Booklist, American Library Association, Sep '98*

"This book will be a useful addition to anyone's library." — *Choice Health Sciences Supplement, Association of College & Research Libraries, May '98*

". . . a good survey of numerous environmentally induced physical disorders . . . a useful addition to anyone's library."
— *Doody's Health Sciences Book Reviews, Jan '98*

Ethnic Diseases Sourcebook

Basic Consumer Health Information for Ethnic and Racial Minority Groups in the United States, Including General Health Indicators and Behaviors, Ethnic Diseases, Genetic Testing, the Impact of Chronic Diseases, Women's Health, Mental Health Issues, and Preventive Health Care Services

Along with a Glossary and a Listing of Additional Resources

Edited by Joyce Brennfleck Shannon. 664 pages. 2001. 978-0-7808-0336-7.

"Recommended for health sciences libraries where public health programs are a priority."
— *E-Streams, Jan '02*

"Not many books have been written on this topic to date, and the *Ethnic Diseases Sourcebook* is a strong addition to the list. It will be an important introductory resource for health consumers, students, health care personnel, and social scientists. It is recommended for public, academic, and large hospital libraries."
— *American Reference Books Annual, 2002*

"Recommended reference source."
— *Booklist, American Library Association, Oct '01*

"Will prove valuable to any library seeking to maintain a current, comprehensive reference collection of health resources. . . . An excellent source of health information about genetic disorders which affect particular ethnic and racial minorities in the U.S."
— *The Bookwatch, Aug '01*

Eye Care Sourcebook, 2nd Edition

Basic Consumer Health Information about Eye Care and Eye Disorders, Including Facts about the Diagnosis, Prevention, and Treatment of Common Refractive Problems Such as Myopia, Hyperopia, Astigmatism, and Presbyopia, and Eye Diseases, Including Glaucoma, Cataract, Age-Related Macular Degeneration, and Diabetic Retinopathy

Along with a Section on Vision Correction and Refractive Surgeries, Including LASIK and LASEK, a Glossary, and Directories of Resources for Additional Help and Information

Edited by Amy L. Sutton. 543 pages. 2003. 978-0-7808-0635-1.

". . . a solid reference tool for eye care and a valuable addition to a collection."
— *American Reference Books Annual, 2004*

Family Planning Sourcebook

Basic Consumer Health Information about Planning for Pregnancy and Contraception, Including Traditional Methods, Barrier Methods, Hormonal Methods, Permanent Methods, Future Methods, Emergency Contraception, and Birth Control Choices for Women at Each Stage of Life

Along with Statistics, a Glossary, and Sources of Additional Information

Edited by Amy Marcaccio Keyzer. 520 pages. 2001. 978-0-7808-0379-4.

"Recommended for public, health, and undergraduate libraries as part of the circulating collection."
— *E-Streams, Mar '02*

"Information is presented in an unbiased, readable manner, and the sourcebook will certainly be a necessary addition to those public and high school libraries where Internet access is restricted or otherwise problematic." — *American Reference Books Annual, 2002*

"Recommended reference source."
— *Booklist, American Library Association, Oct '01*

"Will prove valuable to any library seeking to maintain a current, comprehensive reference collection of health resources. . . . Excellent reference."
— *The Bookwatch, Aug '01*

SEE ALSO *Pregnancy & Birth Sourcebook*

Fitness & Exercise Sourcebook, 3rd Edition

Basic Consumer Health Information about the Physical and Mental Benefits of Fitness, Including Cardiorespiratory Endurance, Muscular Strength, Muscular Endurance, and Flexibility, with Facts about Sports Nutrition and Exercise-Related Injuries and Tips about Physical Activity and Exercises for People of All Ages and for People with Health Concerns

Along with Advice on Selecting and Using Exercise Equipment, Maintaining Exercise Motivation, a Glossary of Related Terms, and a Directory of Resources for More Help and Information

Edited by Amy L. Sutton. 663 pages. 2007. 978-0-7808-0946-8.

"This work is recommended for all general reference collections."
— *American Reference Books Annual, 2002*

"Highly recommended for public, consumer, and school grades fourth through college." — *E-Streams, Nov '01*

"Recommended reference source."
— *Booklist, American Library Association, Oct '01*

"The information appears quite comprehensive and is considered reliable. . . . This second edition is a welcomed addition to the series."
— *Doody's Review Service, Sep '01*

Food Safety Sourcebook

Basic Consumer Health Information about the Safe Handling of Meat, Poultry, Seafood, Eggs, Fruit Juices, and Other Food Items, and Facts about Pesticides, Drinking Water, Food Safety Overseas, and the Onset, Duration, and Symptoms of Foodborne Illnesses, Including Types of Pathogenic Bacteria, Parasitic Protozoa, Worms, Viruses, and Natural Toxins

Along with the Role of the Consumer, the Food Handler, and the Government in Food Safety; a Glossary, and Resources for Additional Help and Information

Edited by Dawn D. Matthews. 339 pages. 1999. 978-0-7808-0326-8.

"This book is recommended for public libraries and universities with home economic and food science programs." — *E-Streams, Nov '00*

"Recommended reference source."
— *Booklist, American Library Association, May '00*

"This book takes the complex issues of food safety and foodborne pathogens and presents them in an easily understood manner. [It does] an excellent job of covering a large and often confusing topic."
— *American Reference Books Annual, 2000*

∎

Forensic Medicine Sourcebook

Basic Consumer Information for the Layperson about Forensic Medicine, Including Crime Scene Investigation, Evidence Collection and Analysis, Expert Testimony, Computer-Aided Criminal Identification, Digital Imaging in the Courtroom, DNA Profiling, Accident Reconstruction, Autopsies, Ballistics, Drugs and Explosives Detection, Latent Fingerprints, Product Tampering, and Questioned Document Examination

Along with Statistical Data, a Glossary of Forensics Terminology, and Listings of Sources for Further Help and Information

Edited by Annemarie S. Muth. 574 pages. 1999. 978-0-7808-0232-2.

"Given the expected widespread interest in its content and its easy to read style, this book is recommended for most public and all college and university libraries."
— *E-Streams, Feb '01*

"Recommended for public libraries."
— *Reference & User Services Quarterly, American Library Association, Spring 2000*

"Recommended reference source."
— *Booklist, American Library Association, Feb '00*

"A wealth of information, useful statistics, references are up-to-date and extremely complete. This wonderful collection of data will help students who are interested in a career in any type of forensic field. It is a great resource for attorneys who need information about types of expert witnesses needed in a particular case. It also offers useful information for fiction and nonfiction writers whose work involves a crime. A fascinating compilation. All levels."
— *Choice, Association of College & Research Libraries, Jan '00*

"There are several items that make this book attractive to consumers who are seeking certain forensic data. . . . This is a useful current source for those seeking general forensic medical answers."
— *American Reference Books Annual, 2000*

Gastrointestinal Diseases & Disorders Sourcebook, 2nd Edition

Basic Consumer Health Information about the Upper and Lower Gastrointestinal (GI) Tract, Including the Esophagus, Stomach, Intestines, Rectum, Liver, and Pancreas, with Facts about Gastroesophageal Reflux Disease, Gastritis, Hernias, Ulcers, Celiac Disease, Diverticulitis, Irritable Bowel Syndrome, Hemorrhoids, Gastrointestinal Cancers, and Other Diseases and Disorders Related to the Digestive Process

Along with Information about Commonly Used Diagnostic and Surgical Procedures, Statistics, Reports on Current Research Initiatives and Clinical Trials, a Glossary, and Resources for Additional Help and Information

Edited by Sandra J. Judd. 681 pages. 2006. 978-0-7808-0798-3.

". . . very readable form. The successful editorial work that brought this material together into a useful and understandable reference makes accessible to all readers information that can help them more effectively understand and obtain help for digestive tract problems."
— *Choice, Association of College & Research Libraries, Feb '97*

SEE ALSO *Diet & Nutrition Sourcebook, Digestive Diseases & Disorders Sourcebook, Eating Disorders Sourcebook*

∎

Genetic Disorders Sourcebook, 3rd Edition

Basic Consumer Health Information about Hereditary Diseases and Disorders, Including Facts about the Human Genome, Genetic Inheritance Patterns, Disorders Associated with Specific Genes, Such as Sickle Cell Disease, Hemophilia, and Cystic Fibrosis, Chromosome Disorders, Such as Down Syndrome, Fragile X Syndrome, and Turner Syndrome, and Complex Diseases and Disorders Resulting from the Interaction of Environmental and Genetic Factors, Such as Allergies, Cancer, and Obesity

Along with Facts about Genetic Testing, Suggestions for Parents of Children with Special Needs, Reports on Current Research Initiatives, a Glossary of Genetic Terminology, and Resources for Additional Help and Information

Edited by Karen Bellenir. 777 pages. 2004. 978-0-7808-0742-6.

"This text is recommended for any library with an interest in providing consumer health resources."
— *E-Streams, Aug '05*

"This is a valuable resource for anyone wishing to have an understandable description of any of the topics or disorders included. The editor succeeds in making complex genetic issues understandable."
— *Doody's Book Review Service, May '05*

"A good acquisition for public libraries."
— *American Reference Books Annual, 2005*

Head Trauma Sourcebook

Basic Information for the Layperson about Open-Head and Closed-Head Injuries, Treatment Advances, Recovery, and Rehabilitation

Along with Reports on Current Research Initiatives

Edited by Karen Bellenir. 414 pages. 1997. 978-0-7808-0208-7.

Headache Sourcebook

Basic Consumer Health Information about Migraine, Tension, Cluster, Rebound and Other Types of Headaches, with Facts about the Cause and Prevention of Headaches, the Effects of Stress and the Environment, Headaches during Pregnancy and Menopause, and Childhood Headaches

Along with a Glossary and Other Resources for Additional Help and Information

Edited by Dawn D. Matthews. 362 pages. 2002. 978-0-7808-0337-4.

Healthy Aging Sourcebook

Basic Consumer Health Information about Maintaining Health through the Aging Process, Including Advice on Nutrition, Exercise, and Sleep, Help in Making Decisions about Midlife Issues and Retirement, and Guidance Concerning Practical and Informed Choices in Health Consumerism

Along with Data Concerning the Theories of Aging, Different Experiences in Aging by Minority Groups, and Facts about Aging Now and Aging in the Future; and Featuring a Glossary, a Guide to Consumer Help, Additional Suggested Reading, and Practical Resource Directory

Edited by Jenifer Swanson. 536 pages. 1999. 978-0-7808-0390-9.

SEE ALSO Physical & Mental Issues in Aging Sourcebook

Healthy Children Sourcebook

Basic Consumer Health Information about the Physical and Mental Development of Children between the Ages of 3 and 12, Including Routine Health Care, Preventative Health Services, Safety and First Aid, Healthy Sleep, Dental Care, Nutrition, and Fitness, and Featuring Parenting Tips on Such Topics as Bedwetting, Choosing Day Care, Monitoring TV and Other Media, and Establishing a Foundation for Substance Abuse Prevention

Along with a Glossary of Commonly Used Pediatric Terms and Resources for Additional Help and Information.

Edited by Chad T. Kimball. 647 pages. 2003. 978-0-7808-0247-6.

SEE ALSO Childhood Diseases & Disorders Sourcebook

Healthy Heart Sourcebook for Women

Basic Consumer Health Information about Cardiac Issues Specific to Women, Including Facts about Major Risk Factors and Prevention, Treatment and Control Strategies, and Important Dietary Issues

Along with a Special Section Regarding the Pros and Cons of Hormone Replacement Therapy and Its Impact on Heart Health, and Additional Help, Including Recipes, a Glossary, and a Directory of Resources

Edited by Dawn D. Matthews. 336 pages. 2000. 978-0-7808-0329-9.

SEE ALSO Cardiovascular Diseases & Disorders Sourcebook, Women's Health Concerns Sourcebook

Hepatitis Sourcebook

Basic Consumer Health Information about Hepatitis A, Hepatitis B, Hepatitis C, and Other Forms of Hepatitis, Including Autoimmune Hepatitis, Alcoholic Hepatitis, Nonalcoholic Steatohepatitis, and Toxic Hepatitis, with

Facts about Risk Factors, Screening Methods, Diagnostic Tests, and Treatment Options

Along with Information on Liver Health, Tips for People Living with Chronic Hepatitis, Reports on Current Research Initiatives, a Glossary of Terms Related to Hepatitis, and a Directory of Sources for Further Help and Information

Edited by Sandra J. Judd. 597 pages. 2005. 978-0-7808-0749-5.

"Highly recommended."
— American Reference Books Annual, 2006

■

Household Safety Sourcebook

Basic Consumer Health Information about Household Safety, Including Information about Poisons, Chemicals, Fire, and Water Hazards in the Home

Along with Advice about the Safe Use of Home Maintenance Equipment, Choosing Toys and Nursery Furniture, Holiday and Recreation Safety, a Glossary, and Resources for Further Help and Information

Edited by Dawn D. Matthews. 606 pages. 2002. 978-0-7808-0338-1.

"This work will be useful in public libraries with large consumer health and wellness departments."
— American Reference Books Annual, 2003

"As a sourcebook on household safety this book meets its mark. It is encyclopedic in scope and covers a wide range of safety issues that are commonly seen in the home." — E-Streams, Jul '02

■

Hypertension Sourcebook

Basic Consumer Health Information about the Causes, Diagnosis, and Treatment of High Blood Pressure, with Facts about Consequences, Complications, and Co-Occurring Disorders, Such as Coronary Heart Disease, Diabetes, Stroke, Kidney Disease, and Hypertensive Retinopathy, and Issues in Blood Pressure Control, Including Dietary Choices, Stress Management, and Medications

Along with Reports on Current Research Initiatives and Clinical Trials, a Glossary, and Resources for Additional Help and Information

Edited by Dawn D. Matthews and Karen Bellenir. 613 pages. 2004. 978-0-7808-0674-0.

"Academic, public, and medical libraries will want to add the Hypertension Sourcebook to their collections."
— E-Streams, Aug '05

"The strength of this source is the wide range of information given about hypertension."
— American Reference Books Annual, 2005

■

Immune System Disorders Sourcebook, 2nd Edition

Basic Consumer Health Information about Disorders of the Immune System, Including Immune System Function and Response, Diagnosis of Immune Disorders, Information about Inherited Immune Disease, Acquired Immune Disease, and Autoimmune Diseases, Including Primary Immune Deficiency, Acquired Immunodeficiency Syndrome (AIDS), Lupus, Multiple Sclerosis, Type 1 Diabetes, Rheumatoid Arthritis, and Graves' Disease

Along with Treatments, Tips for Coping with Immune Disorders, a Glossary, and a Directory of Additional Resources.

Edited by Joyce Brennfleck Shannon. 671 pages. 2005. 978-0-7808-0748-8.

"Highly recommended for academic and public libraries." — American Reference Books Annual, 2006

"The updated second edition is a 'must' for any consumer health library seeking a solid resource covering the treatments, symptoms, and options for immune disorder sufferers. . . . An excellent guide."
— MBR Bookwatch, Jan '06

■

Infant & Toddler Health Sourcebook

Basic Consumer Health Information about the Physical and Mental Development of Newborns, Infants, and Toddlers, Including Neonatal Concerns, Nutrition Recommendations, Immunization Schedules, Common Pediatric Disorders, Assessments and Milestones, Safety Tips, and Advice for Parents and Other Caregivers

Along with a Glossary of Terms and Resource Listings for Additional Help

Edited by Jenifer Swanson. 585 pages. 2000. 978-0-7808-0246-9.

"As a reference for the general public, this would be useful in any library." — E-Streams, May '01

"Recommended reference source."
— Booklist, American Library Association, Feb '01

"This is a good source for general use."
— American Reference Books Annual, 2001

■

Infectious Diseases Sourcebook

Basic Consumer Health Information about Non-Contagious Bacterial, Viral, Prion, Fungal, and Parasitic Diseases Spread by Food and Water, Insects and Animals, or Environmental Contact, Including Botulism, E. Coli, Encephalitis, Legionnaires' Disease, Lyme Disease, Malaria, Plague, Rabies, Salmonella, Tetanus, and Others, and Facts about Newly Emerging Diseases, Such as Hantavirus, Mad Cow Disease, Monkeypox, and West Nile Virus

Along with Information about Preventing Disease Transmission, the Threat of Bioterrorism, and Current Research Initiatives, with a Glossary and Directory of Resources for More Information

Edited by Karen Bellenir. 634 pages. 2004. 978-0-7808-0675-7.

"This reference continues the excellent tradition of the *Health Reference Series* in consolidating a wealth of information on a selected topic into a format that is easy to use and accessible to the general public."
— *American Reference Books Annual, 2005*

"Recommended for public and academic libraries."
— *E-Streams, Jan '05*

Injury & Trauma Sourcebook

Basic Consumer Health Information about the Impact of Injury, the Diagnosis and Treatment of Common and Traumatic Injuries, Emergency Care, and Specific Injuries Related to Home, Community, Workplace, Transportation, and Recreation

Along with Guidelines for Injury Prevention, a Glossary, and a Directory of Additional Resources

Edited by Joyce Brennfleck Shannon. 696 pages. 2002. 978-0-7808-0421-0.

"This publication is the most comprehensive work of its kind about injury and trauma."
— *American Reference Books Annual, 2003*

"This sourcebook provides concise, easily readable, basic health information about injuries. . . . This book is well organized and an easy to use reference resource suitable for hospital, health sciences and public libraries with consumer health collections."
— *E-Streams, Nov '02*

"Practitioners should be aware of guides such as this in order to facilitate their use by patients and their families."
— *Doody's Health Sciences Book Review Journal, Sep-Oct '02*

"Recommended reference source."
— *Booklist, American Library Association, Sep '02*

"Highly recommended for academic and medical reference collections." — *Library Bookwatch, Sep '02*

Kidney & Urinary Tract Diseases & Disorders Sourcebook

SEE *Urinary Tract & Kidney Diseases & Disorders Sourcebook*

Learning Disabilities Sourcebook, 2nd Edition

Basic Consumer Health Information about Learning Disabilities, Including Dyslexia, Developmental Speech and Language Disabilities, Non-Verbal Learning Disorders, Developmental Arithmetic Disorder, Developmental Writing Disorder, and Other Conditions That Impede Learning Such as Attention Deficit/Hyperactivity Disorder, Brain Injury, Hearing Impairment, Klinefelter Syndrome, Dyspraxia, and Tourette's Syndrome

Along with Facts about Educational Issues and Assistive Technology, Coping Strategies, a Glossary of Related Terms, and Resources for Further Help and Information

Edited by Dawn D. Matthews. 621 pages. 2003. 978-0-7808-0626-9.

"The second edition of Learning Disabilities Sourcebook far surpasses the earlier edition in that it is more focused on information that will be useful as a consumer health resource."
— *American Reference Books Annual, 2004*

"Teachers as well as consumers will find this an essential guide to understanding various syndromes and their latest treatments. [An] invaluable reference for public and school library collections alike."
— *Library Bookwatch, Apr '03*

Named "Outstanding Reference Book of 1999."
— *New York Public Library, Feb '00*

"An excellent candidate for inclusion in a public library reference section. It's a great source of information. Teachers will also find the book useful. Definitely worth reading."
— *Journal of Adolescent & Adult Literacy, Feb 2000*

"Readable . . . provides a solid base of information regarding successful techniques used with individuals who have learning disabilities, as well as practical suggestions for educators and family members. Clear language, concise descriptions, and pertinent information for contacting multiple resources add to the strength of this book as a useful tool." — *Choice, Association of College & Research Libraries, Feb '99*

"Recommended reference source."
— *Booklist, American Library Association, Sep '98*

"A useful resource for libraries and for those who don't have the time to identify and locate the individual publications." — *Disability Resources Monthly, Sep '98*

Leukemia Sourcebook

Basic Consumer Health Information about Adult and Childhood Leukemias, Including Acute Lymphocytic Leukemia (ALL), Chronic Lymphocytic Leukemia (CLL), Acute Myelogenous Leukemia (AML), Chronic Myelogenous Leukemia (CML), and Hairy Cell Leukemia, and Treatments Such as Chemotherapy, Radiation Therapy, Peripheral Blood Stem Cell and Marrow Transplantation, and Immunotherapy

Along with Tips for Life During and After Treatment, a Glossary, and Directories of Additional Resources

Edited by Joyce Brennfleck Shannon. 587 pages. 2003. 978-0-7808-0627-6.

"Unlike other medical books for the layperson, . . . the language does not talk down to the reader. . . . This volume is highly recommended for all libraries."
— *American Reference Books Annual, 2004*

". . . a fine title which ranges from diagnosis to alternative treatments, staging, and tips for life during and after diagnosis." — *The Bookwatch, Dec '03*

Liver Disorders Sourcebook

Basic Consumer Health Information about the Liver and How It Works; Liver Diseases, Including Cancer, Cirrhosis, Hepatitis, and Toxic and Drug Related Diseases; Tips for Maintaining a Healthy Liver; Laboratory Tests, Radiology Tests, and Facts about Liver Transplantation

Along with a Section on Support Groups, a Glossary, and Resource Listings

Edited by Joyce Brennfleck Shannon. 591 pages. 2000. 978-0-7808-0383-1.

"A valuable resource."
—American Reference Books Annual, 2001

"This title is recommended for health sciences and public libraries with consumer health collections."
—E-Streams, Oct '00

"Recommended reference source."
—Booklist, American Library Association, Jun '00

■

Lung Disorders Sourcebook

Basic Consumer Health Information about Emphysema, Pneumonia, Tuberculosis, Asthma, Cystic Fibrosis, and Other Lung Disorders, Including Facts about Diagnostic Procedures, Treatment Strategies, Disease Prevention Efforts, and Such Risk Factors as Smoking, Air Pollution, and Exposure to Asbestos, Radon, and Other Agents

Along with a Glossary and Resources for Additional Help and Information

Edited by Dawn D. Matthews. 678 pages. 2002. 978-0-7808-0339-8.

"This title is a great addition for public and school libraries because it provides concise health information on the lungs."
—American Reference Books Annual, 2003

"Highly recommended for academic and medical reference collections."
—Library Bookwatch, Sep '02

SEE ALSO Respiratory Diseases & Disorders Sourcebook

■

Medical Tests Sourcebook, 2nd Edition

Basic Consumer Health Information about Medical Tests, Including Age-Specific Health Tests, Important Health Screenings and Exams, Home-Use Tests, Blood and Specimen Tests, Electrical Tests, Scope Tests, Genetic Testing, and Imaging Tests, Such as X-Rays, Ultrasound, Computed Tomography, Magnetic Resonance Imaging, Angiography, and Nuclear Medicine

Along with a Glossary and Directory of Additional Resources

Edited by Joyce Brennfleck Shannon. 654 pages. 2004. 978-0-7808-0670-2.

"Recommended for hospital and health sciences

libraries with consumer health collections."
—E-Streams, Mar '00

"This is an overall excellent reference with a wealth of general knowledge that may aid those who are reluctant to get vital tests performed."
—Today's Librarian, Jan '00

"A valuable reference guide."
—American Reference Books Annual, 2000

■

Men's Health Concerns Sourcebook, 2nd Edition

Basic Consumer Health Information about the Medical and Mental Concerns of Men, Including Theories about the Shorter Male Lifespan, the Leading Causes of Death and Disability, Physical Concerns of Special Significance to Men, Reproductive and Sexual Concerns, Sexually Transmitted Diseases, Men's Mental and Emotional Health, and Lifestyle Choices That Affect Wellness, Such as Nutrition, Fitness, and Substance Use

Along with a Glossary of Related Terms and a Directory of Organizational Resources in Men's Health

Edited by Robert Aquinas McNally. 644 pages. 2004. 978-0-7808-0671-9.

"A very accessible reference for non-specialist general readers and consumers."
—The Bookwatch, Jun '04

"This comprehensive resource and the series are highly recommended."
—American Reference Books Annual, 2000

"Recommended reference source."
—Booklist, American Library Association, Dec '98

■

Mental Health Disorders Sourcebook, 3rd Edition

Basic Consumer Health Information about Mental and Emotional Health and Mental Illness, Including Facts about Depression, Bipolar Disorder, and Other Mood Disorders, Phobias, Post-Traumatic Stress Disorder (PTSD), Obsessive-Compulsive Disorder, and Other Anxiety Disorders, Impulse Control Disorders, Eating Disorders, Personality Disorders, and Psychotic Disorders, Including Schizophrenia and Dissociative Disorders

Along with Statistical Information, a Special Section Concerning Mental Health Issues in Children and Adolescents, a Glossary, and Directories of Resources for Additional Help and Information

Edited by Karen Bellenir. 661 pages. 2005. 978-0-7808-0747-1.

"Recommended for public libraries and academic libraries with an undergraduate program in psychology."
—American Reference Books Annual, 2006

"Recommended reference source."
—Booklist, American Library Association, Jun '00

Mental Retardation Sourcebook

Basic Consumer Health Information about Mental Retardation and Its Causes, Including Down Syndrome, Fetal Alcohol Syndrome, Fragile X Syndrome, Genetic Conditions, Injury, and Environmental Sources

Along with Preventive Strategies, Parenting Issues, Educational Implications, Health Care Needs, Employment and Economic Matters, Legal Issues, a Glossary, and a Resource Listing for Additional Help and Information

Edited by Joyce Brennfleck Shannon. 642 pages. 2000. 978-0-7808-0377-0.

"Public libraries will find the book useful for reference and as a beginning research point for students, parents, and caregivers."
— American Reference Books Annual, 2001

"The strength of this work is that it compiles many basic fact sheets and addresses for further information in one volume. It is intended and suitable for the general public. This sourcebook is relevant to any collection providing health information to the general public."
— E-Streams, Nov '00

"From preventing retardation to parenting and family challenges, this covers health, social and legal issues and will prove an invaluable overview."
— Reviewer's Bookwatch, Jul '00

Movement Disorders Sourcebook

Basic Consumer Health Information about Neurological Movement Disorders, Including Essential Tremor, Parkinson's Disease, Dystonia, Cerebral Palsy, Huntington's Disease, Myasthenia Gravis, Multiple Sclerosis, and Other Early-Onset and Adult-Onset Movement Disorders, Their Symptoms and Causes, Diagnostic Tests, and Treatments

Along with Mobility and Assistive Technology Information, a Glossary, and a Directory of Additional Resources

Edited by Joyce Brennfleck Shannon. 655 pages. 2003. 978-0-7808-0628-3.

". . . a good resource for consumers and recommended for public, community college and undergraduate libraries." *— American Reference Books Annual, 2004*

Muscular Dystrophy Sourcebook

Basic Consumer Health Information about Congenital, Childhood-Onset, and Adult-Onset Forms of Muscular Dystrophy, Such as Duchenne, Becker, Emery-Dreifuss, Distal, Limb-Girdle, Facioscapulohumeral (FSHD), Myotonic, and Ophthalmoplegic Muscular Dystrophies, Including Facts about Diagnostic Tests, Medical and Physical Therapies, Management of Co-Occurring Conditions, and Parenting Guidelines

Along with Practical Tips for Home Care, a Glossary, and Directories of Additional Resources

Edited by Joyce Brennfleck Shannon. 577 pages. 2004. 978-0-7808-0676-4.

"This book is highly recommended for public and academic libraries as well as health care offices that support the information needs of patients and their families."
— E-Streams, Apr '05

"Excellent reference." *— The Bookwatch, Jan '05*

Obesity Sourcebook

Basic Consumer Health Information about Diseases and Other Problems Associated with Obesity, and Including Facts about Risk Factors, Prevention Issues, and Management Approaches

Along with Statistical and Demographic Data, Information about Special Populations, Research Updates, a Glossary, and Source Listings for Further Help and Information

Edited by Wilma Caldwell and Chad T. Kimball. 376 pages. 2001. 978-0-7808-0333-6.

"The book synthesizes the reliable medical literature on obesity into one easy-to-read and useful resource for the general public."
— American Reference Books Annual, 2002

"This is a very useful resource book for the lay public."
— Doody's Review Service, Nov '01

"Well suited for the health reference collection of a public library or an academic health science library that serves the general population." *— E-Streams, Sep '01*

"Recommended reference source."
— Booklist, American Library Association, Apr '01

"Recommended pick both for specialty health library collections and any general consumer health reference collection." *— The Bookwatch, Apr '01*

Oral Health Sourcebook

SEE Dental Care & Oral Health Sourcebook

Osteoporosis Sourcebook

Basic Consumer Health Information about Primary and Secondary Osteoporosis and Juvenile Osteoporosis and Related Conditions, Including Fibrous Dysplasia, Gaucher Disease, Hyperthyroidism, Hypophosphatasia, Myeloma, Osteopetrosis, Osteogenesis Imperfecta, and Paget's Disease

Along with Information about Risk Factors, Treatments, Traditional and Non-Traditional Pain Management, a Glossary of Related Terms, and a Directory of Resources

Edited by Allan R. Cook. 584 pages. 2001. 978-0-7808-0239-1.

"This would be a book to be kept in a staff or patient library. The targeted audience is the layperson, but the therapist who needs a quick bit of information on a particular topic will also find the book useful."
— Physical Therapy, Jan '02

"This resource is recommended as a great reference source for public, health, and academic libraries, and is another triumph for the editors of Omnigraphics."
— *American Reference Books Annual, 2002*

"Recommended for all public libraries and general health collections, especially those supporting patient education or consumer health programs."
— *E-Streams, Nov '01*

"Will prove valuable to any library seeking to maintain a current, comprehensive reference collection of health resources. . . . From prevention to treatment and associated conditions, this provides an excellent survey."
— *The Bookwatch, Aug '01*

"Recommended reference source."
— *Booklist, American Library Association, Jul '01*

SEE ALSO *Healthy Aging Sourcebook, Physical & Mental Issues in Aging Sourcebook, Women's Health Concerns Sourcebook*

Pain Sourcebook, 2nd Edition

Basic Consumer Health Information about Specific Forms of Acute and Chronic Pain, Including Muscle and Skeletal Pain, Nerve Pain, Cancer Pain, and Disorders Characterized by Pain, Such as Fibromyalgia, Shingles, Angina, Arthritis, and Headaches

Along with Information about Pain Medications and Management Techniques, Complementary and Alternative Pain Relief Options, Tips for People Living with Chronic Pain, a Glossary, and a Directory of Sources for Further Information

Edited by Karen Bellenir. 670 pages. 2002. 978-0-7808-0612-2.

"A source of valuable information. . . . This book offers help to nonmedical people who need information about pain and pain management. It is also an excellent reference for those who participate in patient education."
— *Doody's Review Service, Sep '02*

"Highly recommended for academic and medical reference collections." — *Library Bookwatch, Sep '02*

"The text is readable, easily understood, and well indexed. This excellent volume belongs in all patient education libraries, consumer health sections of public libraries, and many personal collections."
— *American Reference Books Annual, 1999*

"The information is basic in terms of scholarship and is appropriate for general readers. Written in journalistic style . . . intended for non-professionals. Quite thorough in its coverage of different pain conditions and summarizes the latest clinical information regarding pain treatment." — *Choice, Association of College and Research Libraries, Jun '98*

"Recommended reference source."
— *Booklist, American Library Association, Mar '98*

Pediatric Cancer Sourcebook

Basic Consumer Health Information about Leukemias, Brain Tumors, Sarcomas, Lymphomas, and Other Cancers in Infants, Children, and Adolescents, Including Descriptions of Cancers, Treatments, and Coping Strategies

Along with Suggestions for Parents, Caregivers, and Concerned Relatives, a Glossary of Cancer Terms, and Resource Listings

Edited by Edward J. Prucha. 587 pages. 1999. 978-0-7808-0245-2.

"An excellent source of information. Recommended for public, hospital, and health science libraries with consumer health collections." — *E-Streams, Jun '00*

"Recommended reference source."
— *Booklist, American Library Association, Feb '00*

"A valuable addition to all libraries specializing in health services and many public libraries."
— *American Reference Books Annual, 2000*

SEE ALSO *Childhood Diseases & Disorders Sourcebook, Healthy Children Sourcebook*

Physical & Mental Issues in Aging Sourcebook

Basic Consumer Health Information on Physical and Mental Disorders Associated with the Aging Process, Including Concerns about Cardiovascular Disease, Pulmonary Disease, Oral Health, Digestive Disorders, Musculoskeletal and Skin Disorders, Metabolic Changes, Sexual and Reproductive Issues, and Changes in Vision, Hearing, and Other Senses

Along with Data about Longevity and Causes of Death, Information on Acute and Chronic Pain, Descriptions of Mental Concerns, a Glossary of Terms, and Resource Listings for Additional Help

Edited by Jenifer Swanson. 660 pages. 1999. 978-0-7808-0233-9.

"This is a treasure of health information for the layperson." — *Choice Health Sciences Supplement, Association of College & Research Libraries, May '00*

"Recommended for public libraries."
— *American Reference Books Annual, 2000*

"Recommended reference source."
— *Booklist, American Library Association, Oct '99*

SEE ALSO *Healthy Aging Sourcebook*

Podiatry Sourcebook, 2nd Edition

Basic Consumer Health Information about Disorders, Diseases, Deformities, and Injuries that Affect the Foot and Ankle, Including Sprains, Corns, Calluses, Bunions, Plantar Warts, Plantar Fasciitis, Neuromas, Clubfoot, Flat Feet, Achilles Tendonitis, and Much More

Along with Information about Selecting a Foot Care Specialist, Foot Fitness, Shoes and Socks, Diagnostic Tests and Corrective Procedures, Financial Assistance for Corrective Devices, a Glossary of Related Terms, and a Directory of Resources for Additional Help and Information

Edited by Ivy L. Alexander. 543 pages. 2007. 978-0-7808-0944-4.

"Recommended reference source."
— *Booklist, American Library Association, Feb '02*

"There is a lot of information presented here on a topic that is usually only covered sparingly in most larger comprehensive medical encyclopedias."
— *American Reference Books Annual, 2002*

Pregnancy & Birth Sourcebook, 2nd Edition

Basic Consumer Health Information about Conception and Pregnancy, Including Facts about Fertility, Infertility, Pregnancy Symptoms and Complications, Fetal Growth and Development, Labor, Delivery, and the Postpartum Period, as Well as Information about Maintaining Health and Wellness during Pregnancy and Caring for a Newborn

Along with Information about Public Health Assistance for Low-Income Pregnant Women, a Glossary, and Directories of Agencies and Organizations Providing Help and Support

Edited by Amy L. Sutton. 626 pages. 2004. 978-0-7808-0672-6.

"Will appeal to public and school reference collections strong in medicine and women's health. . . . Deserves a spot on any medical reference shelf."
— *The Bookwatch, Jul '04*

"A well-organized handbook. Recommended."
— *Choice, Association of College & Research Libraries, Apr '98*

"Recommended reference source."
— *Booklist, American Library Association, Mar '98*

"Recommended for public libraries."
— *American Reference Books Annual, 1998*

SEE ALSO *Breastfeeding Sourcebook, Congenital Disorders Sourcebook, Family Planning Sourcebook*

Prostate & Urological Disorders Sourcebook

Basic Consumer Health Information about Urogenital and Sexual Disorders in Men, Including Prostate and Other Andrological Cancers, Prostatitis, Benign Prostatic Hyperplasia, Testicular and Penile Trauma, Cryptorchidism, Peyronie Disease, Erectile Dysfunction, and Male Factor Infertility, and Facts about Commonly Used Tests and Procedures, Such as Prostatectomy, Vasectomy, Vasectomy Reversal, Penile Implants, and Semen Analysis

Along with a Glossary of Andrological Terms and a Directory of Resources for Additional Information

Edited by Karen Bellenir. 631 pages. 2005. 978-0-7808-0797-6.

Prostate Cancer Sourcebook

Basic Consumer Health Information about Prostate Cancer, Including Information about the Associated Risk Factors, Detection, Diagnosis, and Treatment of Prostate Cancer

Along with Information on Non-Malignant Prostate Conditions, and Featuring a Section Listing Support and Treatment Centers and a Glossary of Related Terms

Edited by Dawn D. Matthews. 358 pages. 2001. 978-0-7808-0324-4.

"Recommended reference source."
— *Booklist, American Library Association, Jan '02*

"A valuable resource for health care consumers seeking information on the subject. . . . All text is written in a clear, easy-to-understand language that avoids technical jargon. Any library that collects consumer health resources would strengthen their collection with the addition of the *Prostate Cancer Sourcebook*."
— *American Reference Books Annual, 2002*

SEE ALSO *Men's Health Concerns Sourcebook*

Reconstructive & Cosmetic Surgery Sourcebook

Basic Consumer Health Information on Cosmetic and Reconstructive Plastic Surgery, Including Statistical Information about Different Surgical Procedures, Things to Consider Prior to Surgery, Plastic Surgery Techniques and Tools, Emotional and Psychological Considerations, and Procedure-Specific Information

Along with a Glossary of Terms and a Listing of Resources for Additional Help and Information

Edited by M. Lisa Weatherford. 374 pages. 2001. 978-0-7808-0214-8.

"An excellent reference that addresses cosmetic and medically necessary reconstructive surgeries. . . . The style of the prose is calm and reassuring, discussing the many positive outcomes now available due to advances in surgical techniques."
— *American Reference Books Annual, 2002*

"Recommended for health science libraries that are open to the public, as well as hospital libraries that are open to the patients. This book is a good resource for the consumer interested in plastic surgery."
— *E-Streams, Dec '01*

"Recommended reference source."
— *Booklist, American Library Association, Jul '01*

Rehabilitation Sourcebook

Basic Consumer Health Information about Rehabilitation for People Recovering from Heart Surgery, Spinal Cord Injury, Stroke, Orthopedic Impairments, Amputation, Pulmonary Impairments, Traumatic Injury, and More, Including Physical Therapy, Occupational Therapy, Speech/Language Therapy, Massage Therapy, Dance Therapy, Art Therapy, and Recreational Therapy

Along with Information on Assistive and Adaptive Devices, a Glossary, and Resources for Additional Help and Information

Edited by Dawn D. Matthews. 531 pages. 1999. 978-0-7808-0236-0.

"This is an excellent resource for public library reference and health collections."
— *American Reference Books Annual, 2001*

"Recommended reference source."
— *Booklist, American Library Association, May '00*

■

Respiratory Diseases & Disorders Sourcebook

Basic Information about Respiratory Diseases and Disorders, Including Asthma, Cystic Fibrosis, Pneumonia, the Common Cold, Influenza, and Others, Featuring Facts about the Respiratory System, Statistical and Demographic Data, Treatments, Self-Help Management Suggestions, and Current Research Initiatives

Edited by Allan R. Cook and Peter D. Dresser. 771 pages. 1995. 978-0-7808-0037-3.

"Designed for the layperson and for patients and their families coping with respiratory illness. . . . an extensive array of information on diagnosis, treatment, management, and prevention of respiratory illnesses for the general reader." — *Choice, Association of College & Research Libraries, Jun '96*

"A highly recommended text for all collections. It is a comforting reminder of the power of knowledge that good books carry between their covers."
— *Academic Library Book Review, Spring '96*

"A comprehensive collection of authoritative information presented in a nontechnical, humanitarian style for patients, families, and caregivers."
— *Association of Operating Room Nurses, Sep/Oct '95*

SEE ALSO Lung Disorders Sourcebook

■

Sexually Transmitted Diseases Sourcebook, 3rd Edition

Basic Consumer Health Information about Chlamydial Infections, Gonorrhea, Hepatitis, Herpes, HIV/AIDS, Human Papillomavirus, Pubic Lice, Scabies, Syphilis, Trichomoniasis, Vaginal Infections, and Other Sexually Transmitted Diseases, Including Facts about Risk Factors, Symptoms, Diagnosis, Treatment, and the Prevention of Sexually Transmitted Infections

Along with Updates on Current Research Initiatives, a Glossary of Related Terms, and Resources for Additional Help and Information

Edited by Amy L. Sutton. 629 pages. 2006. 978-0-7808-0824-9.

"Recommended for consumer health collections in public libraries, and secondary school and community college libraries."
— *American Reference Books Annual, 2002*

"Every school and public library should have a copy of this comprehensive and user-friendly reference book."
— *Choice, Association of College & Research Libraries, Sep '01*

"This is a highly recommended book. This is an especially important book for all school and public libraries."
— *AIDS Book Review Journal, Jul-Aug '01*

"Recommended reference source."
— *Booklist, American Library Association, Apr '01*

■

Sleep Disorders Sourcebook, 2nd Edition

Basic Consumer Health Information about Sleep and Sleep Disorders, Including Insomnia, Sleep Apnea, Restless Legs Syndrome, Narcolepsy, Parasomnias, and Other Health Problems That Affect Sleep, Plus Facts about Diagnostic Procedures, Treatment Strategies, Sleep Medications, and Tips for Improving Sleep Quality

Along with a Glossary of Related Terms and Resources for Additional Help and Information

Edited by Amy L. Sutton. 567 pages. 2005. 978-0-7808-0743-3.

"This book will be useful for just about everybody, especially the 40 million Americans with sleep disorders."
— *American Reference Books Annual, 2006*

"Recommended for public libraries and libraries supporting health care professionals." — *E-Streams, Sep '05*

". . . key medical library acquisition."
— *The Bookwatch, Jun '05*

■

Smoking Concerns Sourcebook

Basic Consumer Health Information about Nicotine Addiction and Smoking Cessation, Featuring Facts about the Health Effects of Tobacco Use, Including Lung and Other Cancers, Heart Disease, Stroke, and Respiratory Disorders, Such as Emphysema and Chronic Bronchitis

Along with Information about Smoking Prevention Programs, Suggestions for Achieving and Maintaining a Smoke-Free Lifestyle, Statistics about Tobacco Use, Reports on Current Research Initiatives, a Glossary of Related Terms, and Directories of Resources for Additional Help and Information

Edited by Karen Bellenir. 621 pages. 2004. 978-0-7808-0323-7.

"Provides everything needed for the student or general reader seeking practical details on the effects of tobacco use." — *The Bookwatch, Mar '05*

"Public libraries and consumer health care libraries will find this work useful."
— *American Reference Books Annual, 2005*

Sports Injuries Sourcebook, 3rd Edition

Basic Consumer Health Information about Sprains and Strains, Fractures, Growth Plate Injuries, Overtraining

Injuries, and Injuries to the Head, Face, Shoulders, Elbows, Hands, Spinal Column, Knees, Ankles, and Feet, and with Facts about Heat-Related Illness, Steroids and Sport Supplements, Protective Equipment, Diagnostic Procedures, Treatment Options, and Rehabilitation

Along with a Glossary of Related Terms and a Directory of Resources for Additional Help and Information

Edited by Sandra J. Judd. 614 pages. 2007. 978-0-7808-0949-9.

"This is an excellent reference for consumers and it is recommended for public, community college, and undergraduate libraries."
— American Reference Books Annual, 2003

"Recommended reference source."
— Booklist, American Library Association, Feb '03

Stress-Related Disorders Sourcebook

Basic Consumer Health Information about Stress and Stress-Related Disorders, Including Stress Origins and Signals, Environmental Stress at Work and Home, Mental and Emotional Stress Associated with Depression, Post-Traumatic Stress Disorder, Panic Disorder, Suicide, and the Physical Effects of Stress on the Cardiovascular, Immune, and Nervous Systems

Along with Stress Management Techniques, a Glossary, and a Listing of Additional Resources

Edited by Joyce Brennfleck Shannon. 610 pages. 2002. 978-0-7808-0560-6.

"Well written for a general readership, the Stress-Related Disorders Sourcebook is a useful addition to the health reference literature."
— American Reference Books Annual, 2003

"I am impressed by the amount of information. It offers a thorough overview of the causes and consequences of stress for the layperson. . . . A well-done and thorough reference guide for professionals and nonprofessionals alike."
— Doody's Review Service, Dec '02

Stroke Sourcebook

Basic Consumer Health Information about Stroke, Including Ischemic, Hemorrhagic, Transient Ischemic Attack (TIA), and Pediatric Stroke, Stroke Triggers and Risks, Diagnostic Tests, Treatments, and Rehabilitation Information

Along with Stroke Prevention Guidelines, Legal and Financial Information, a Glossary, and a Directory of Additional Resources

Edited by Joyce Brennfleck Shannon. 606 pages. 2003. 978-0-7808-0630-6.

"This volume is highly recommended and should be in every medical, hospital, and public library."
— American Reference Books Annual, 2004

"Highly recommended for the amount and variety of topics and information covered." — Choice, Nov '03

Surgery Sourcebook

Basic Consumer Health Information about Inpatient and Outpatient Surgeries, Including Cardiac, Vascular, Orthopedic, Ocular, Reconstructive, Cosmetic, Gynecologic, and Ear, Nose, and Throat Procedures and More

Along with Information about Operating Room Policies and Instruments, Laser Surgery Techniques, Hospital Errors, Statistical Data, a Glossary, and Listings of Sources for Further Help and Information

Edited by Annemarie S. Muth and Karen Bellenir. 596 pages. 2002. 978-0-7808-0380-0.

"Large public libraries and medical libraries would benefit from this material in their reference collections."
— American Reference Books Annual, 2004

"Invaluable reference for public and school library collections alike." — Library Bookwatch, Apr '03

Thyroid Disorders Sourcebook

Basic Consumer Health Information about Disorders of the Thyroid and Parathyroid Glands, Including Hypothyroidism, Hyperthyroidism, Graves Disease, Hashimoto Thyroiditis, Thyroid Cancer, and Parathyroid Disorders, Featuring Facts about Symptoms, Risk Factors, Tests, and Treatments

Along with Information about the Effects of Thyroid Imbalance on Other Body Systems, Environmental Factors That Affect the Thyroid Gland, a Glossary, and a Directory of Additional Resources

Edited by Joyce Brennfleck Shannon. 599 pages. 2005. 978-0-7808-0745-7.

"Recommended for consumer health collections."
— American Reference Books Annual, 2006

"Highly recommended pick for basic consumer health reference holdings at all levels."
— The Bookwatch, Aug '05

Transplantation Sourcebook

Basic Consumer Health Information about Organ and Tissue Transplantation, Including Physical and Financial Preparations, Procedures and Issues Relating to Specific Solid Organ and Tissue Transplants, Rehabilitation, Pediatric Transplant Information, the Future of Transplantation, and Organ and Tissue Donation

Along with a Glossary and Listings of Additional Resources

Edited by Joyce Brennfleck Shannon. 628 pages. 2002. 978-0-7808-0322-0.

"Along with these advances [in transplantation technology] have come a number of daunting questions for potential transplant patients, their families, and their health care providers. This reference text is the best single tool to address many of these questions. . . . It will be a much-needed addition to the reference collections in health care, academic, and large public libraries."
— American Reference Books Annual, 2003

Traveler's Health Sourcebook

Basic Consumer Health Information for Travelers, Including Physical and Medical Preparations, Transportation Health and Safety, Essential Information about Food and Water, Sun Exposure, Insect and Snake Bites, Camping and Wilderness Medicine, and Travel with Physical or Medical Disabilities

Along with International Travel Tips, Vaccination Recommendations, Geographical Health Issues, Disease Risks, a Glossary, and a Listing of Additional Resources

Edited by Joyce Brennfleck Shannon. 613 pages. 2000. 978-0-7808-0384-8.

SEE ALSO *Worldwide Health Sourcebook*

Urinary Tract & Kidney Diseases & Disorders Sourcebook, 2nd Edition

Basic Consumer Health Information about the Urinary System, Including the Bladder, Urethra, Ureters, and Kidneys, with Facts about Urinary Tract Infections, Incontinence, Congenital Disorders, Kidney Stones, Cancers of the Urinary Tract and Kidneys, Kidney Failure, Dialysis, and Kidney Transplantation

Along with Statistical and Demographic Information, Reports on Current Research in Kidney and Urologic Health, a Summary of Commonly Used Diagnostic Tests, a Glossary of Related Terms, and a Directory of Resources for Additional Help and Information

Edited by Ivy L. Alexander. 649 pages. 2005. 978-0-7808-0750-1.

Vegetarian Sourcebook

Basic Consumer Health Information about Vegetarian Diets, Lifestyle, and Philosophy, Including Definitions of Vegetarianism and Veganism, Tips about Adopting Vegetarianism, Creating a Vegetarian Pantry, and Meeting Nutritional Needs of Vegetarians, with Facts Regarding Vegetarianism's Effect on Pregnant and Lactating Women, Children, Athletes, and Senior Citizens

Along with a Glossary of Commonly Used Vegetarian Terms and Resources for Additional Help and Information

Edited by Chad T. Kimball. 360 pages. 2002. 978-0-7808-0439-5.

SEE ALSO *Diet & Nutrition Sourcebook*

Women's Health Concerns Sourcebook, 2nd Edition

Basic Consumer Health Information about the Medical and Mental Concerns of Women, Including Maintaining Health and Wellness, Gynecological Concerns, Breast Health, Sexuality and Reproductive Issues, Menopause, Cancer in Women, Leading Causes of Death and Disability among Women, Physical Concerns of Special Significance to Women, and Women's Mental and Emotional Health

Along with a Glossary of Related Terms and Directories of Resources for Additional Help and Information

Edited by Amy L. Sutton. 746 pages. 2004. 978-0-7808-0673-3.

SEE ALSO *Breast Cancer Sourcebook, Cancer Sourcebook for Women, Healthy Heart Sourcebook for Women, Osteoporosis Sourcebook*

Workplace Health & Safety Sourcebook

Basic Consumer Health Information about Workplace Health and Safety, Including the Effect of Workplace Hazards on the Lungs, Skin, Heart, Ears, Eyes, Brain,

Reproductive Organs, Musculoskeletal System, and Other Organs and Body Parts

Along with Information about Occupational Cancer, Personal Protective Equipment, Toxic and Hazardous Chemicals, Child Labor, Stress, and Workplace Violence

Edited by Chad T. Kimball. 626 pages. 2000. 978-0-7808-0231-5.

"As a reference for the general public, this would be useful in any library." — *E-Streams, Jun '01*

"Provides helpful information for primary care physicians and other caregivers interested in occupational medicine. . . . General readers; professionals." — *Choice, Association of College & Research Libraries, May '01*

"Recommended reference source." — *Booklist, American Library Association, Feb '01*

"Highly recommended." — *The Bookwatch, Jan '01*

Worldwide Health Sourcebook

Basic Information about Global Health Issues, Including Malnutrition, Reproductive Health, Disease Dispersion and Prevention, Emerging Diseases, Risky Health Behaviors, and the Leading Causes of Death

Along with Global Health Concerns for Children, Women, and the Elderly, Mental Health Issues, Research and Technology Advancements, and Economic, Environmental, and Political Health Implications, a Glossary, and a Resource Listing for Additional Help and Information

Edited by Joyce Brennfleck Shannon. 614 pages. 2001. 978-0-7808-0330-5.

"Named an Outstanding Academic Title." — *Choice, Association of College & Research Libraries, Jan '02*

"Yet another handy but also unique compilation in the extensive *Health Reference Series*, this is a useful work because many of the international publications reprinted or excerpted are not readily available. Highly recommended." — *Choice, Association of College & Research Libraries, Nov '01*

"Recommended reference source." — *Booklist, American Library Association, Oct '01*

SEE ALSO *Traveler's Health Sourcebook*

Teen Health Series
Helping Young Adults Understand, Manage, and Avoid Serious Illness

List price $65 per volume. **School and library price $58 per volume.**

Alcohol Information for Teens
Health Tips about Alcohol and Alcoholism

Including Facts about Underage Drinking, Preventing Teen Alcohol Use, Alcohol's Effects on the Brain and the Body, Alcohol Abuse Treatment, Help for Children of Alcoholics, and More

Edited by Joyce Brennfleck Shannon. 370 pages. 2005. 978-0-7808-0741-9.

"Boxed facts and tips add visual interest to the well-researched and clearly written text."
— *Curriculum Connection, Apr '06*

Allergy Information for Teens
Health Tips about Allergic Reactions Such as Anaphylaxis, Respiratory Problems, and Rashes

Including Facts about Identifying and Managing Allergies to Food, Pollen, Mold, Animals, Chemicals, Drugs, and Other Substances

Edited by Karen Bellenir. 410 pages. 2006. 978-0-7808-0799-0.

Asthma Information for Teens
Health Tips about Managing Asthma and Related Concerns

Including Facts about Asthma Causes, Triggers, Symptoms, Diagnosis, and Treatment

Edited by Karen Bellenir. 386 pages. 2005. 978-0-7808-0770-9.

"Highly recommended for medical libraries, public school libraries, and public libraries."
— *American Reference Books Annual, 2006*

"It is so clearly written and well organized that even hesitant readers will be able to find the facts they need, whether for reports or personal information. . . . A succinct but complete resource."
— *School Library Journal, Sep '05*

Body Information for Teens
Health Tips about Maintaining Well-Being for a Lifetime

Including Facts about the Development and Functioning of the Body's Systems, Organs, and Structures and the Health Impact of Lifestyle Choices

Edited by Sandra Augustyn Lawton. 458 pages. 2007. 978-0-7808-0443-2.

Cancer Information for Teens
Health Tips about Cancer Awareness, Prevention, Diagnosis, and Treatment

Including Facts about Frequently Occurring Cancers, Cancer Risk Factors, and Coping Strategies for Teens Fighting Cancer or Dealing with Cancer in Friends or Family Members

Edited by Wilma R. Caldwell. 428 pages. 2004. 978-0-7808-0678-8.

"Recommended for school libraries, or consumer libraries that see a lot of use by teens."
— *E-Streams, May '05*

"A valuable educational tool."
— *American Reference Books Annual, 2005*

"Young adults and their parents alike will find this new addition to the *Teen Health Series* an important reference to cancer in teens."
— *Children's Bookwatch, Feb '05*

Complementary and Alternative Medicine Information for Teens
Health Tips about Non-Traditional and Non-Western Medical Practices

Including Information about Acupuncture, Chiropractic Medicine, Dietary and Herbal Supplements, Hypnosis, Massage Therapy, Prayer and Spirituality, Reflexology, Yoga, and More

Edited by Sandra Augustyn Lawton. 405 pages. 2006. 978-0-7808-0966-6.

Diabetes Information for Teens
Health Tips about Managing Diabetes and Preventing Related Complications

Including Information about Insulin, Glucose Control, Healthy Eating, Physical Activity, and Learning to Live with Diabetes

Edited by Sandra Augustyn Lawton. 410 pages. 2006. 978-0-7808-0811-9.

Diet Information for Teens, 2nd Edition

Health Tips about Diet and Nutrition

Including Facts about Dietary Guidelines, Food Groups, Nutrients, Healthy Meals, Snacks, Weight Control, Medical Concerns Related to Diet, and More

Edited by Karen Bellenir. 432 pages. 2006. 978-0-7808-0820-1.

"Full of helpful insights and facts throughout the book. ... An excellent resource to be placed in public libraries or even in personal collections."
— *American Reference Books Annual, 2002*

"Recommended for middle and high school libraries and media centers as well as academic libraries that educate future teachers of teenagers. It is also a suitable addition to health science libraries that serve patrons who are interested in teen health promotion and education." — *E-Streams, Oct '01*

"This comprehensive book would be beneficial to collections that need information about nutrition, dietary guidelines, meal planning, and weight control. ... This reference is so easy to use that its purchase is recommended." — *The Book Report, Sep-Oct '01*

"This book is written in an easy to understand format describing issues that many teens face every day, and then provides thoughtful explanations so that teens can make informed decisions. This is an interesting book that provides important facts and information for today's teens." — *Doody's Health Sciences Book Review Journal, Jul-Aug '01*

"A comprehensive compendium of diet and nutrition. The information is presented in a straightforward, plain-spoken manner. This title will be useful to those working on reports on a variety of topics, as well as to general readers concerned about their dietary health."
— *School Library Journal, Jun '01*

Drug Information for Teens, 2nd Edition

Health Tips about the Physical and Mental Effects of Substance Abuse

Including Information about Marijuana, Inhalants, Club Drugs, Stimulants, Hallucinogens, Opiates, Prescription and Over-the-Counter Drugs, Herbal Products, Tobacco, Alcohol, and More

Edited by Sandra Augustyn Lawton. 468 pages. 2006. 978-0-7808-0862-1.

"A clearly written resource for general readers and researchers alike." — *School Library Journal*

"This book is well-balanced. ... a must for public and school libraries."
— *VOYA: Voice of Youth Advocates, Dec '03*

"The chapters are quick to make a connection to their teenage reading audience. The prose is straightforward and the book lends itself to spot reading. It should be useful both for practical information and for research, and it is suitable for public and school libraries."
— *American Reference Books Annual, 2003*

"Recommended reference source."
— *Booklist, American Library Association, Feb '03*

"This is an excellent resource for teens and their parents. Education about drugs and substances is key to discouraging teen drug abuse and this book provides this much needed information in a way that is interesting and factual." — *Doody's Review Service, Dec '02*

Eating Disorders Information for Teens

Health Tips about Anorexia, Bulimia, Binge Eating, and Other Eating Disorders

Including Information on the Causes, Prevention, and Treatment of Eating Disorders, and Such Other Issues as Maintaining Healthy Eating and Exercise Habits

Edited by Sandra Augustyn Lawton. 337 pages. 2005. 978-0-7808-0783-9.

"An excellent resource for teens and those who work with them."
— *VOYA: Voice of Youth Advocates, Apr '06*

"A welcome addition to high school and undergraduate libraries." — *American Reference Books Annual, 2006*

"This book covers the topic in a lucid manner but delves deeper into every aspect of an eating disorder. A solid addition for any nonfiction or reference collection." — *School Library Journal, Dec '05*

Fitness Information for Teens

Health Tips about Exercise, Physical Well-Being, and Health Maintenance

Including Facts about Aerobic and Anaerobic Conditioning, Stretching, Body Shape and Body Image, Sports Training, Nutrition, and Activities for Non-Athletes

Edited by Karen Bellenir. 425 pages. 2004. 978-0-7808-0679-5.

"Another excellent offering from Omnigraphics in their *Teen Health Series*. ... This book will be a great addition to any public, junior high, senior high, or secondary school library."
— *American Reference Books Annual, 2005*

Learning Disabilities Information for Teens

Health Tips about Academic Skills Disorders and Other Disabilities That Affect Learning

Including Information about Common Signs of Learning Disabilities, School Issues, Learning to Live with a Learning Disability, and Other Related Issues

Edited by Sandra Augustyn Lawton. 337 pages. 2005. 978-0-7808-0796-9.

"This book provides a wealth of information for any reader interested in the signs, causes, and consequences

of learning disabilities, as well as related legal rights and educational interventions. . . . Public and academic libraries should want this title for both students and general readers."
— American Reference Books Annual, 2006

■

Mental Health Information for Teens, 2nd Edition

Health Tips about Mental Wellness and Mental Illness

Including Facts about Mental and Emotional Health, Depression and Other Mood Disorders, Anxiety Disorders, Behavior Disorders, Self-Injury, Psychosis, Schizophrenia, and More

Edited by Karen Bellenir. 400 pages. 2006. 978-0-7808-0863-8.

"In both language and approach, this user-friendly entry in the *Teen Health Series* is on target for teens needing information on mental health concerns."
— Booklist, American Library Association, Jan '02

"Readers will find the material accessible and informative, with the shaded notes, facts, and embedded glossary insets adding appropriately to the already interesting and succinct presentation."
— School Library Journal, Jan '02

"This title is highly recommended for any library that serves adolescents and parents/caregivers of adolescents." — E-Streams, Jan '02

"Recommended for high school libraries and young adult collections in public libraries. Both health professionals and teenagers will find this book useful."
— American Reference Books Annual, 2002

"This is a nice book written to enlighten the society, primarily teenagers, about common teen mental health issues. It is highly recommended to teachers and parents as well as adolescents."
— Doody's Review Service, Dec '01

■

Sexual Health Information for Teens

Health Tips about Sexual Development, Human Reproduction, and Sexually Transmitted Diseases

Including Facts about Puberty, Reproductive Health, Chlamydia, Human Papillomavirus, Pelvic Inflammatory Disease, Herpes, AIDS, Contraception, Pregnancy, and More

Edited by Deborah A. Stanley. 391 pages. 2003. 978-0-7808-0445-6.

"This work should be included in all high school libraries and many larger public libraries. . . . highly recommended."
— American Reference Books Annual, 2004

"*Sexual Health* approaches its subject with appropriate seriousness and offers easily accessible advice and information." — School Library Journal, Feb '04

Skin Health Information for Teens

Health Tips about Dermatological Concerns and Skin Cancer Risks

Including Facts about Acne, Warts, Hives, and Other Conditions and Lifestyle Choices, Such as Tanning, Tattooing, and Piercing, That Affect the Skin, Nails, Scalp, and Hair

Edited by Robert Aquinas McNally. 429 pages. 2003. 978-0-7808-0446-3.

"This volume, as with others in the series, will be a useful addition to school and public library collections." — American Reference Books Annual, 2004

"There is no doubt that this reference tool is valuable."
— VOYA: Voice of Youth Advocates, Feb '04

"This volume serves as a one-stop source and should be a necessity for any health collection."
— Library Media Connection

■

Sports Injuries Information for Teens

Health Tips about Sports Injuries and Injury Protection

Including Facts about Specific Injuries, Emergency Treatment, Rehabilitation, Sports Safety, Competition Stress, Fitness, Sports Nutrition, Steroid Risks, and More

Edited by Joyce Brennfleck Shannon. 405 pages. 2003. 978-0-7808-0447-0.

"This work will be useful in the young adult collections of public libraries as well as high school libraries."
— American Reference Books Annual, 2004

■

Suicide Information for Teens

Health Tips about Suicide Causes and Prevention

Including Facts about Depression, Risk Factors, Getting Help, Survivor Support, and More

Edited by Joyce Brennfleck Shannon. 368 pages. 2005. 978-0-7808-0737-2.

■

Tobacco Information for Teens

Health Tips about the Hazards of Using Cigarettes, Smokeless Tobacco, and Other Nicotine Products

Including Facts about Nicotine Addiction, Immediate and Long-Term Health Effects of Tobacco Use, Related Cancers, Smoking Cessation, Tobacco Use Prevention, and Tobacco Use Statistics

Edited by Karen Bellenir. 440 pages. 2007. 978-0-7808-0976-5.

Health Reference Series